HORIZONS IN WORLD CARDIOVASCULAR RESEARCH

VOLUME 6

Horizons in World Cardiovascular Research

Additional books in this series can be found on Nova's website
under the Series tab.

Additional e-books in this series can be found on Nova's website
under the e-book tab.

HORIZONS IN WORLD CARDIOVASCULAR RESEARCH

VOLUME 6

ELEANOR H. BENNINGTON
EDITOR

New York

Library of Congress Cataloging-in-Publication Data

ISBN: 978-1-63321-298-5

ISSN: 2157-6130

Published by Nova Science Publishers, Inc. † New York

Contents

Preface

Cardiovascular disease refers to the class of diseases that involve the heart or blood vessels. While the term technically refers to any disease that affects the cardiovascular system, it is usually used to refer to those related to atherosclerosis. Chronic heart failure (CHF) has emerged as a major worldwide epidemic. This book gathers the latest research in cardiovascular disease with a focus on such topics as cardiac sarcoidosis; heart failure and acute phase proteins; endothelial dysfunction in hypertension; treatment of unprotected left main coronary artery; cholesterol and coronary atherosclerosis; pulse decomposition for artery pressure waveforms; and multidetector computed tomography as a potential modality to detect subclinical atherosclerosis.

Chapter 1 – Sarcoidosis is an elusive multisystem disease characterized by granulomatous inflammation of affected tissue. Originally named in 1899 by Norwegian dermatologist Caesar Boeck, the term "sarcoid" came from his observation of nodular skin lesions that resembled sarcoma. Boeck's description of "epithelioid cells with large pale nuclei and also a few giant cells," typifies the distinguishing pathological feature of this disease. The presence of noncaseating granulomas is pathognomonic for sarcoidosis regardless of the tissue involved. Most commonly, sarcoidosis is associated with lung and lymph node involvement but may also affect the heart, liver, spleen, skin, eyes, pharyngeal bones and parotid glands. The nervous, musculoskeletal, renal, and endocrine systems may also be involved. Although some variations of the disease can be self-limited or take a benign course, sarcoidosis of the heart deserves special consideration as cardiac involvement portends a poor prognosis. Despite efforts to standardize diagnostic criteria and advancements in imaging technology, cardiac sarcoidosis remains to be difficult to diagnose owing both to its highly variable clinical course and unpredictable manifestations. Patient presentation extends from asymptomatic to sudden death with heart failure, arrhythmia, and syncope filling the gap between. Thus, a high index of clinical suspicion is necessary both in patients with extracardiac sarcoid and those who present with a sudden onset of unexplained cardiac phenomena.

Chapter 2 – Heart failure (HF) describes a complex clinical syndrome, where the heart is incapable of providing the body with an adequate amount of blood to meet metabolic requirements. It is a major public health concern, affecting about 6 million Americans, with rates expected to nearly triple over the next 3 decades as the population ages. But HF is not limited to industrialized, developed countries; instead it is a global burden rising in developing countries paralleling increases in cardiovascular risk factors such as hypertension, diabetes and obesity. HF is a progressive disease with various stages and a number of risk factors contributing to the onset of HF symptoms with the inflammatory cascade as one of the key players in each stage of HF. This chapter reviews a number of these key inflammatory mediators with the aim of further understanding their role in the transition from disease risk factors to development and advancement of HF.

Chapter 3 – *Introduction:* The vascular endothelium plays an important rule in vascular homeostasis, tone and as a consequence, vascular health. Impairment in endothelial function or endothelial dysfunction translates to increased vascular tone and possibly to high blood pressure. Although is still debatable whether endothelial dysfunction remains a cause or consequence of essential hypertension, reversal of this target organ damage undoubtedly leads to improved cardiovascular prognosis. Not unreasonably, reversal of endothelial dysfunction has become therefore an ambitious treatment target. In this article, after exploring and providing evidence for the presence of endothelial dysfunction in hypertension, the authorsalso provide a systemic literature search review of endothelial dysfunction reversal in essential hypertension.

Methods: The authors conducted a MEDLINE, EMBASE etc. search of all of published studies referring to endothelial dysfunction reversal or improvement in hypertension from 1989 to 2012. Studies involving placebo were also included.

Results: The authors identified several pharmacologic and non-pharmacologic approaches favourably affecting endothelial function. Interestingly, blood pressure reduction per se did not affect vascular function. Modulators of the renin-angiotensin-aldosterone system (RAAS) appeared to have a consistent and a powerful effect in ameliorating or even reversing endothelial dysfunction in comparison to other antihypertensive agents for the same blood pressure control.

Conclusions: Reducing blood pressure without specific antihypertensive drugs does not seem to improve endothelial dysfunction. Modulators of the RAAS appear to have a long lasting beneficial effect on endothelial function perhaps providing a mechanistic link to their favourable effects on hypertensive cardiovascular prognosis.

Chapter 4 – When considering the significance of a left main coronary artery (LMCA) obstruction, one should take into account lesions that obstruct 50% or more of the luminal diameter. The literature shows that, when defined by this criterion, they appear in less than 6% of all patients sent for coronary angiography and 30% of the group submitted to a coronary artery bypass graft surgery (CABG). Although it is not such a prevalent disease, it is important because of the catastrophic results of LMCA occlusion.

Most of the time LMCA disease occurs in combination with multivessel disease and by itself only in less than 8-18%. Randomized trials comparing percutaneous coronary intervention (PCI) and CABG have shown more favorable results for CABG compared to PCI using only balloon angioplasty or bare metal stents (BMS), especially regarding the target lesion revascularization endpoint.

Chapter 5 – The hypothesis that total cholesterol or LDL cholesterol is a risk factor or causative factor for coronary atherosclerosis was advanced without supporting evidence but rather was based on what appeared to be an association between serum cholesterol and acute coronary events. This observation was then extrapolated backwards since it was assumed that atherosclerosis was a prerequisite precursor of myocardial infarction or unstable angina. But this ignored several autopsy studies that showed no correlation between coronary atherosclerosis and circulating cholesterol in healthy accident victims, studies that were prior to or contemporary with the early evolution of the cholesterol-atherosclerosis hypothesis. Atherosclerosis frequently starts at a relatively young age and progresses to eventually generate plaque, atheromas and stenosis with an impact on coronary circulation, and this pathology increases dramatically with age. To study the cholesterol-atherosclerosis hypothesis, it seems reasonable that one must actually observe the associated arterial manifestations and progression and how they relate to cholesterol levels, rather than focus on acute coronary events or one or two selected atheromas. However, for a considerable period, this was not or could not be done, but the cholesterol-atherosclerosis hypothesis still evolved to become a dogma as did the cholesterol-heart disease hypothesis.

Chapter 6 – An early return of the reflection wave of the artery pressure waveform has been widely accepted as an important risk indicator of cardiovascular diseases. Waveform fitting method using Gaussian functions has been proven as a useful tool for decomposing the pressure waveform into sub-waves and hence assessing and quantifying the wave reflection. However, different researches employed different number of Gaussian functions and the appropriate number is still not determined. So the comparison for the parameters of Gaussian functions between using different Gaussian functions is essentially important for this Gaussian fitting method. The aim of this study is to compare the parameters differences between using three and four Gaussian functions. Fifty-six normal subjects and 51 heart failure subjects (New York Heart Association class II or III) were studied by noninvasive techniques applied to acquire the carotid artery pressure waveforms (CAPW) and radial artery pressure waveforms (RAPW). Then CAPW and RAPW signals were analyzed using Gaussian fitting and two-stage particle swarm optimizer to determine the parameters for each Gaussian function: peak time, peak amplitude and half-width. The results showed that for both normal and heart failure subjects, as well as for both CAPW and RAPW signals, the parameters from the first and second Gaussian functions have no significant statistical differences between using three and four Gaussians fitting (all $P>0.05$) whereas the parameters from the third Gaussian function have (all $P<0.01$). Further analysis showed that for both using three and four Gaussians fitting, as well as for both CAPW and RAPW signals, in comparison with normal subjects, heart failure subjects had significantly decreased peak amplitude of the first Gaussian function ($P<0.01$), significantly increased peak amplitude and significantly shorter peak times of the second Gaussian function (both $P<0.01$). This study is therefore an important step to further understand the underlying physiological mechanisms of the artery pressure waveform features using Gaussian functions.

Chapter 7 – Coronary artery disease is a leading cause of mortality and morbidity in the developing and developed countries. In approximately 50% of patients with newly diagnosed coronary artery disease, the first presentation is either acute myocardial infarction or sudden cardiac death. Global risk scores are developed to stratify the risk of coronary artery disease. However recent research has revealed that the global risk score significantly underestimates or misclassifies risk in key subsets of the population. Many data also demonstrate that the major determinant of risk for atherosclerotic cardiovascular disease in asymptomatic adults is the presence of the underlying disease itself, namely subclinical atherosclerosis.

Multidetector computed tomography (MDCT) has emerged as a promising modality to evaluate coronary artery disease. MDCT has an excellent capacity to detect hemodynamically relevant stenosis and its ability to detect and characterize coronary plaque noninvasively is increasingly recognized. Recent studies using MDCT demonstrate that the prevalence of subclinical atherosclerosis in asymptomatic patients with low to intermediate risk is high.

Especially, asymptomatic diabetic patients and asymptomatic patients with abnormal carotid finding have high prevalence of subclinical atherosclerosis. Also recent studies demonstrate that the coronary plaques that are prone to subsequent acute coronary syndrome are often associated with positive remodeling and low attenuation plaque, suggesting that once a patient is identified to be at high risk of having an adverse cardiac event by clinical risk assessment, imaging with MDCT would help better identify those at greater risk of acute coronary events. Thus it is time to change the paradigm for testing for coronary artery disease from detection of a symptomatic luminal obstruction to preclinical arterial wall atherosclerosis. There is increasing need to detect disease at earlier stages so that asymptomatic patients with atherosclerosis in need of aggressive medical management can be identified. The authors believe that MDCT has a potential to fulfill these needs.

In: Horizons in World Cardiovascular Research. Vol. 6
Editor: Eleanor H. Bennington
ISBN: 978-1-63321-298-5

Chapter 1

Cardiac Sarcoidosis

Bernard Kadosh and Igor Mamkin*
New York Methodist Hospital, Division of Cardiology, Brooklyn, NY, US

Introduction

Sarcoidosis is an elusive multisystem disease characterized by granulomatous inflammation of affected tissue. Originally named in 1899 by Norwegian dermatologist Caesar Boeck, the term "sarcoid" came from his observation of nodular skin lesions that resembled sarcoma. [1] Boeck's description of "epithelioid cells with large pale nuclei and also a few giant cells," [2] typifies the distinguishing pathological feature of this disease. The presence of noncaseating granulomas is pathognomonic for sarcoidosis regardless of the tissue involved. Most commonly, sarcoidosis is associated with lung and lymph node involvement but may also affect the heart, liver, spleen, skin, eyes, pharyngeal bones and parotid glands. [3] The nervous, musculoskeletal, renal, and endocrine systems may also be involved. [4]

Although some variations of the disease can be self-limited or take a benign course, sarcoidosis of the heart deserves special consideration as cardiac involvement portends a poor prognosis. Despite efforts to standardize diagnostic criteria and advancements in imaging technology, cardiac sarcoidosis remains to be difficult to diagnose owing both to its highly variable clinical course and unpredictable manifestations. Patient presentation extends from asymptomatic to sudden death with heart failure, arrhythmia, and syncope filling the gap between. [5-7] Thus, a high index of clinical suspicion is necessary both in patients with extracardiac sarcoid and those who present with a sudden onset of unexplained cardiac phenomena.

* Corresponding author: Igor Mamkin, MD FACC, New York Methodist Hospital, Division of Cardiology, 506 Sixth Street, Brooklyn, NY 11215, Email: igor_mamkin@yahoo.com.

Epidemiology

The global incidence of sarcoidosis varies widely. Although the disease affects people of all racial and ethnic groups, trends have been demonstrated to indicate susceptibility in certain populations. In the United States, the estimated annual incidence of sarcoidosis ranges from 10.9 per 100,000 in Caucasians to 35.5 per 100,000 in African Americans. African American females have the highest rates at 107 per 100,000. [8] In Europe, the highest incidence is among Scandinavian countries estimated by some studies at 50-60 per 100,000 whereas South American, Middle Eastern, and Japanese rates range anywhere from 0.8-5 per 100,000. [8-11] The age of onset also varies between populations, but usually falls between the 3rd and 5th decade of life. [12]

It has been demonstrated that at least 25% of patients in the United States have evidence of cardiac involvement at autopsy. [13-15] Cardiac sarcoidosis is responsible for 13% to 25% of mortality from the disease in the United States, however in Japan the rates are much higher particularly in older women, accounting for 58% to 85% of deaths. [8,14,16] Diagnosis is challenging due to the variable clinical presentation of cardiac sarcoidosis. As a result, only 40% to 50% of patients with myocardial involvement confirmed at autopsy have ever had clinical evidence of the disease throughout their lifetime. [15] In one Japanese study of 320 autopsied cases, 46.9% of deaths were attributable to cardiac sarcoidosis, but a clinical diagnosis was only made in 26.7% of cases. [16] This was consistent with a more recent epidemiological study in Japan demonstrating only 23% of sarcoid patients with any abnormal cardiac laboratory findings. [17] In the United States, cardiac sarcoidosis is clinically apparent in only 5% of cases. [2]

Pathophysiology

The inciting event that leads to sarcoidosis currently remains unknown. However, granulomatous inflammation is the fundamental lesion of this disease process. In general, granulomas form in order to "wall off" pathogens and limit damage to surrounding tissues. Macrophages, in response to chronic stimulation from inflammatory cytokines, organize and differentiate into epithelioid cells. These cells merge to form multinucleated giant cells. Once granulomas form they may either regress and resolve, or progress to fibrosis in 20% to 25% of patients. [2] As granulomas progress, fibroblasts and collagen encase these cells leading to sclerosis, eventually disturbing the architecture of the tissue and function of the involved organ. [2,18-20] At the center of this interaction is the presence of CD4+ cells which interact with antigen presenting cells to drive this process and maintain granuloma formation. Activated CD4+ cells differentiate into type 1 helper T cells and secrete interleukin-2 and interferon-γ. This augments TNF-α production by macrophages and amplifies the local cellular immune response (Figure 1). [18] The oligoclonal activation of these T-cells suggests a response to a classical antigenic peptide rather than a superantigen which would initiate a polyclonal response. [19] Still, the nature of this antigenic trigger remains elusive with infectious (*Mycobacterium* tuberculosis, *Mycoplasma* species, *Corynebacteria* species, spirochetes), environmental agents (insecticides, mold, aluminium, pollen, clay, talc, wood-burning stoves) and occupational exposure (navy servicemen, metal workers, building material suppliers, educators, firefighters) all implicated as potential offenders. [4,6,12,21,22]

The geographical, seasonal, and occupational patterns in the prevalence of sarcoidosis suggest an environmental etiology to the disease; however genetic predisposition plays an equally important role. Familial clusters occur in roughly 19% of African American cases and 5% in Caucasian cases. First degree relatives of sarcoidosis patients have almost five times the risk of developing the disease compared to those with no family history. Moreover, monozygotic twins are affected more commonly than dizygotic twins. [23,24] The effects of several genes including human leukocyte antigens (HLA), cytokines such as tumor necrosis factor (TNF), and immunoglobulin receptors have been recognized as predisposing factors. HLA-DRB1*1101 is well known for its positive association with both white and African American sarcoidosis patients in the United States. [25,26] In cardiac sarcoid specifically, HLA-DQB1*0601 has been recognized as a marker and may confer increased risk for cardiac involvement. [4,27,28] HLA genotype associations do not always necessarily indicate risk for the disease. Some studies suggest predisposition to phenotype rather than susceptibility. For example, HLA-DRB1*0301 and HLA-DQB*0201 have been strongly associated with mild disease and good prognosis. [29,30] Among cytokine genes, TNF-308A and TNF-857T polymorphisms have been linked with British and Dutch sarcoidosis patients. [31] The TNFA2 allele is associated with cardiac sarcoidosis in Japanese patients, particularly females. [12,28,32] Butyrophilinlike-2 (BTNL2) is an immunoglobulin receptor gene, one of many that are responsible for regulation of immune responses. Recently, BTNL2 has been found to moderately influence disease risk in Caucasians and African Americans in the United States. [33] This association was confirmed by another study of German populations. [34] Whether BTNL2 is an independent risk factor, however, is not entirely clear due to its proximity to HLA-DRB1 alleles. [35] Since 2001, several genome-wide studies have been conduced showing strong associations to sarcoid phenotypes. Strong linkages at chromosomes 3p and 6p in Germans as well as 5p and 5q in African Americans have been demonstrated. [36,37] Subsequent studies have confirmed these linkages and identified new loci, notably on chromosome 10p associated with advanced-stage sarcoidosis [38,39] and 18q22 in patients with cardiac and renal involvement. [27]

What is clear from these studies is that susceptibility to sarcoidosis depends on an intricate interaction between genetic polymorphisms and environmental exposures. [40] One such interaction has been identified between HLA-DQB1 and humid work environments in African American patients. [29] Further identification of interactions between susceptibility-loci, genetic modifiers, and environmental exposures will help reveal much more about the etiology of sarcoidosis and why it expresses itself so differently between individuals.

Clinical Manifestations

The clinical presentation of cardiac sarcoidosis is highly inconsistent. The clinical picture depends entirely on whether the pathology involves the myocardium, the conduction system, the valves, or secondary to advanced pulmonary sarcoid. From asymptomatic electrocardiographic (ECG) findings to sudden death, the initial presentation of cardiac sarcoidosis lacks the clinical *sine qua non* of other diseases and often becomes ruled in by exclusion. Chest pain, palpitations, dyspnea, orthopnea, dizziness, syncope, or peripheral edema are all possible, making cardiac sarcoid a great mimic of common diseases of the heart. The factors that account for this variability between patients are not fully understood, but likely depend on a combination of genetic predisposition, sex, and the duration of the illness.

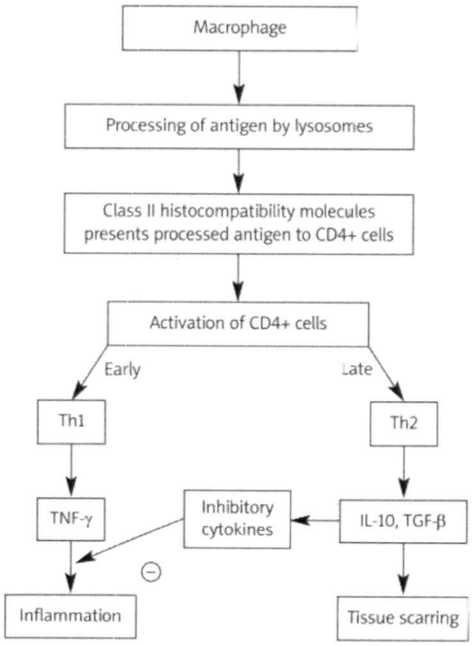

Figure 1. Pathogenesis of sarcoidosis. Reprinted with permission of Termedia & Banach. Copyright 2011. [23].

Signs and symptoms of congestive heart failure are often seen in sarcoid patients, but result from assorted etiologies. Direct granulomatous inflammation of the myocardium can lead to both systolic and diastolic ventricular failure. Chronic granulation and fibrosis leads to a pathological thickening or thinning of the ventricular walls. In rare cases thinning of the ventricular free wall results in aneurysm or spontaneous rupture. [41] Of note, ventricular aneurysms in cardiac sarcoidosis are distinct from ischemic causes of aneurysm as they do not follow the territorial distribution of the coronary arteries. Though direct involvement of sarcoid granulomas have been reported in all four valves, [3,42-44] mitral regurgitation is the most common consequence of valvular involvement, leading to left atrial dilatation and pulmonary congestion. The pericardium is not safe from granulomatous inflammation either, having been reported usually in the context of pericarditis, small effusions and, rarely, tamponade. [3,45-48] Extensive fibrosis of the lungs has an indirect affect on the heart by increasing pulmonary vascular resistance. Cor pulmonale may eventually result from chronic pulmonary hypertension, though this diagnosis can be overlooked by the clinician focused on the primary parenchymal disease of the lungs. [49,50]

Conduction abnormalities collectively constitute the greatest proportion of abnormal findings in cardiac sarcoidosis. With a prevalence of up to 62%, disturbances in the conduction system can manifest as a result of scaring or granulomas in the atria and ventricles, or as a result of ischemic change to the nodal artery. [4] Complete heart block, often presenting as syncope, is the most common conduction abnormality. However, AV block, complete or incomplete bundle branch block, and sinus arrest are all possible. Sarcoid granulomas involving the ventricular myocardium can become foci for abnormal automaticity or disperse ventricular activation and recovery, increasing the risk for re-entrant tachyarrhythmia. [23] Ventricular tachycardia is the most common arrhythmia seen in cardiac sarcoidosis with a prevalence ranging from 2% to 42% (Figure 2A). [3,45,51,52] Sudden death due to ventricular arrhythmia or complete heart block is the most feared complication in these patients, responsible for up to 65% of all cardiac sarcoid related deaths. One study found that sudden death was the initial presenting symptom in 17% of cases. [42]

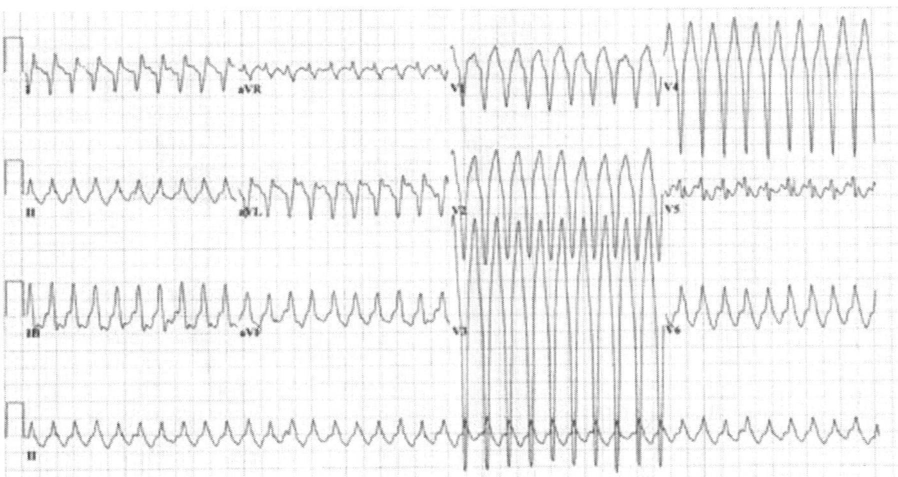

Figure 2A. A 12-lead electrocardiogram shows monomorphic ventricular tachycardia. Reprinted with permission of Texas Heart Institute.Copyright 2011. [145].

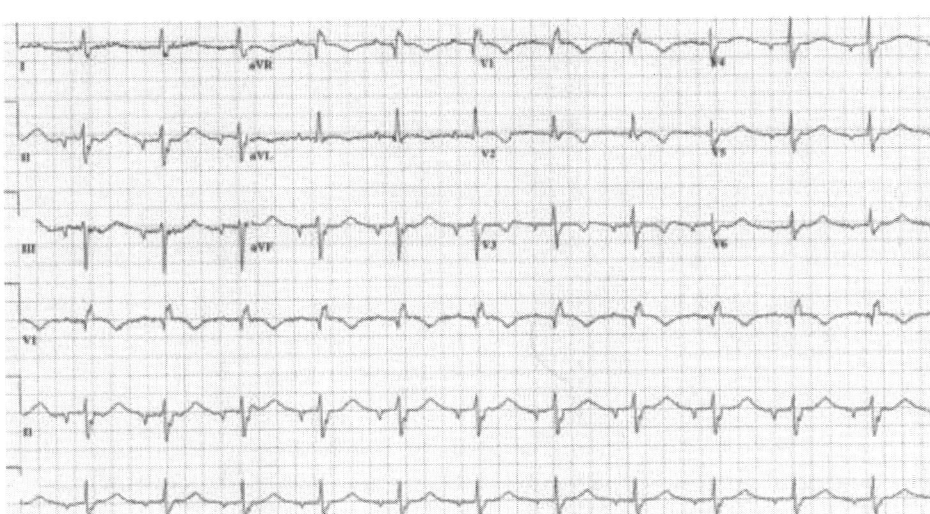

Figure 2B. A 12-lead surface electrocardiogram shows ectopic atrial rhythm with 1st-degree atrioventricular block, right bundle branch block, and left anterior fascicular block. Reprinted with permission of Texas Heart Institute. Copyright 2009. [146].

In contrast to the ventricles, supraventricular arrhythmias such as atrial ectopy, atrial flutter, atrial fibrillation, and atrial tachycardia usually result from atrial dilatation rather than direct granulomatous involvement. These occur less commonly than ventricular arrhythmias, accounting for 15% to 17% of conduction abnormalities. [3]

Diagnosis

In light of the multitude of clinical presentations possible in cardiac sarcoidosis, it is not surprising that diagnosis of the disease is extremely challenging. The diagnostic approach has not yet been standardized and has, to date, relied largely on clinical criteria proposed by the Japanese Ministry of Health and Welfare (JMHW) in 1993 (Table 1). [53] These guidelines have been used as a gold standard for clinical diagnosis despite recent advances in imaging technology such as positron emission tomography (PET) and magnetic resonance imaging (MRI). [6] Proposals to replace the Japanese guidelines, such the Sarcoidosis Three-Dimensional Assessment Instrument, include newer imaging modalities to assess the probability of sarcoid involvement in each organ system. [54] Though promising, this instrument has not yet been validated and the optimal diagnostic strategy remains elusive since most tests have a low sensitivity, specificity, or both.

Despite the difficulty of definitively diagnosing cardiac sarcoidosis, the disease is both potentially fatal and treatable, thus warranting thorough investigation and frequent screening. Any patient with known sarcoidosis should be screened for cardiac involvement by detailed history and physical exam as well as a routine ECG. Patients with symptoms or significant ECG findings should be evaluated further by 24 to 48 hours of Holter or up to 30 days of event monitoring and/or echocardiography. [5,55] Abnormal results should prompt investigation with more advanced imaging techniques such as PET and MRI. There is no consensus on follow-up intervals for patients with negative findings, but 6 to 12 month screenings are considered a reasonable approach. [56] More controversial is the question of how aggressive these screenings should be. Since many cardiac sarcoidosis patients do not have any symptoms or ECG abnormalities, cardiac involvement may remain undetected without additional testing. The clinical benefit of chasing a diagnosis in asymptomatic patients has been called into question by studies suggesting that an absence of symptoms predicts a benign course. [5] Furthermore, the utility of noninvasive testing is as of yet undetermined, complicating the picture of cost effectiveness or clinical benefit studies.

Electrocardiography

Up to 70% of cardiac sarcoid patients will have some type of abnormality on ECG, most commonly conduction abnormalities (Figure 2B). As a screening tool, ECGs are favored for their affordability and non-invasiveness. Overall, however, sarcoid related ECG findings may be transient or subtle which impairs the test's sensitivity. [57] In isolation, ECG abnormalities may not have any clinical significance, but in the patient with known sarcoidosis conduction abnormalities and arrhythmias should prompt high clinical suspicion for cardiac involvement.

Table 1. Japanese Ministry of Health and Welfare Guidelines

Histologic diagnosis group
Cardiac sarcoidosis is confirmed when histologic analysis of operative or endomyocardial biopsy specimens demonstrates epithelioid granuloma without caseating granuloma
Clinical diagnosis group
In patients with a histologic diagnosis of extracardiac sarcoidosis, cardiac sarcoidosis is suspected when item (a) and one or more of items (b) though (e) are present:
(a) Complete right bundle branch block, left axis deviation, atrioventricular block, ventricular tachycardia, premature ventricular contraction (≥ Lown 2), or abnormal Q or ST-T change on the ECG or ambulatory ECG
(b) Abnormal wall motion, regional wall thinning, or dilation of the left ventricle
(c) Perfusion defect by thallium-201 myocardial scintigraphy or abnormal accumulation by gallium-67 or technetium-99m myocardial scintigraphy
(d) Abnormal intracardiac pressure, low cardiac output, or abnormal wall motion or depressed ejection fraction of the left ventricle
(e) Interstitial fibrosis or cellular infiltration over moderate grade even if the findings are non-specific

Table 2. Comparison of the utility of imaging modalities in the diagnosis of cardiac sarcoidosis

Modality	Advantages	Disadvantages	Sensitivity	Specificity
Echocardiography	• Good for evaluation of LV and diastolic function	• Low sensitivity for small defects • Operator dependant	Low to moderate	Low
^{201}Tl or ^{99m}Tc scintigraphy	• Effective in evaluation of ischemic heart disease	• Low specificity • Abnormalities do not correlate with survival rates in asymptomatic patients • Radiation exposure	Moderate	Moderate
^{67}Ga scintigraphy	• Shows areas of active inflammation • May predict response to corticosteroid treatment	• Low spatial resolution • Radiation exposure	Low	High
FDG-PET	• High sensitivity for active lesions and scar • May be used to monitor treatment	• Diffuse FDG uptake may occur physiologically • Radiation exposure	High	Moderate to high
Cardiac MRI	• High spatial and temporal resolution • Accurately shows active lesions and myocardial scar • Evaluates LV and RV function as well as regional wall motion abnormalities • May use to guide EMB • May be used to monitor treatment	• Contraindicated in patients with certain implantable devices • Contraindicated in severe renal failure • Image quality varies depending on scan protocol	Moderate to high	High

^{67}Ga, gallium-67; ^{99m}Tc, technetium-99m; ^{201}Tl, thallium-201; EMB, endomyocardial biopsy; FDG, fluorodeoxyglucose; LV, left ventricle; PET, positron emission tomography; RV, right ventricle. Adapted from Ayyala et al. [55] and Kim et al. [6].

Holter monitoring improves the sensitivity of ECG by detecting transient anomalies that would otherwise be missed. One study demonstrated that Holter detected >100 extrasystoles in up to 67% of confirmed cardiac sarcoid patients compared with 8% of control patients. [58] Heart rate variability (HRV) analysis obtained through Holter monitoring gives a measure of autonomic activity. Decreased HRV is seen in both systemic and cardiac sarcoid patients, but more markedly in the latter group. HRV can be helpful in evaluating the probability of cardiac involvement, but the clinical significance of this finding has yet to be fully evaluated. [59]

Electrophysiology Study

The role of electrophysiology study (EPS) in cardiac sarcoidosis is controversial. EPS is used to identify patients with coronary artery disease who are at risk for reentrant ventricular arrhythmias and sudden death, however its role in nonischemic cardiomyopathy is limited. With the exception of right ventricular dysplasia, programmed ventricular stimulation in order to induce sustained ventricular arrhythmia has too low a sensitivity for proper risk-stratification of these patients. [6] Studies evaluating the usefulness of EPS to identify candidates for an implantable cardioverter-defibrillator (ICD) are not concordant. Inducible ventricular arrhythmias were seen in 67% of patients in one study and predicted future life-threatening arrhythmia in all patients despite the use of antiarrhythmic drugs. [45] Conversely, another study demonstrated inducible arrhythmias in only 2 of 17 patients, none of whom died within the 2-year follow-up. [60] The specificity of EPS is not known and difficult to evaluate in cardiac sarcoidosis. The progressive nature of the disease is such that non-inducibility at one point in time cannot predict the effects of future myocardial involvement. [6] The use of EPS to risk-stratify patients for ICD therapy requires more prospective studies before its role in cardiac sarcoidosis is clearly defined.

Endomyocardial Biopsy

The presence of noncaseating granulomas on endomyocardial biopsy allows for confirmatory evidence of cardiac sarcoidosis (Figure 3). In the past, a tissue diagnosis confirming cardiac involvement was not possible. With the exception of rare trans-thoracic needle biopsies of the heart in the 1950s'[61] diagnosis was possible in only a small percentage of patients based on clinical grounds alone. [62] Despite its specificity, however, endomyocardial biopsy is highly insensitive due to the patchy, multifocal nature of sarcoid granulomas (Figure 4). While sarcoid granulomas tend to favor the basal septum and left ventricular free wall, endomyocardial biopsy is usually obtained from the apical septum. [3,63,64] As a result, positive biopsy is only obtained in 20% to 25% of patients with a clinical diagnosis of cardiac sarcoidosis and less than 10% of patients with arrhythmia alone. [64,65]

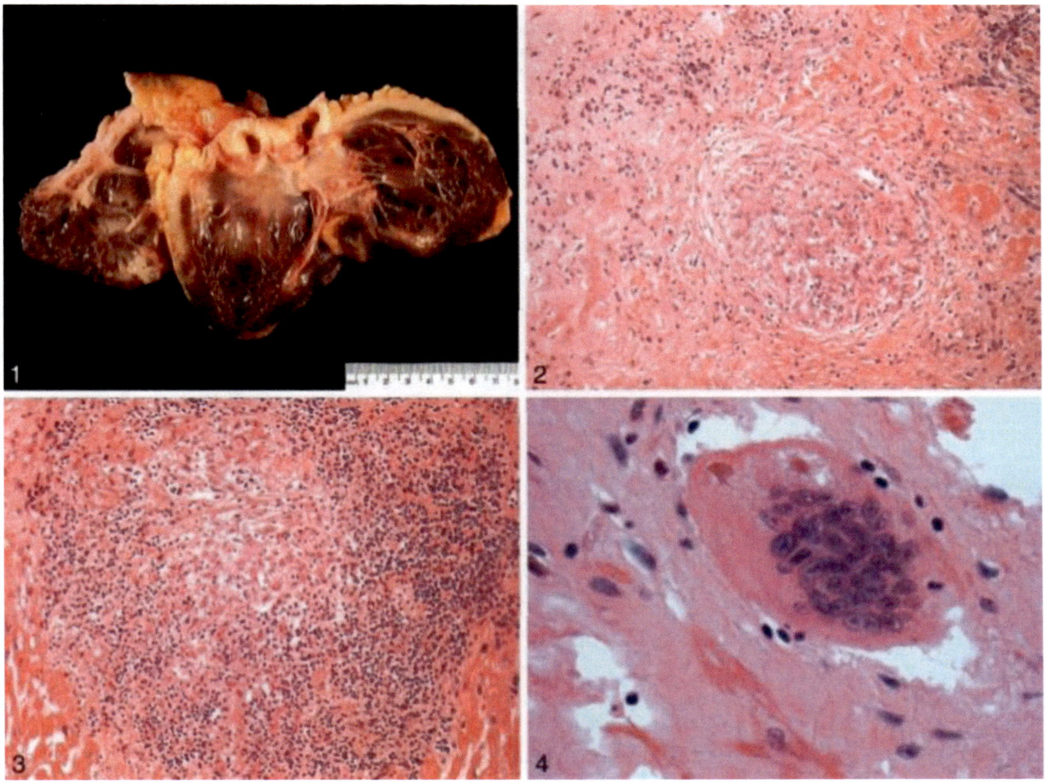

Figure 3. 1) Heart of a patient who underwent transplantation showing advanced tan to yellow-white fibrotic areas in endocardium, myocardium and epicardium, with a gradient of involvement, more severe toward the base of the heart. Note the heavy involvement of the epicardium in the anterior left ventricle (upper right of the picture) and endocardium of the right ventricle (lower left of the picture). 2) Low-power view of a typical tight, naked, non-necrotizing a epithelioid granuloma in the myocardium of an explanted heart from a 43-year-old man with sarcoidosis and heart failure (hematoxylin-eosin, original magnification x10). 3) Low-power view of a less typical, looser granuloma with rare giant cells at the periphery and surrounding lymphoplasmacytic infiltrate in the myocardium of the same patient (hematoxyllin-eosin, original magnification x10). 4) High-power view of an asteroid body within the multinucleated giant cell in the top right area above the nuclei. Note the stellate shape and cytoplasmic clearing. Also note the nuclei are clustered in a configuration more commonly thought to represent a foreign body-type giant cell (hematoxylin-eosin, original magnification x40). Reprinted with permission of College of American Pathologists. Copyright 2010. [147].

A useful consequence of this is that a positive biopsy is a valuable prognostic indicator associated with a shorter mean survival time. [65] This is likely a function of the test's low sensitivity: a biopsy is more likely to catch granulomatous inflammation in a heart with more extensively affected myocardium.

On the other hand, patients who are highly suspicious for myocardial involvement are treated despite a negative biopsy, begging the question of whether the benefits outweigh the risks of an invasive test. [64] Endomyocardial biopsy is most useful to rule out other diagnoses in cases of unexplained cardiomyopathy, but should not be used to exclude cardiac sarcoidosis if the test is negative.

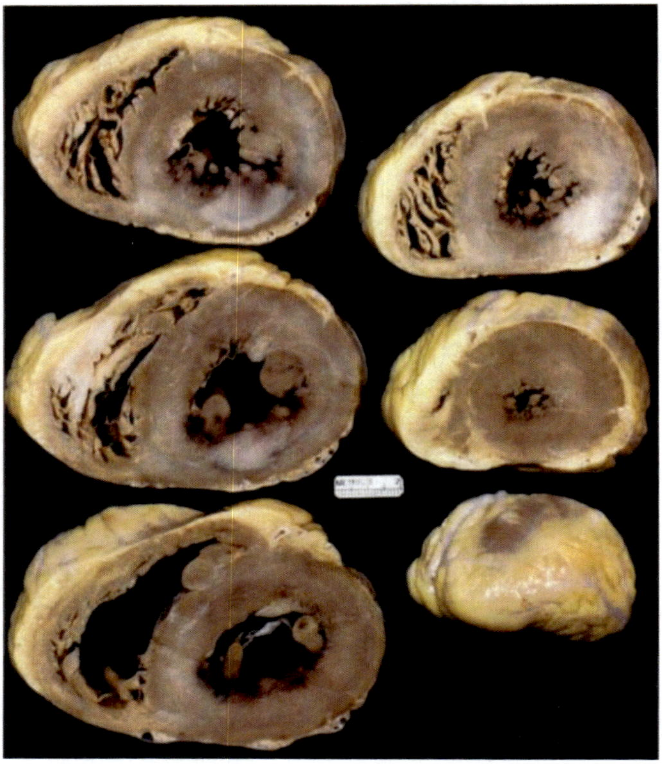

Figure 4. Cross-sections of the ventricular walls and cavities showing multiple sarcoid granulomas. Reprinted with permission of Baylor University Medical Center. Copyright 2009. [148].

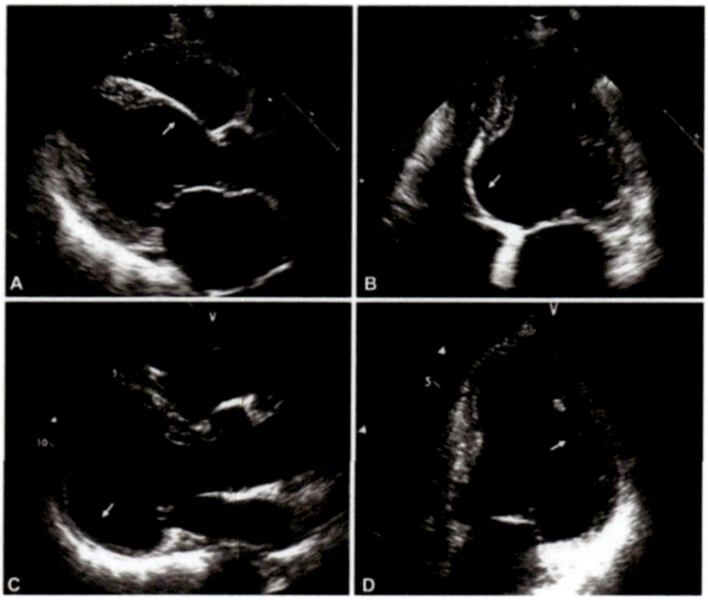

Figure 5. Representative echocardiographic images suggestive of cardiac involvement of sarcoidosis. Type 1 morphologic change is characterized by thinning and akinesia of the basal septum (A and B). Aneurysmal dilatation involving inferior or posterolateral wall is classified as type 2 (C and D). Reprinted with permission of The Korean Society of Cardiology. Copyright 2011. [149].

Imaging

Echocardiography

Abnormalities seen on echocardiography include septal thinning or thickening, left ventricular regional systolic dysfunction, left ventricular diastolic dysfunction, pericardial effusion, ventricular aneurysms, and valvular abnormalities (Figure 5 and 6). Usually these are seen in advanced disease, detectable in anywhere from 14% to 56% of sarcoid patients. [66-71] In addition, this modality lacks the sensitivity to detect small defects associated with early cardiac involvement. [68] Echocardiographic findings are not specific, but wall motion abnormalities or thin myocardium in areas not associated with a coronary artery distribution can suggest a sarcoid etiology. Smedema and colleagues found that positive echocardiographic findings correlated with the degree of involvement on MRI. [5] Impaired diastolic relaxation, however, was observed in 35% of patients without MRI evidence of cardiac sarcoidosis. Studies have shown improved sensitivity in early disease with the use of ultrasonic tissue characterization with integrated backscatter, which measures acoustic properties of the basal septum. [72,73] It has also been suggested that techniques such as transesophageal echocardiography [74] and tissue strain imaging [75] may increase detection rates in patients with known sarcoidosis, but these techniques have not been fully investigated yet.

Radionuclide Imaging

Single-photon emission computed tomography (SPECT) with thallium-201 (^{201}Tl) and technetium-99m (^{99m}Tc) have been extensively studied for their utility in detecting cardiac sarcoidosis. [4] Perfusion scanning at rest typically shows regions of decreased uptake, similar to what is seen in coronary artery disease. The pathophysiological explanation of this is not entirely clear. Decreased uptake on scintigraphy in sarcoidosis may result from the replacement of myocardium with granulomas and scarring[76], microvascular vasoconstriction [77], or regional metabolic abnormalities. [78] Two features on scintigraphy in cardiac sarcoidosis, however, help to differentiate this disease entity from the other. First, the appearance of myocardial defects tends to be patchy in sarcoidosis and not as clearly delineated along arterial distributions as is seen in coronary artery disease (Figure 7). Second, antithetical to stenosis of the coronary arteries, perfusion defects in cardiac sarcoidosis actually improve or disappear with exercise or vasodilation with dipyridamole. [77,79-81] This phenomenon, called "reverse distribution," is characteristic of sarcoid involvement of the heart, but not specific enough to be pathognomonic. Reported sensitivity for ^{201}Tl ranges from 35% to 58%. [82,83] ^{99m}Tc performs a little better with a sensitivity of 65% compared to 46% for ^{201}Tl in one study. [78] More recently, Okumura et al. [84] reported a sensitivity of 64% for ^{99m}Tc using the Japanese Ministry of Heath and Welfare guidelines as a diagnostic gold standard. The sensitivities of SPECT are intermediate and the findings are not specific enough to conclude a diagnosis. Additionally, abnormalities on scintigraphy have not been shown to correlate with survival rates especially in asymptomatic patients. [66,85] Thus, thallium and technetium scintigraphy should be interpreted with caution and are not recommended for screening sarcoid patients without cardiac symptoms. [4,85] Interestingly, a correlation has been found between the amount of reverse distribution and responsiveness to corticosteroids, [78] but the practical utility of using ^{201}Tl and ^{99m}Tc to guide management has not been evaluated.

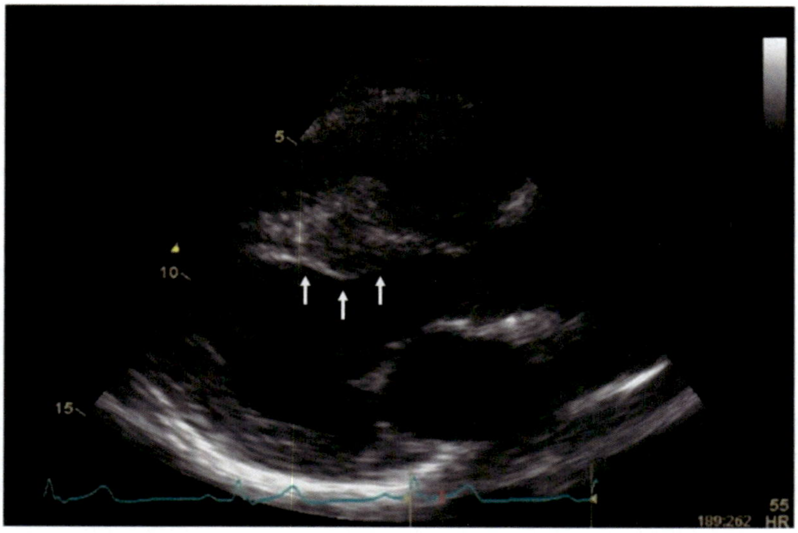

Figure 6. Transthoracic echocardiogram from a patient with cardiac sarcoidosis. Parasternal long axis view demonstrating marked thickening of the mid-basal anteroseptal wall of the left ventricle (arrows). Marked hypokinesis of the anteroseptal wall was also present.

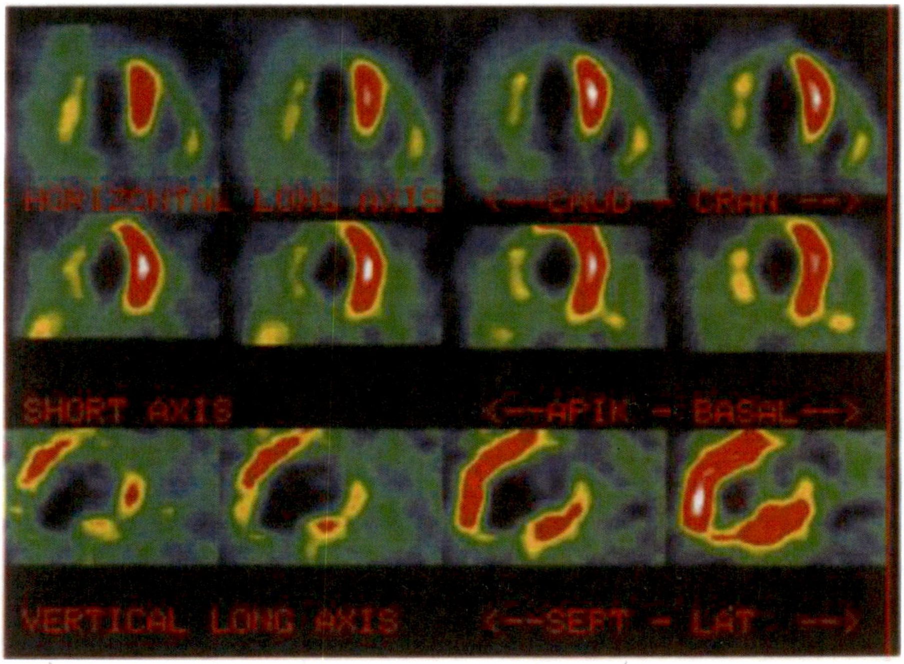

Figure 7. Rest thallium-201 SPECT scintigraphy on a 31 year old man with cardiac sarcoidosis shows patchy tracer uptake defects in the apex, septum, and inferior wall of the left ventricle. Reprinted with permission of BMJ Publishing Group Ltd. Copyright 2010. [150].

Gallium 67 (^{67}Ga) is a radionuclide that accumulates in areas of active granulomatous inflammation. Gallium scanning has typically been used to assess disease activity in pulmonary and systemic sarcoidosis, but lacks the spatial resolution to evaluate individual organs in detail. SPECT can be used with ^{67}Ga in order to differentiate the heart from surrounding lung tissue; however, fibrotic lesions without associated inflammation may be missed. As a result, the specificity of ^{67}Ga in the detection of cardiac sarcoidosis is substantially lower than that of ^{201}Tl and ^{99m}Tc, ranging from 18% to 50%. [63,81,83] While gallium scanning is clearly not suitable as a diagnostic tool, its predilection for areas of active inflammation can help guide medical treatment. Since the test is only positive when the disease is active, ^{67}Ga can predict response to corticosteroids. Several reports have shown improvement in ^{67}Ga scintigraphy after treatment with corticosteroids. [86-88] Even when used in combination with SPECT, cardiac and lung uptake are difficult to distinguish from one another on gallium scanning. In order to improve overall diagnostic and therapeutic utility, several multimodality imaging approaches have been suggested including combination of ^{67}Ga with ^{201}Tl, ^{99m}Tc or MRI imaging. [63,86-88] The benefit to a multimodal approach requires further investigation. However, in general, gallium scanning has fallen out of favor for the purposes of screening in cardiac sarcoidosis. [56]

Positron Emission Tomography

The utility of positron emission tomography with ^{18}F-fluorodeoxyglucose (FDG-PET) has been studied for diagnosis of cardiac sarcoidosis. FDG accumulates in inflammatory cells such as leukocytes, lymphocytes and macrophages, particularly in the lung and hilar lymph nodes of sarcoid patients. Moreover, this accumulation correlates with the histologic activity of the disease. [89,90] FDG uptake in the myocardium can be focal or have a focal-on-diffuse pattern presumably indicating areas of granulomatous inflammation. [82,83,91,92] In addition, PET has the added capability of perfusion imaging which, when combined with FDG uptake, affords a measure of disease activity as well as irreversible fibrotic changes (Figure 8). [81] Several small studies have compared FDG-PET to ^{201}Tl, ^{99m}Tc, and ^{67}Ga in patients diagnosed with cardiac sarcoidosis on the basis of the JMHW guidelines. Superiority for PET has been reported with sensitivities between 82% and 100%. [81,83,84,91,93,94] The reported diagnostic specificity is about 91% and 82% in 2 small studies, [84,91] and 90% in a larger study of PET. [94] In contrast, Ohira et al. [93] reported a specificity of only 39% for PET. One possible explanation for this discrepancy proposed by the authors is the ability of PET to detect subclinical myocardial involvement, suggesting that the JMHW guidelines are not an appropriate gold standard. Nevertheless, nonspecific FDG uptake is known to occur in patients with idiopathic dilated cardiomyopathies. [92,95]

There are several other confounding factors that impede the use of FDG-PET. Diffuse myocardial uptake of FDG can occur physiologically in many healthy subjects. Efforts to minimize this background uptake include a long fasting period or administration of intravenous heparin prior to scanning, but these techniques have not been rigorously tested. [91,93,94] Focal uptake of FDG can also be seen in the papillary muscles or in the lateral left ventricular wall. In addition, right ventricular and interventricular septum uptake of FDG is seen in cases of pulmonary hypertension due to increased mechanical load. [56]

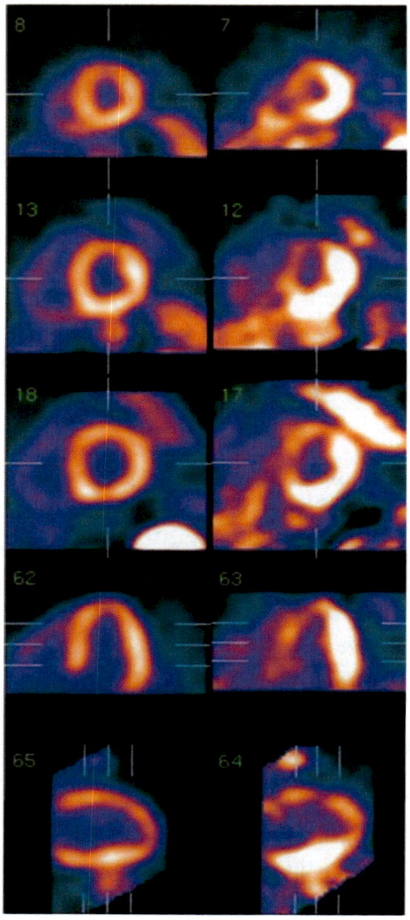

Figure 8. A cardiac PET imaging study, featuring rubidium-82 myocardial perfusion (left column) and glucose-loaded FDG metabolic images (right column). The PET images demonstrate normal myocardial perfusion and increased FDG uptake in the inferior and lateral walls consistent with hypermetabolism/inflammation, often seen in cardiac sarcoidosis. Although perfusion defects may also be seen with cardiac sarcoidosis, this patient had no significant perfusion defects. Reprinted from American Heart Journal, 157(1), Kim JS, Judson MA, Donnino R, Gold M, Cooper LT, Prystowsky EN, Prystowsky S, Cardiac Sarcoidosis, Pages 9-21, Copyright (2009), with permission from Elsevier. [6].

Analyses comparing FDG-PET to SPECT with technetium-99m have shown regional defects both in concordance and discordance between these two modalities. [84,91] This suggests that PET and SPECT may recognize separate features of the disease on a continuum of granulomatous inflammation to fibrotic replacement of myocardium. Note that the added clinical benefit of PET over conventional scintigraphy has not been validated. FDG uptake correlates with serum angiotensin levels, but not with left ventricular dysfunction. [84,93] PET may be used to monitor treatment with FDG uptake having been shown to diminish or disappear after corticosteroid therapy. [82] Currently there are no pathological correlation studies, nor have any longitudinal studies of patients with positive PET findings and negative scintigraphy been conducted to date. Systematic evaluation of FDG-PET in the diagnosis of cardiac sarcoidosis is still required, especially in comparison to newer modalities such as cardiac magnetic resonance imaging, discussed below.

Magnetic Resonance Imaging

Cardiac involvement of sarcoidosis can be suggested by several findings on MRI. As a high spatial and temporal resolution modality, MRI offers unique advantages such as detailed anatomical information and measures of both global and regional ventricular function with cine sequences. [56,96] Delayed gadolinium enhancement (also known as late gadolinium enhancement) on T1-weighted images 5 to 10 minutes after injection of gadolinium is central to a diagnosis of cardiac sarcoidosis and has been shown to more than double the detection rate as compared with the JMHW guidelines. [97] In acute disease, segmental wall motion abnormalities with associated myocardial thickening are typical. Increased signal intensity on both T2-weighted imaging and early gadolinium enhancement indicate areas of inflammation associated with edema. [96,98-101] Older lesions appear as focal regions of wall thinning due to scar formation. In contrast to acute lesions, chronic stage granulomas tend to persist on delayed gadolinium enhancement. The high-resolution capability of MRI allows for detection of non-transmural lesions as well as small, nodular foci in patchy distributions. [102] The typical pattern on late gadolinium enhancement (LGE) is midmyocardial, most commonly in the basal segments of the septum and lateral walls (Figure 9). [63,96,98,103] This is in contrast to coronary atherosclerosis which shows LGE of the subendocardium in the distribution of the coronary arteries. [104]

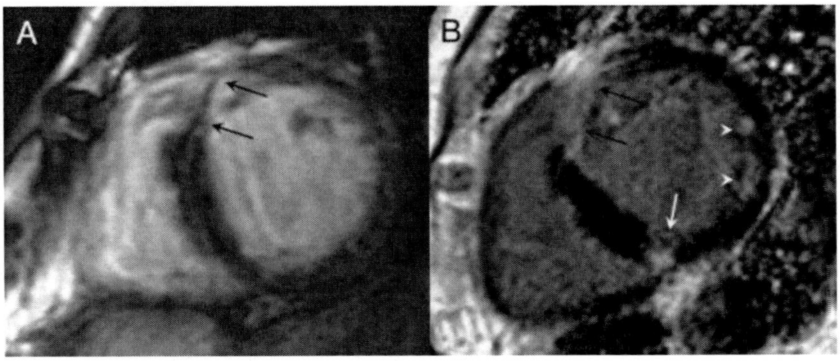

Figure 9. (A) Still frame from short-axis cine sequence showing an area of marked thinning the anterior septum. (B) Same view after gadolinium administration showing 3 different patterns of fibrosis. Transmural hyperenhancement corresponding to the area of septal thinning (black arrows), subepicardial hyperenhancement in the inferior right ventricular insertion point (white arrow), and midwall enhancement in the inferolateral wall (white arrowheads). Reprinted from Journal of the American College of Cardiology, 54(15), Karamitsos TD, Francis JM, Myerson S, Selvanayagam JB, Neubauer S, The role of cardiovascular magnetic resonance imaging in heart failure, Pages 1407-1424, Copyright (2009), with permission from Elsevier. [102].

Using the JMHW guidelines as a gold standard, MRI performed with a sensitivity and specificity of 100% and 78% respectively in a study of 58 patients. [103] Another study of 21 patients found a sensitivity of 75% and specificity of 77% against the JMHW gold standard. [93] MRI was found to be more sensitive for cardiac sarcoidosis than either ^{201}Tl or ^{67}Ga scintigraphy, [72] however comparisons with FDG-PET are less clear. Though PET performs with better sensitivity, MRI may be more specific. [60,93,105] Abnormal findings overlap between these two modalities, but may be distributed differently in the myocardium. Theoretically, this difference in performance underscores two different pathological processes with inflammation and necrosis depicted by PET, and scarring with edema depicted by MRI. [93]

The clinical utility of MRI has been demonstrated in several studies. The clinical severity of cardiac involvement correlates well with the extent of gadolinium enhancement. [106,107] Furthermore, abnormalities on MRI have been shown to decrease after corticosteroid treatment (Figure 10). [99,106-108] In a study of follow-up changes on MRI, Vignaux et al. demonstrated a strong correlation between MRI findings and clinical outcomes; patients with an improved or cleared MRI had improved symptoms, whereas those with worse MRI findings worsened clinically as well. [107] Patients with irreversible scar show slight decreases or no change on enhancement after treatment. [97,109] Patel and colleagues conducted the first prospective study evaluating the utility of cardiac MRI in asymptomatic patients with biopsy-proven extracardiac sarcoidosis. [97] As mentioned previously, MRI was more than twice as sensitive as the JMHW guidelines for cardiac sarcoidosis, likely due to detection of early disease. More importantly, patients with myocardial findings on MRI had a 9-fold higher rate of adverse events and 11.5-fold higher rate of death than those with negative MRI studies. This was the first study to demonstrate the outcome of cardiac sarcoid patients diagnosed with MRI, who would have no evidence of the disease on standard evaluation.

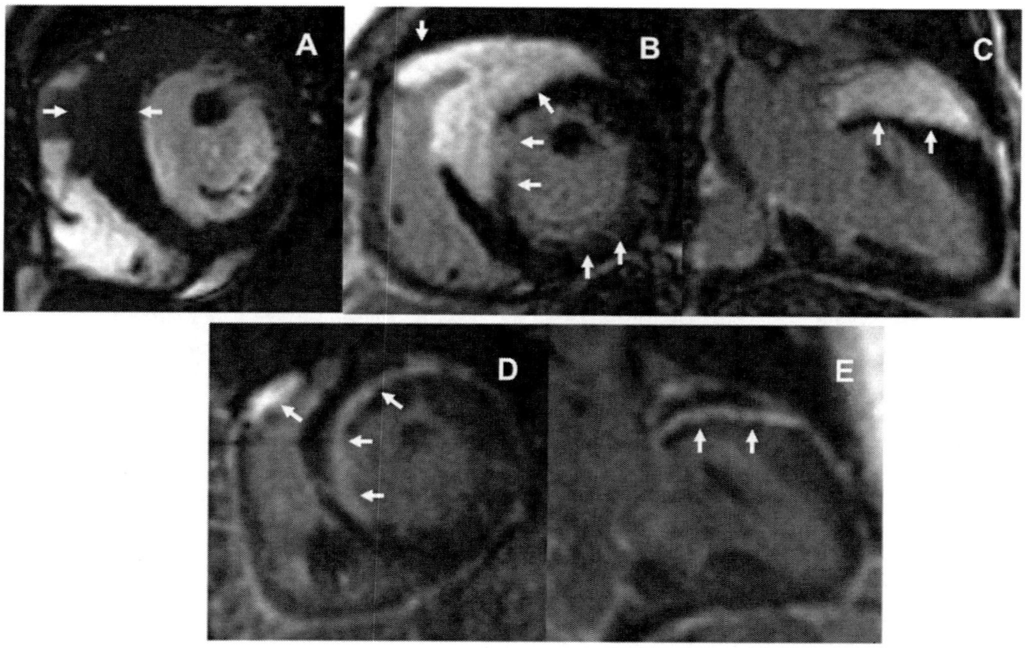

Figure 10. Cardiac MRI of a patient at diagnosis and at 3-month follow-up after treatment with corticosteroids. (A) Cine steady-state free precession short axis image shows increased thickness of the mid-basal left ventricular anterior and anteroseptal walls (arrows). (B) Gadolinium DE-CMR shows transmural hyperenhancement of the anterior, anteroseptal and anterosuperior right ventricular free walls (arrows). (C) Gadolinium DE-CMR shows nearly transmural hyperenhancement of the basal anterior wall in the 2-chamber view (arrows). Significant decrease in hyperenhancement is seen in both (D) short axis and (E) 2-chamber views as compared to the previous study. Reprinted from Journal of the American College of Cardiology, 61(14), Kadosh B, Steele J, Gulkarov I, Mamkin I, Cardiac Sarcoidosis, Page 1548, Copyright (2013), with permission from Elsevier. [108].

MRI does not expose patients to radiation, which is an advantage over other radionuclide studies. As a result of its increased spatial resolution capabilities, MRI can be used to guide endomyocardial biopsies, thus improving the sensitivity of that test. [110] MRI is also less costly than PET and is more widely available, though this varies between institutions. [6] There are, however, several limitations to MRI as well. Image quality varies considerably between different techniques.

Subtle abnormalities such as low-intensity enhancements may be difficult to distinguish from artifact to which MRI is particularly prone. [56] Inter-observer reliability in the context of cardiac sarcoidosis has yet to be evaluated. Another drawback to MRI is its contraindication with implantable cardiac devices, though this is not an absolute contraindication especially with the advent of MRI-safe pacemakers. In addition, gadolinium may be contraindicated in patients with renal failure due to the risk of nephrogenic systemic fibrosis.

Case reports describing late enhancement with nonionic iodinated contrast agent have shown similar findings to MRI in both location and extent of enhancement. [111,112] Future directions in cardiac MRI include the use of diffusion weighted imaging (DWI) in order to characterize tissue without the use of contrast injection. Magnetic resonance tractography, a derivative of DWI, may make it possible to directly evaluate myofiber architecture as well. [56]

Prognosis

The evolution of diagnosis and management of cardiac sarcoidosis has greatly altered prognosis for patients with the disease. Though prognosis is not well defined, outcomes for patients with symptoms are known to be poor compared with asymptomatic patients. Autopsy studies conducted in the 1970s showed that most patients died within 2 years of symptom onset. [3]

In later studies, outcomes improved with 5-year survival rates from 55% and 75% in steroid treated patients and up to 90% in treated patients with preserved systolic function. [42,113,114] In untreated patients, however, outcomes were grim with only 10% survival after 5 years. [114] As diagnostic techniques improve, cardiac sarcoidosis is identified earlier in the disease course allowing for more aggressive therapy and improved long-term outcomes. [5,7,60,97]

The three most powerful prognostic indicators for mortality in cardiac sarcoidosis are the New York Heart Association functional class, left ventricular enlargement on echocardiography, and sustained ventricular tachycardia. [114] As discussed previously, the prognostic value cardiac MRI has been studied prospectively, [97] demonstrating a cardiac death rate of 11.5% per year in MRI-positive patients versus 1% per year in MRI-negative patients. This was contrasted with a death rate of 9.7% versus 2.5% per year in JHMW-positive versus JHMW-negative patients.

Management

Corticosteroids

Corticosteroid therapy is the mainstay of treatment for cardiac sarcoidosis. Corticosteroids suppress inflammation and slow the progression of fibrosis by suppressing pro-inflammatory cytokines and chemokines that are involved in cell-mediated immune responses. [115] They have been shown to improve sarcoid manifestations such as atrioventricular blocks, ventricular arrhythmia, and left ventricular function as well as longterm survival. [7,114,116-118] One report examined therapeutic response by looking at left ventricular ejection fractions. [118] Patients with ejection fractions less than 30% did not respond to corticosteroids and had a 10-year survival of 19%. Those with ejection fractions of 30% to 50% significantly improved with treatment and survived at a rate of 67% after 5 years. Finally, patients with ejection fractions above 50% had a 100% survival rate at 10 years. These results suggest that early intervention with corticosteroids, before irreversible scar formation compromises cardiac function, is critical.

Although corticosteroids are used with confidence, timing, initial dosing, and duration of treatment is still debatable. Immediate high dose therapy with prednisone (1 mg/kg/day) in symptomatic patients is common; [7,98] however in the asymptomatic patient the benefit of high dose treatment is not clear. One Japanese study failed to find any significant difference in outcomes between patients receiving greater than 40 mg/day of prednisone versus those receiving 30 mg/day or less. [114] Typically treatment is tapered to an equivalent of 5 to 15 mg of prednisone for 12 months. [6] This duration of treatment, however, remains controversial. Case reports on sudden death after withdrawal of corticosteroids have influenced some authors to recommend indefinite treatment at minimal doses, [7,119] whereas others recommend a duration of 24 months. [56] In any case, there is consensus for close surveillance of these patients with complete history, physical exam, and ECG studies every 3 months during the steroid taper. Follow-up imaging can guide treatment as well, first at the initial 3 month visit and then less frequently, every 4 to 6 months as needed. After the taper, follow-up imaging can be conducted at 3 and 6 months in the first year, when relapses are most common, and then annually as long as there is no interval change. [6] Though most clinicians agree that this is a reasonable approach to routine management of cardiac sarcoidosis, this method has not been studied systematically.

Immunosuppressive Drugs

Some patients are unresponsive to steroid therapy, while others may not tolerate their side effects. Immunosuppressive medications can be used in both scenarios as well as steroid-sparing agents in an attempt to mitigate the side effects of corticosteroids by maintaining patients on lower doses. [56] A number of agents including infliximab, methotrexate, azathioprine, cyclophosphamide, antimalarials, pentoxifylline, and thalidomide have been used in systemic sarcoidosis with varying degrees of success. [120-127] Evidence for the use of these agents in cardiac sarcoidosis is minimal and treatment choice is usually based on clinical experience. Cyclophosphamide has been used in conjunction with methotrexate for limited duration (usually between 6 to 12 months) in refractory cardiac sarcoidosis. [7,122,128] The response can be rapid, however severe side effects such as sterility and increased risk of malignancies is cause for concern. Infliximab, a TNF-alpha antagonist, has been shown to be effective in pulmonary and systemic sarcoid manifestations. [127] Paradoxically, infliximab has the potential to actually induce cardiac dysfunction, warranting extreme caution for use in cardiac sarcoidosis. Nevertheless, one case report has demonstrated efficacy [120] which suggests that this agent may be considered for salvage therapy in certain cases. More studies are needed to properly evaluate the potential risks and benefits for cardiac sarcoidosis patients.

Cardiologic Treatment

The sequelae of cardiac sarcoidosis require special attention and treatment to prevent morbidity and mortality in these patients. Heart failure and arrhythmia should be addressed, but never in lieu of optimal treatment of the underlying sarcoidosis. [6,118,129] Therapies for these conditions have no impact on the progression of the disease and therefore do not affect the increased risk of death in cardiac sarcoidosis. [129]

Heart failure due to cardiac sarcoidosis should be treated in the same manner as heart failure from other causes. Angiotensin-converting enzyme inhibitors and diuretics should be used as indicated. In the setting of heart failure, β-blockers are also appropriate but should be used with caution as these patients are prone to heart block. Antiarrhythmic drugs are used to control ventricular arrhythmias in patients who have good atrioventricular nodal function. [56] Currently there are no recommendations on drugs of choice for this purpose, though it should be noted that amiodarone is to be used with caution as it could exacerbate restrictive lung disease in pulmonary sarcoidosis. [4]

There is evidence suggesting that sustained ventricular tachycardia due to cardiac sarcoidosis is particularly resistant to antiarrhythmic drugs. [52] Radiofrequency catheter ablation has been used with mixed results in these patients. [130,131] ICD implantation, however, can be a life saving measure. Likewise in patients with syncope, heart block, or ventricular fibrillation, ICD placement is recommended to circumvent sudden death. [132] Whether to use ICDs as primary prevention in patients without spontaneous arrhythmias or decreased myocardial function is less clear. Some practitioners prefer ICD placement in patients with known cardiac involvement and either ECG abnormalities or ventricular wall motion abnormalities on echocardiogram. [6] The American College of Cardiology/American Heart Association/Heart Rhythm Society guidelines for device-based therapy considers cardiac sarcoidosis as an indication for pacemaker placement, but defers to the judgment of clinicians regarding ICD therapy. [132]

Recent efforts by the American College of Cardiology Foundation, the Heart Rhythm Society and other key subspecialty societies have outlined guidelines for appropriate use of ICD therapies. [133] Myocardial sarcoidosis was deemed an appropriate indication for secondary prevention of ventricular fibrillation or hemodynamically unstable ventricular tachycardia. ICD therapy was graded as "maybe appropriate" for nonischemic cardiomyopathy due to sarcoidosis, and "definitely appropriate" in patients who have a left ventricular ejection fraction (LVEF) of 35% or less. Since the evidence is variable on ICD therapy in patients with LVEF greater than 35%, the decision whether to proceed with an ICD implantation or not should be based on a particular clinical scenario.

More challenging are those asymptomatic patients with no ECG or echocardiographic findings, but with cardiac involvement detected on advanced imaging. Since sudden death is known to be a presenting symptom in some patients, this population may be at risk. Kron and colleagues conducted the largest study to date evaluating ICD efficacy and safety in cardiac sarcoid patients. [134] Of 235 patients with ICDs followed over 4 years, 36% received appropriate shocks and/or anti-tachycardia pacing at an event rate of 8.6% per year. Thirty percent of patients received appropriate shocks alone at an event rate of 7.1% per year.

Patients who received appropriate therapy were more likely to be male, have a history of syncope, have a lower mean LVEF, an indication for secondary prevention with an ICD, and have ventricular pacing on baseline ECG. On the other hand, 24% of patients experienced inappropriate shocks or pacing and 18% suffered from device complications such as lead dislodgement and fracture as well as infection.

The results illustrate the cost/benefit conundrum of ICD therapy and offered some direction towards risk stratification in these patients. However, prospective randomized trials have yet to be conducted on this population. Consequently the data demonstrates some benefit to ICD therapy in general, but is lacking to support ICD implantation in asymptomatic patients.

Surgery

Directed surgical intervention can be helpful for cardiac sarcoidosis patients with certain clinical presentations. Massive pericardial effusions presenting as tamponade require drainage via pericardiocentesis or pericardectomy. [128,135] Surgical resection of sarcoid-associated left ventricular aneurysm was shown to cure refractory ventricular tachycardia in one case. [136]

Another case described surgical removal of a ball-like left ventricular thrombus associated with cardiac sarcoidosis. [137] Left ventricular exclusion and restoration procedures have been performed with variable success. [138-140]

Cardiac transplantation is rare in sarcoidosis, but can be successful for these patients. [141] Advanced and refractory disease is debilitating with a high risk of mortality due to heart failure or ventricular arrhythmias. Cardiac transplantation must be considered in these cases despite the spreading nature of the disease. [116] Recurrence of sarcoidosis in the transplanted heart is rare but has been reported in several cases, occurring between 24 weeks and 19 months postoperatively. [141-143]

In one case, transmission of sarcoidosis occurred from an allograft donor to its recipient. [144] Though concerns have been raised over issues of relapse, the evidence suggests that recurrent disease is responsive to steroids with good outcome. [142,143] It has also been shown that sarcoidosis patients undergoing heart transplantation have survival rates at least as good as patients who receive heart transplants for other causes. [143]

Conclusion

Cardiac sarcoidosis is a relatively rare disease with the potential for devastating complications. Owing to its unknown etiology and unpredictable manifestations including sudden cardiac death, patients with systemic sarcoidosis deserve a thorough search for evidence of cardiac involvement. Additionally, cardiac sarcoidosis should remain in the differential for those patients presenting with unexplained cardiac phenomena as this disease may mimic other common conditions. Advances in imaging techniques such as FDG-PET and MRI have improved the detection rate of this disease, revealing that cardiac involvement is likely more common in sarcoidosis than we know. Prognosis is not well defined, but known to be poor in symptomatic patients and those who do not receive treatment. Corticosteroids are considered the drug of choice for first-line therapy. Other immunosuppressive drugs and antiarrhythmics may be considered depending on specific clinical scenarios. Implantable pacemakers and defibrillators should be considered early in the disease due to the risk of sudden cardiac death, especially in the presence of ventricular arrhythmias. Surgical intervention and transplantation are a last resort, but may improve outcomes in advanced disease. Future goals for research are to conduct more prospective trials evaluating PET and MRI for the early detection of cardiac sarcoidosis as well as the development of diagnostic and therapeutic guidelines. The advancement of newer imaging protocols and tissue characterization techniques may improve the capability of these tests to differentiate cardiac sarcoidosis from other cardiomyopathies.

References

[1] Boeck, C., Multiple, Benign, Sarcoid of the Skin. *J Cutan Genitourin Dis.*, 1899, 17, 543.

[2] Iannuzzi, MC; Rybicki, BA; Teirstein, AS. Sarcoidosis. *The New England journal of medicine.*, Nov 22 2007, 357(21), 2153-2165.

[3] Roberts, WC; McAllister, HA; Jr.; Ferrans, VJ. Sarcoidosis of the heart. A clinicopathologic study of 35 necropsy patients (group 1) and review of 78 previously described necropsy patients (group 11). *The American journal of medicine*, Jul 1977, 63(1), 86-108.

[4] Doughan, AR; Williams, BR. Cardiac sarcoidosis. *Heart*, Feb 2006, 92(2), 282-288.

[5] Smedema, JP; Snoep, G; van Kroonenburgh, MP; et al. Cardiac involvement in patients with pulmonary sarcoidosis assessed at two university medical centers in the Netherlands. *Chest*, Jul 2005, 128(1), 30-35.

[6] Kim, JS; Judson, MA; Donnino, R; et al. Cardiac sarcoidosis. *American heart journal.*, Jan 2009, 157(1), 9-21.

[7] Chapelon-Abric, C; de Zuttere, D; Duhaut, P; et al. Cardiac sarcoidosis: a retrospective study of 41 cases. *Medicine*, Nov 2004, 83(6), 315-334.

[8] Rybicki, BA; Major, M; Popovich, J; Jr. Maliarik, MJ; Iannuzzi, MC. Racial differences in sarcoidosis incidence: a 5-year study in a health maintenance organization. *American journal of epidemiology*, Feb 1 1997, 145(3), 234-241.

[9] Bresnitz, EA; Strom, BL. Epidemiology of sarcoidosis. *Epidemiologic reviews*, 1983, 5, 124-156.

[10] Yigla, M; Badarna-Abu-Ria, N; Tov, N; Ravell-Weiller, D; Rubin, AH. Sarcoidosis in northern Israel: clinical characteristics of 120 patients. *Sarcoidosis, vasculitis, and diffuse lung diseases: official journal of WASOG / World Association of Sarcoidosis and Other Granulomatous Disorders*, Oct 2002, 19(3), 220-226.

[11] Pietinalho, A; Hiraga, Y; Hosoda, Y; Lofroos, AB; Yamaguchi, M; Selroos, O. The frequency of sarcoidosis in Finland and Hokkaido, Japan. A comparative epidemiological study. *Sarcoidosis*, Mar 1995, 12(1), 61-67.

[12] Rybicki, BA; Iannuzzi, MC. Epidemiology of sarcoidosis, recent advances and future prospects. *Seminars in respiratory and critical care medicine*, Feb 2007, 28(1), 22-35.

[13] Perry, A; Vuitch, F. Causes of death in patients with sarcoidosis. A morphologic study of 38 autopsies with clinicopathologic correlations. *Archives of pathology & laboratory medicine*, Feb 1995, 119(2), 167-172.

[14] Iwai, K; Sekiguti, M; Hosoda, Y; et al. Racial difference in cardiac sarcoidosis incidence observed at autopsy. *Sarcoidosis*, Mar 1994, 11(1), 26-31.

[15] Silverman, KJ; Hutchins, GM; Bulkley, BH. Cardiac sarcoid, a clinicopathologic study of 84 unselected patients with systemic sarcoidosis. *Circulation*, Dec 1978, 58(6), 1204-1211.

[16] Iwai, K; Tachibana, T; Takemura, T; Matsui, Y; Kitaichi, M; Kawabata, Y. Pathological studies on sarcoidosis autopsy. I. Epidemiological features of 320 cases in Japan. *Acta pathologica japonica*, Jul-Aug 1993, 43(7-8), 372-376.

[17] Morimoto, T; Azuma, A; Abe, S; et al. Epidemiology of sarcoidosis in Japan. *The European respiratory journal: official journal of the European Society for Clinical Respiratory Physiology*, Feb 2008, 31(2), 372-379.

[18] Zissel, G; Prasse, A; Muller-Quernheim, J. Sarcoidosis--immunopathogenetic concepts. *Seminars in respiratory and critical care medicine*, Feb 2007, 28(1), 3-14.

[19] Silver, RF; Crystal, RG; Moller, DR. Limited heterogeneity of biased T-cell receptor V beta gene usage in lung but not blood T cells in active pulmonary sarcoidosis. *Immunology*, Aug 1996, 88(4), 516-523.

[20] Agostini, C; Adami, F; Semenzato, G. New pathogenetic insights into the sarcoid granuloma. *Current opinion in rheumatology*, Jan 2000, 12(1), 71-76.

[21] Semenzato, G. ACCESS: A Case Control Etiologic Study of Sarcoidosis. *Sarcoidosis, vasculitis, and diffuse lung diseases: official journal of WASOG / World Association of Sarcoidosis and Other Granulomatous Disorders*, Jun 2005, 22(2), 83-86.

[22] Barnard, J; Rose, C; Newman, L; et al. Job and industry classifications associated with sarcoidosis in A Case-Control Etiologic Study of Sarcoidosis (ACCESS). *Journal of occupational and environmental medicine/American College of Occupational and Environmental Medicine*, Mar 2005, 47(3), 226-234.

[23] Sekhri, V; Sanal, S; Delorenzo, LJ; Aronow, WS; Maguire, GP. Cardiac sarcoidosis: a comprehensive review. *Archives of medical science: AMS*, Aug 2011, 7(4), 546-554.

[24] Rybicki, BA; Iannuzzi, MC; Frederick, MM, et al. Familial aggregation of sarcoidosis. A case-control etiologic study of sarcoidosis (ACCESS). *American journal of respiratory and critical care medicine*., Dec 1 2001, 164(11), 2085-2091.

[25] Rossman, MD; Thompson, B; Frederick, M; et, al. HLA-DRB1*1101: a significant risk factor for sarcoidosis in blacks and whites. *American journal of human genetics*, Oct 2003, 73(4), 720-735.

[26] Iannuzzi, MC; Rybicki, BA. Genetics of sarcoidosis: candidate genes and genome scans. *Proceedings of the American Thoracic Society*, Jan 2007, 4(1), 108-116.

[27] Rybicki, BA; Sinha, R; Iyengar, S; Gray-McGuire, C; Elston, RC; Iannuzzi, MC. Genetic linkage analysis of sarcoidosis phenotypes: the sarcoidosis genetic analysis (SAGA) study. *Genes and immunity*, Jul 2007, 8(5), 379-386.

[28] Naruse, TK; Matsuzawa, Y; Ota, M; et al. HLA-DQB1*0601 is primarily associated with the susceptibility to cardiac sarcoidosis. *Tissue antigens*, Jul 2000, 56(1), 52-57.

[29] Iannuzzi, MC; Maliarik, MJ; Poisson, LM; Rybicki, BA. Sarcoidosis susceptibility and resistance HLA-DQB1 alleles in African Americans. *American journal of respiratory and critical care medicine*, May 1 2003, 167(9), 1225-1231.

[30] Sato, H; Grutters, JC; Pantelidis, P; et al. HLA-DQB1*0201: a marker for good prognosis in British and Dutch patients with sarcoidosis. *American journal of respiratory cell and molecular biology*, Oct 2002, 27(4), 406-412.

[31] Grutters, JC; Sato, H; Pantelidis, P; et, al. Increased frequency of the uncommon tumor necrosis factor -857T allele in British and Dutch patients with sarcoidosis. *American journal of respiratory and critical care medicine*., Apr 15 2002, 165(8), 1119-1124.

[32] Takashige, N; Naruse, TK; Matsumori, A; et al. Genetic polymorphisms at the tumour necrosis factor loci (TNFA and TNFB) in cardiac sarcoidosis. *Tissue antigens*, Aug 1999, 54(2), 191-193.

[33] Rybicki, BA; Walewski, JL; Maliarik, MJ; Kian, H; Iannuzzi, MC. The BTNL2 gene and sarcoidosis susceptibility in African Americans and Whites. *American journal of human genetics*, Sep 2005, 77(3), 491-499.

[34] Valentonyte, R; Hampe, J; Huse, K; et al. Sarcoidosis is associated with a truncating splice site mutation in BTNL2. *Nature genetics*, Apr 2005, 37(4), 357-364.

[35] Iannuzzi, MC. Genetics of sarcoidosis. *Seminars in respiratory and critical care medicine*, Feb 2007, 28(1), 15-21.

[36] Schurmann, M; Reichel, P; Muller-Myhsok, B; Schlaak, M; Muller-Quernheim, J; Schwinger, E. Results from a genome-wide search for predisposing genes in sarcoidosis. *American journal of respiratory and critical care medicine*, Sep 1 2001, 164(5), 840-846.

[37] Iannuzzi, MC; Iyengar, SK; Gray-McGuire, C; et al. Genome-wide search for sarcoidosis susceptibility genes in African Americans. *Genes and immunity*, Sep 2005, 6(6), 509-518.

[38] Franke, A; Fischer, A; Nothnagel, M; et al. Genome-wide association analysis in sarcoidosis and Crohn's disease unravels a common susceptibility locus on 10p12.2. *Gastroenterology*, Oct 2008, 135(4), 1207-1215.

[39] Rybicki, BA; Levin, AM; McKeigue, P; et al. A genome-wide admixture scan for ancestry-linked genes predisposing to sarcoidosis in African-Americans. *Genes and immunity*, Mar 2011, 12(2), 67-77.

[40] Culver, DA; Newman, LS; Kavuru, MS. Gene-environment interactions in sarcoidosis: challenge and opportunity. *Clinics in dermatology*, May-Jun 2007, 25(3), 267-275.

[41] Halushka, MK; Yuh, DD; Russell, SD. Right ventricle-dominant cardiac sarcoidosis with sparing of the left ventricle. *The Journal of heart and lung transplantation: the*

official publication of the International Society for Heart Transplantation, Apr 2006, 25(4), 479-482.

[42] Fleming, HA; Bailey, SM. Sarcoid heart disease. *Journal of the Royal College of Physicians of London*, Oct 1981, 15(4), 245-246, 249-253.

[43] Gasparovic, H; Bueno, R; Rybicki, FJ; et al. Sarcoidosis of the aortic root. *The Journal of thoracic and cardiovascular surgery*, Nov 2004, 128(5), 761-762.

[44] Goyal, SB; Aragam, JR. Cardiac sarcoidosis with primary involvement of the tricuspid valve. *Cardiology in review*, Sep-Oct 2006, 14(5), e12-13.

[45] Aizer, A; Stern, EH; Gomes, JA; Teirstein, AS; Eckart, RE; Mehta, D. Usefulness of programmed ventricular stimulation in predicting future arrhythmic events in patients with cardiac sarcoidosis. *The American journal of cardiology*, Jul 15 2005, 96(2), 276-282.

[46] Garrett, J; O'Neill, H; Blake, S. Constrictive pericarditis associated with sarcoidosis. *American heart journal*, Feb 1984, 107(2), 394.

[47] Kinney, E; Murthy, R; Ascunce, G; Donohoe, R; Zelis, R. Pericardial effusions in sarcoidosis. *Chest*, Oct 1979, 76(4), 476-478.

[48] Zelcer, AA; LeJemtel, TH; Jones, J; Stahl, J. Pericardial tamponade in sarcoidosis. *The Canadian journal of cardiology*, Jan-Feb 1987, 3(1), 12-13.

[49] Handa, T; Nagai, S; Miki, S; et al. Incidence of pulmonary hypertension and its clinical relevance in patients with sarcoidosis. *Chest*, May 2006, 129(5), 1246-1252.

[50] Shigemitsu, H; Nagai, S; Sharma, OP. Pulmonary hypertension and granulomatous vasculitis in sarcoidosis. *Current opinion in pulmonary medicine*, Sep 2007, 13(5), 434-438.

[51] Sekiguchi, M; Hiroe, M; Take, M; Hirosawa, K. Clinical and histopathological profile of sarcoidosis of the heart and acute idiopathic myocarditis. Concepts through a study employing endomyocardial biopsy. II. Myocarditis. *Japanese circulation journal*, Apr 1980, 44(4), 264-273.

[52] Winters, SL; Cohen, M; Greenberg, S; et al. Sustained ventricular tachycardia associated with sarcoidosis: assessment of the underlying cardiac anatomy and the prospective utility of programmed ventricular stimulation, drug therapy and an implantable antitachycardia device. *Journal of the American College of Cardiology*, Oct 1991, 18(4), 937-943.

[53] Hiraga, H; Yuwai, K; Hiroe, M. *Guideline for diagnosis of cardiac sarcoidosis: study report on diffuse pulmonary diseases from the Japanese Ministry of Health and Welfare*, Tokyo: Japanese Ministry of Health and Welfare, 1993.

[54] Judson, MA. A proposed solution to the clinical assessment of sarcoidosis: the sarcoidosis three-dimensional assessment instrument (STAI). *Medical hypotheses*, 2007, 68(5), 1080-1087.

[55] Ayyala, US; Nair, AP; Padilla, ML. Cardiac sarcoidosis. *Clinics in chest medicine*, Sep 2008, 29(3), 493-508, ix.

[56] Nunes, H; Freynet, O; Naggara, N; et al. Cardiac sarcoidosis. *Seminars in respiratory and critical care medicine*, Aug 2010, 31(4), 428-441.

[57] Sekiguchi, M; Yazaki, Y; Isobe, M; Hiroe, M. Cardiac sarcoidosis: diagnostic, prognostic, and therapeutic considerations. *Cardiovascular drugs and therapy/ sponsored by the International Society of Cardiovascular Pharmacotherapy*, Nov 1996, 10(5), 495-510.

[58] Suzuki, T; Kanda, T; Kubota, S; Imai, S; Murata, K. Holter monitoring as a noninvasive indicator of cardiac involvement in sarcoidosis. *Chest*, Oct 1994, 106(4), 1021-1024.

[59] Judson, MA; Baughman, RP; Teirstein, AS; Terrin, ML; Yeager, H; Jr. Defining organ involvement in sarcoidosis: the ACCESS proposed instrument. ACCESS Research Group. A Case Control Etiologic Study of Sarcoidosis. *Sarcoidosis, vasculitis, and diffuse lung diseases: official journal of WASOG/World Association of Sarcoidosis and Other Granulomatous Disorders*, Mar 1999, 16(1), 75-86.

[60] Mehta, D; Lubitz, SA; Frankel, Z; et al. Cardiac involvement in patients with sarcoidosis: diagnostic and prognostic value of outpatient testing. *Chest*, Jun 2008, 133(6), 1426-1435.

[61] Weinberg, M; Fell, EH; Lynfield, J. Diagnostic biopsy of the pericardium and myocardium. *A.M.A. archives of surgery*, May 1958, 76(5), 825-829.

[62] Ratner, SJ; Fenoglio, JJ; Jr. Ursell, PC. Utility of endomyocardial biopsy in the diagnosis of cardiac sarcoidosis. *Chest*, Oct 1986, 90(4), 528-533.

[63] Tadamura, E; Yamamuro, M; Kubo, S; et al. Effectiveness of delayed enhanced MRI for identification of cardiac sarcoidosis, comparison with radionuclide imaging. *AJR. American journal of roentgenology*, Jul 2005, 185(1), 110-115.

[64] Uemura, A; Morimoto, S; Hiramitsu, S; Kato, Y; Ito, T; Hishida, H. Histologic diagnostic rate of cardiac sarcoidosis, evaluation of endomyocardial biopsies. *American heart journal*, Aug 1999, 138(2 Pt 1), 299-302.

[65] Ardehali, H; Howard, DL; Hariri, A; et al. A positive endomyocardial biopsy result for sarcoid is associated with poor prognosis in patients with initially unexplained cardiomyopathy. *American heart journal*, Sep 2005, 150(3), 459-463.

[66] Kinney, EL; Jackson, GL; Reeves, WC; Zelis, R. Thallium-scan myocardial defects and echocardiographic abnormalities in patients with sarcoidosis without clinical cardiac dysfunction. An analysis of 44 patients. *The American journal of medicine*, Apr 1980, 68(4), 497-503.

[67] Lewin, RF; Mor, R; Spitzer, S; Arditti, A; Hellman, C; Agmon, J. Echocardiographic evaluation of patients with systemic sarcoidosis. *American heart journa.*, Jul 1985, 110(1 Pt 1), 116-122.

[68] Burstow, DJ; Tajik, AJ; Bailey, KR; DeRemee, RA; Taliercio, CP. Two-dimensional echocardiographic findings in systemic sarcoidosis. *The American journal of cardiology*, Feb 15 1989, 63(7), 478-482.

[69] Gibbons, WJ; Levy, RD; Nava, S; et al. Subclinical cardiac dysfunction in sarcoidosis. *Chest*, Jul 1991, 100(1), 44-50.

[70] Angomachalelis, N; Hourzamanis, A; Vamvalis, C; Gavrielides, A. Doppler echocardiographic evaluation of left ventricular diastolic function in patients with systemic sarcoidosis. *Postgraduate medical journal*, 1992, 68 Suppl 1, S52-56.

[71] Fahy, GJ; Marwick, T; McCreery, CJ; Quigley, PJ; Maurer, BJ. Doppler echocardiographic detection of left ventricular diastolic dysfunction in patients with pulmonary sarcoidosis. *Chest*, Jan 1996, 109(1), 62-66.

[72] Hyodo, E; Hozumi, T; Takemoto, Y; et al. Early detection of cardiac involvement in patients with sarcoidosis by a non-invasive method with ultrasonic tissue characterisation. *Heart*, Nov 2004, 90(11), 1275-1280.

[73] Yasutake, H; Seino, Y; Kashiwagi, M; Honma, H; Matsuzaki, T; Takano, T. Detection of cardiac sarcoidosis using cardiac markers and myocardial integrated backscatter. *International journal of cardiology*, Jul 10 2005, 102(2), 259-268.

[74] Hourigan, LA; Burstow, DJ; Pohlner, P; Clarke, BE; Donnelly, JE. Transesophageal echocardiographic abnormalities in a case of cardiac sarcoidosis. *Journal of the American Society of Echocardiography: official publication of the American Society of Echocardiography*, May 2001, 14(5), 399-402.

[75] Weidemann, F; Strotmann, JM. Use of tissue Doppler imaging to identify and manage systemic diseases. *Clinical research in cardiology: official journal of the German Cardiac Society*, Feb 2008, 97(2), 65-73.

[76] Bulkley, BH; Rouleau, JR; Whitaker, JQ; Strauss, HW; Pitt, B. The use of 201thallium for myocardial perfusion imaging in sarcoid heart disease. *Chest*, Jul 1977, 72(1), 27-32.

[77] Tellier, P; Paycha, F; Antony, I; et al. Reversibility by dipyridamole of thallium-201 myocardial scan defects in patients with sarcoidosis. *The American journal of medicine*, Aug 1988, 85(2), 189-193.

[78] Le, Guludec, D; Menad, F; Faraggi, M; Weinmann, P; Battesti, JP; Valeyre, D. Myocardial sarcoidosis. Clinical value of technetium-99m sestamibi tomoscintigraphy. *Chest*, Dec 1994, 106(6), 1675-1682.

[79] Haywood, LJ; Sharma, OP; Siegel, ME; et al. Detection of myocardial sarcoidosis by thallium 201 imaging. *Journal of the National Medical Association*, Oct 1982, 74(10), 959-964.

[80] Tellier, P; Valeyre, D; Nitenberg, A; Foult, JM; Bedig, G; Battesti, JP. Cardiac sarcoidosis: reversion of myocardial perfusion abnormalities by dipyridamole. *European journal of nuclear medicine*, 1985, 11(6-7), 201-204.

[81] Fields, CL; Ossorio, MA; Roy, TM; Denny, DM; Varga, DW. Thallium-201 scintigraphy in the diagnosis and management of myocardial sarcoidosis. *Southern medical journal*, Mar 1990, 83(3), 339-342.

[82] Yamagishi, H; Shirai, N; Takagi, M; et al. Identification of cardiac sarcoidosis with (13)N-NH(3)/(18)F-FDG PET. *Journal of nuclear medicine: official publication, Society of Nuclear Medicine*, Jul 2003, 44(7), 1030-1036.

[83] Kaminaga, T; Takeshita, T; Yamauchi, T; Kawamura, H; Yasuda, M. The role of iodine-123-labeled 15-(p-iodophenyl)-3R,S-methylpentadecanoic acid scintigraphy in the detection of local myocardial involvement of sarcoidosis. *International journal of cardiology*, Mar 2004, 94(1), 99-103.

[84] Okumura, W; Iwasaki, T; Toyama, T; et al. Usefulness of fasting 18F-FDG PET in identification of cardiac sarcoidosis. *Journal of nuclear medicine: official publication, Society of Nuclear Medicine*, Dec 2004, 45(12), 1989-1998.

[85] Kinney, EL; Caldwell, JW. Do thallium myocardial perfusion scan abnormalities predict survival in sarcoid patients without cardiac symptoms? *Angiology*, Jul 1990, 41(7), 573-576.

[86] Okayama, K; Kurata, C; Tawarahara, K; Wakabayashi, Y; Chida, K; Sato, A. Diagnostic and prognostic value of myocardial scintigraphy with thallium-201 and gallium-67 in cardiac sarcoidosis. *Chest*, Feb 1995, 107(2), 330-334.

[87] Nakazawa, A; Ikeda, K; Ito, Y; et al. Usefulness of dual 67Ga and 99mTc-sestamibi single-photon-emission CT scanning in the diagnosis of cardiac sarcoidosis. *Chest*, Oct 2004, 126(4), 1372-1376.

[88] Kiuchi, S; Teraoka, K; Koizumi, K; Takazawa, K; Yamashina, A. Usefulness of late gadolinium enhancement combined with MRI and 67-Ga scintigraphy in the diagnosis of cardiac sarcoidosis and disease activity evaluation. *The international journal of cardiovascular imaging*, Apr 2007, 23(2), 237-241.

[89] Lewis, PJ; Salama, A. Uptake of fluorine-18-fluorodeoxyglucose in sarcoidosis. *Journal of nuclear medicine: official publication, Society of Nuclear Medicine*, Oct 1994, 35(10), 1647-1649.

[90] Brudin, LH; Valind, SO; Rhodes, CG; et al. Fluorine-18 deoxyglucose uptake in sarcoidosis measured with positron emission tomography. *European journal of nuclear medicine*, Apr 1994, 21(4), 297-305.

[91] Ishimaru, S; Tsujino, I; Takei, T; et al. Focal uptake on 18F-fluoro-2-deoxyglucose positron emission tomography images indicates cardiac involvement of sarcoidosis. *European heart journal*, Aug 2005, 26(15), 1538-1543.

[92] Yokoyama, I; Momomura, S; Ohtake, T; et al. Role of positron emission tomography using fluorine-18 fluoro-2-deoxyglucose in predicting improvement in left ventricular function in patients with idiopathic dilated cardiomyopathy. *European journal of nuclear medicine*, Jul 1998, 25(7), 736-743.

[93] Ohira, H; Tsujino, I; Ishimaru, S; et al. Myocardial imaging with 18F-fluoro-2-deoxyglucose positron emission tomography and magnetic resonance imaging in sarcoidosis. *European journal of nuclear medicine and molecular imaging*, May 2008, 35(5), 933-941.

[94] Langah, R; Spicer, K; Gebregziabher, M; Gordon, L. Effectiveness of prolonged fasting 18f-FDG PET-CT in the detection of cardiac sarcoidosis. *Journal of nuclear cardiology: official publication of the American Society of Nuclear Cardiology*, Sep-Oct 2009, 16(5), 801-810.

[95] van den Heuvel, AF; van, Veldhuisen, DJ; van, der, Wall, EE; et al. Regional myocardial blood flow reserve impairment and metabolic changes suggesting myocardial ischemia in patients with idiopathic dilated cardiomyopathy. *Journal of the American College of Cardiology*, Jan 2000, 35(1), 19-28.

[96] Vignaux, O. Cardiac sarcoidosis, spectrum of MRI features. *AJR, American journal of roentgenology*, Jan 2005, 184(1), 249-254.

[97] Patel, MR; Cawley, PJ; Heitner, JF; et al. Detection of myocardial damage in patients with sarcoidosis. *Circulation*, Nov 17 2009, 120(20), 1969-1977.

[98] Vignaux, O; Dhote, R; Duboc, D; et al. Detection of myocardial involvement in patients with sarcoidosis applying T2-weighted, contrast-enhanced, and cine magnetic resonance imaging: initial results of a prospective study. *Journal of computer assisted tomography*, Sep-Oct 2002, 26(5), 762-767.

[99] Inoue, S; Shimada, T; Murakami, Y. Clinical significance of gadolinium-DTPA-enhanced MRI for detection of myocardial lesions in a patient with sarcoidosis. *Clinical radiology*, Jan 1999, 54(1), 70-72.

[100] Matsuki, M; Matsuo, M. MR findings of myocardial sarcoidosis. *Clinical radiology*, Apr 2000, 55(4), 323-325.

[101] Shimada, T; Shimada, K; Sakane, T; et al. Diagnosis of cardiac sarcoidosis and evaluation of the effects of steroid therapy by gadolinium-DTPA-enhanced magnetic resonance imaging. *The American journal of medicine*, May 2001, 110(7), 520-527.

[102] Karamitsos, TD; Francis, JM; Myerson, S; Selvanayagam, JB; Neubauer, S. The role of cardiovascular magnetic resonance imaging in heart failure. *Journal of the American College of Cardiology*, Oct 6 2009, 54(15), 1407-1424.

[103] Smedema, JP; Snoep, G; van, Kroonenburgh, MP; et al. Evaluation of the accuracy of gadolinium-enhanced cardiovascular magnetic resonance in the diagnosis of cardiac sarcoidosis. *Journal of the American College of Cardiology*, May 17 2005, 45(10), 1683-1690.

[104] Kim, RJ; Fieno, DS; Parrish, TB; et al. Relationship of MRI delayed contrast enhancement to irreversible injury, infarct age, and contractile function. *Circulation*, Nov 9 1999, 100(19), 1992-2002.

[105] Tadamura, E; Yamamuro, M; Kubo, S; et al. Images in cardiovascular medicine. Multimodality imaging of cardiac sarcoidosis before and after steroid therapy. *Circulation*, May 23 2006, 113(20), e771-773.

[106] Doherty, MJ; Kumar, SK; Nicholson, AA; McGivern, DV. Cardiac sarcoidosis: the value of magnetic resonance imaging in diagnosis and assessment of response to treatment. *Respiratory medicine*, Apr 1998, 92(4), 697-699.

[107] Vignaux, O; Dhote, R; Duboc, D; et al. Clinical significance of myocardial magnetic resonance abnormalities in patients with sarcoidosis: a 1-year follow-up study. *Chest*, Dec 2002, 122(6), 1895-1901.

[108] Kadosh, B; Steele, J; Gulkarov, I; Mamkin, I. Cardiac sarcoidosis. *Journal of the American College of Cardiology*, Apr 9 2013, 61(14), 1548.

[109] Matoh, F; Satoh, H; Shiraki, K; et al. The usefulness of delayed enhancement magnetic resonance imaging for diagnosis and evaluation of cardiac function in patients with cardiac sarcoidosis. *Journal of cardiology*, Jun 2008, 51(3), 179-188.

[110] Niida, T; Isoda, K; Sasaki, M; Horikawa, M; Hayashi, K; Ohsuzu, F. Late gadolinium enhanced high resolution magnetic resonance imaging reveals pathophysiological condition of cardiac sarcoidosis. *International heart journal*, Mar 2009, 50(2), 263-266.

[111] Kanao, S; Tadamura, E; Yamamuro, M; et al. Demonstration of cardiac involvement of sarcoidosis by contrast-enhanced multislice computed tomography and delayed-enhanced magnetic resonance imaging. *Journal of computer assisted tomography*, Nov-Dec 2005, 29(6), 745-748.

[112] Smedema, JP; Truter, R; de, Klerk, PA; Zaaiman, L; White, L; Doubell, AF. Cardiac sarcoidosis evaluated with gadolinium-enhanced magnetic resonance and contrast-enhanced 64-slice computed tomography. *International journal of cardiology*, Sep 20 2006, 112(2), 261-263.

[113] Okura, Y; Dec, GW; Hare, JM; et al. A clinical and histopathologic comparison of cardiac sarcoidosis and idiopathic giant cell myocarditis. *Journal of the American College of Cardiology*, Jan 15 2003, 41(2), 322-329.

[114] Yazaki, Y; Isobe, M; Hiroe, M; et al. Prognostic determinants of long-term survival in Japanese patients with cardiac sarcoidosis treated with prednisone. *The American journal of cardiology*, Nov 1 2001, 88(9), 1006-1010.

[115] Grutters, JC; van, den, Bosch, JM. Corticosteroid treatment in sarcoidosis. *The European respiratory journal: official journal of the European Society for Clinical Respiratory Physiology*, Sep 2006, 28(3), 627-636.
[116] Valantine, HA; Tazelaar, HD; Macoviak, J; et al. Cardiac sarcoidosis: response to steroids and transplantation. *The Journal of heart transplantation*, Jul-Aug 1987, 6(4), 244-250.
[117] Ishikawa, T; Kondoh, H; Nakagawa, S; Koiwaya, Y; Tanaka, K. Steroid therapy in cardiac sarcoidosis. Increased left ventricular contractility concomitant with electrocardiographic improvement after prednisolone. *Chest*, Mar 1984, 85(3), 445-447.
[118] Chiu, CZ; Nakatani, S; Zhang, G; et al. Prevention of left ventricular remodeling by long-term corticosteroid therapy in patients with cardiac sarcoidosis. *The American journal of cardiology*, Jan 1 2005, 95(1), 143-146.
[119] Bargout, R; Kelly, RF. Sarcoid heart disease: clinical course and treatment. *International journal of cardiology*, Nov 2004, 97(2), 173-182.
[120] Uthman, I; Touma, Z; Khoury, M. Cardiac sarcoidosis responding to monotherapy with infliximab. *Clinical rheumatology*, Nov 2007, 26(11), 2001-2003.
[121] Baughman, RP; Judson, MA; Teirstein, AS; Moller, DR; Lower, EE. Thalidomide for chronic sarcoidosis. *Chest*, Jul 2002, 122(1), 227-232.
[122] Demeter, SL. Myocardial sarcoidosis unresponsive to steroids. Treatment with cyclophosphamide. *Chest*, Jul 1988, 94(1), 202-203.
[123] Muller-Quernheim, J; Kienast, K; Held, M; Pfeifer, S; Costabel, U. Treatment of chronic sarcoidosis with an azathioprine/prednisolone regimen. *The European respiratory journal: official journal of the European Society for Clinical Respiratory Physiology*, Nov 1999, 14(5), 1117-1122.
[124] Baltzan, M; Mehta, S; Kirkham, TH; Cosio, MG. Randomized trial of prolonged chloroquine therapy in advanced pulmonary sarcoidosis. *American journal of respiratory and critical care medicine*, Jul 1999, 160(1), 192-197.
[125] Baughman, RP; Ohmichi, M; Lower, EE. Combination therapy for sarcoidosis. *Sarcoidosis, vasculitis, and diffuse lung diseases: official journal of WASOG / World Association of Sarcoidosis and Other Granulomatous Disorders*, Jun 2001, 18(2), 133-137.
[126] Baughman, RP; Costabel, U; du Bois, RM. Treatment of sarcoidosis. *Clinics in chest medicine*, Sep 2008, 29(3), 533-548, ix-x.
[127] Baughman, RP; Drent, M; Kavuru, M; et al. Infliximab therapy in patients with chronic sarcoidosis and pulmonary involvement. *American journal of respiratory and critical care medicine*, Oct 1 2006, 174(7), 795-802.
[128] Israel, RH; Poe, RH. Massive pericardial effusion in sarcoidosis. *Respiration: international review of thoracic diseases*, 1994, 61(3), 176-180.
[129] Kato, Y; Morimoto, S; Uemura, A; Hiramitsu, S; Ito, T; Hishida, H. Efficacy of corticosteroids in sarcoidosis presenting with atrioventricular block. *Sarcoidosis, vasculitis, and diffuse lung diseases: official journal of WASOG / World Association of Sarcoidosis and Other Granulomatous Disorders*, Jun 2003, 20(2), 133-137.
[130] Koplan, BA; Soejima, K; Baughman, K; Epstein, LM; Stevenson, WG. Refractory ventricular tachycardia secondary to cardiac sarcoid: electrophysiologic characteristics, mapping, and ablation. *Heart rhythm: the official journal of the Heart Rhythm Society*, Aug 2006, 3(8), 924-929.

[131] Jefic, D; Joel, B; Good, E; et al. Role of radiofrequency catheter ablation of ventricular tachycardia in cardiac sarcoidosis, report from a multicenter registry. *Heart rhythm: the official journal of the Heart Rhythm Society*, Feb 2009, 6(2), 189-195.

[132] Epstein, AE; DiMarco, JP; Ellenbogen, KA; et al. ACC/AHA/HRS 2008 Guidelines for Device-Based Therapy of Cardiac Rhythm Abnormalities: a report of the American College of Cardiology/American Heart Association Task Force on Practice Guidelines (Writing Committee to Revise the ACC/AHA/NASPE 2002 Guideline Update for Implantation of Cardiac Pacemakers and Antiarrhythmia Devices): developed in collaboration with the American Association for Thoracic Surgery and Society of Thoracic Surgeons. *Circulation*, May 27 2008, 117(21), e350-408.

[133] Russo, AM; Stainback, RF; Bailey, SR; et al. ACCF/HRS/AHA/ASE/HFSA/SCAI/ SCCT/SCMR 2013 appropriate use criteria for implantable cardioverter-defibrillators and cardiac resynchronization therapy: a report of the American College of Cardiology Foundation appropriate use criteria task force, Heart Rhythm Society, American Heart Association, American Society of Echocardiography, Heart Failure Society of America, Society for Cardiovascular Angiography and Interventions, Society of Cardiovascular Computed Tomography, and Society for Cardiovascular Magnetic Resonance. *Journal of the American College of Cardiology*, Mar 26 2013, 61(12), 1318-1368.

[134] Kron, J; Sauer, W; Schuller, J; et al. Efficacy and safety of implantable cardiac defibrillators for treatment of ventricular arrhythmias in patients with cardiac sarcoidosis. *Europace: European pacing, arrhythmias, and cardiac electrophysiology: journal of the working groups on cardiac pacing, arrhythmias, and cardiac cellular electrophysiology of the European Society of Cardiology*, Mar 2013, 15(3), 347-354.

[135] Rubinstein, I; Baum, GL; Hiss, Y. Cardiac tamponade as the presenting symptom of sarcoidosis. *American heart journal*, Jun 1985, 109(6), 1387-1388.

[136] Lull, RJ; Dunn, BE; Gregoratos, G; Cox, WA; Fisher, GW. Ventricular aneurysm due to cardiac sarcoidosis with surgical cure of refractory ventricular tachycardia. *The American journal of cardiology*, Aug 1972, 30(3), 282-287.

[137] Kanemitsu, S; Miyake, Y; Okabe, M. Surgical removal of a left ventricular thrombus associated with cardiac sarcoidosis. *Interactive cardiovascular and thoracic surgery*, Apr 2008, 7(2), 333-335.

[138] Daimon, M; Sasaki, T; Woo, E; Ozawa, H; Morimoto, T; Katsumata, T. Successful surgical treatment for dilated cardiomyopathy with cardiac sarcoidosis. *The Annals of thoracic surgery*, Aug 2007, 84(2), e12-13.

[139] Miyahara, S; Mukohara, N; Morimoto, N; Murakami, H; Nakagiri, K; Yoshida, M. Left ventricular restoration for cardiac sarcoidosis, report of two cases. *Surgery today*, Dec 28 2012.

[140] Jain, A; Starek, PJ; Delany, DL. Ventricular tachycardia and ventricular aneurysm due to unrecognized sarcoidosis. *Clinical cardiology*, Oct 1990, 13(10), 738-740.

[141] Oni, AA; Hershberger, RE; Norman, DJ; et al. Recurrence of sarcoidosis in a cardiac allograft, control with augmented corticosteroids. *The Journal of heart and lung transplantation: the official publication of the International Society for Heart Transplantation*, Mar-Apr 1992, 11(2 Pt 1), 367-369.

[142] Yager, JE; Hernandez, AF; Steenbergen, C; et al. Recurrence of cardiac sarcoidosis in a heart transplant recipient. *The Journal of heart and lung transplantation: the official*

publication of the International Society for Heart Transplantation, Nov 2005, 24(11), 1988-1990.

[143] Zaidi, AR; Zaidi, A; Vaitkus, PT. Outcome of heart transplantation in patients with sarcoid cardiomyopathy. *The Journal of heart and lung transplantation: the official publication of the International Society for Heart Transplantation*, Jul 2007, 26(7), 714-717.

[144] Burke, WM; Keogh, A; Maloney, PJ; Delprado, W; Bryant, DH; Spratt, P. Transmission of sarcoidosis via cardiac transplantation. *Lancet*, Dec 22-29 1990, 336(8730), 1579.

[145] Dhadham, GC; Gupta, N; Parikh, R; Bikkina, M. Cardiac sarcoidosis with a rare initial manifestation, sustained monomorphic ventricular tachycardia. *Texas Heart Institute journal/from the Texas Heart Institute of St. Luke's Episcopal Hospital, Texas Children's Hospital*, 2011, 38(1), 74-76.

[146] Alam, M; Virani, SS; Simpson, L; Williams, SB; Wilson, JM. Cardiac sarcoidosis: a clinical entity uncommonly recognized. *Texas Heart Institute journal / from the Texas Heart Institute of St. Luke's Episcopal Hospital, Texas Children's Hospital*, 2009, 36(5), 501-503.

[147] Lagana, SM; Parwani, AV; Nichols, LC. Cardiac sarcoidosis: a pathology-focused review. *Archives of pathology & laboratory medicine*, Jul 2010, 134(7), 1039-1046.

[148] Sharma, PS; Lubahn, JG; Donsky, AS; et al. Diagnosing cardiac sarcoidosis clinically without tissue confirmation. *Proc (Bayl Univ Med Cent)*, Jul 2009, 22(3), 236-238.

[149] Sun, BJ; Lee, PH; Choi, HO; et al. Prevalence of echocardiographic features suggesting cardiac sarcoidosis in patients with pacemaker or implantable cardiac defibrillator. *Korean circulation journal*, Jun 2011, 41(6), 313-320.

[150] Zimmermann, R; Haunstetter, A; Kubler, W. Images in cardiology. Cardiac sarcoidosis. *Heart*, Jul 1997, 78(1), 6.

In: Horizons in World Cardiovascular Research. Vol. 6 ISBN: 978-1-63321-298-5
Editor: Eleanor H. Bennington

Chapter 2

Heart Failure and Acute Phase Proteins

Katherine Wachmann,[1,2] Johann Altenberger[2] and Paul J. Mills[1]

[1]Department of Psychiatry, Behavioral Medicine Program, University of California, San Diego, La Jolla, CA, US

[2]SKA-RZ Großgmain, Rehabilitation Center for Cardiac and Neurological diseases, Großgmain, Austria

Abstract

Heart failure (HF) describes a complex clinical syndrome, where the heart is incapable of providing the body with an adequate amount of blood to meet metabolic requirements. It is a major public health concern, affecting about 6 million Americans, with rates expected to nearly triple over the next 3 decades as the population ages. But HF is not limited to industrialized, developed countries; instead it is a global burden rising in developing countries paralleling increases in cardiovascular risk factors such as hypertension, diabetes and obesity. HF is a progressive disease with various stages and a number of risk factors contributing to the onset of HF symptoms with the inflammatory cascade as one of the key players in each stage of HF. This chapter reviews a number of these key inflammatory mediators with the aim of further understanding their role in the transition from disease risk factors to development and advancement of HF.

Introduction

Heart failure (HF) describes a complex clinical syndrome, where the heart is incapable of providing the body with an adequate amount of blood to meet metabolic requirements. It is a major public health concern, affecting about 6 million Americans, and with rates expected to nearly triple over the next 3 decades as the population ages [1, 2]. At present, the annual number of hospitalizations exceeds 1 million, and US direct costs exceed $40 billion/year [2, 3]. But HF is not limited to industrialized, developed countries; instead it is a global burden rising in developing countries paralleling increases in cardiovascular risk factors such as hypertension, diabetes and obesity.

The outlook is in general gloomy, with about fifty percent of patients dying at four years post-diagnosis [4]. Worldwide, cardiovascular diseases (CVD) are the number one cause of death, with an estimated 17.3 million people dying from CVDs in 2008, representing 30% of all global deaths [5]. It is disheartening to read that 80% of premature heart disease and stroke is preventable yet the diseases are still so widespread [6].

So how do we get from a healthy happy heart to a heart that is struggling and fighting for its survival? And what do acute phase proteins have to do with it? We will be focusing on these two questions on the following pages.

HF Classifications and Cardiac Pathophysiology and Symptoms

HF is a progressive disease with various stages and a number of risk factors contributing to the onset of HF symptoms. Stages of HF are commonly classified by using the New York Heart Association (NYHA) classification system [7, 8], and in more recent years, the American College of Cardiology/American Heart Association (ACC/AHA) classification system (Table 1).

In 2001, the ACC in conjunction with the AHA proposed a new staging system for individuals with, or at risk for, HF [9]. The goal of this classification system, which includes stages A, B, C, and D, is to emphasize both the evolution and the progressive nature of chronic HF and the need for early implementation of interventions to prevent progression and ultimately to reduce morbidity and mortality.

Stage A patients are people who have a high probability to develop HF but who neither show structural or functional abnormalities nor symptoms of HF. Among the risk factors are hypertension, diabetes, obesity and coronary artery disease (CAD). All of these risk factors have a component of chronic low-grade inflammation which is purportedly involved in HF disease progression.

Controlling these risk factors can reduce the incidence of later cardiovascular events by 30 to 50 percent [1]. It is important to raise awareness in the population about this crucial stage where it is still possible to protect the heart from structural damage, often by measures as "simple" as lifestyle modifications. People should be encouraged to lose excess weight, to improve their physical condition, stay away from smoking and alcohol and reduce stress in their daily lives. This can be accompanied by medical therapies.

As a main contributor in stage A for the development of HF, hypertension is commonly referred to as blood pressure above 140/90 mmHg. The heart has to pump harder in order to overcome the elevated arterial pressure and over time this extra workload induces remodeling of the myocardium, the cardiac muscle.

Hypertension is a chronic condition which does not announce itself with obvious symptoms but is often overlooked until maybe diagnosed at a doctor's appointment for an unrelated cause. In many cases it is associated with obesity and diabetes. The impact of the immune system on the genesis of hypertension has been studied since the 1960's in experimental animals and in the past decade several studies have strengthened the concept that hypertension has an immunologic basis with both the innate and adaptive immune system involved [10-12].

Table 1. Functional Classifications and Disease Progression Stages of Heart Failure

New York Heart Association Functional (NYHA) Classes		
	Definition	Examples
NYHA Class I	No limitation of physical activity	Ordinary physical activity does not cause undue fatigue, palpitation, or dyspnea (shortness of breath)
NYHA Class II	Slight limitation of physical activity	Comfortable at rest, but ordinary physical activity results in fatigue, palpitation, or dyspnea
NYHA Class III	Marked limitation of physical activity	Comfortable at rest, but less than ordinary activity causes fatigue, palpitation, or dyspnea
NYHA Class IV	Unable to carry out any physical activity without discomfort	Symptoms of cardiac insufficiency at rest. If any physical activity is undertaken, discomfort is increased
American College of Cardiology/American Heart Association Stages of Heart Failure		
	Definition	Examples
Stage A	High risk for developing HF, but without structural heart disease or symptoms of HF	Hypertension, diabetes mellitus, CAD, family history of cardiomyopathy
Stage B	Structural heart disease, but asymptomatic	Previous myocardial infarction, left ventricular dysfunction, valvular heart disease
Stage C	Structural heart disease with previous or current symptoms, but managed with medical treatment	Structural heart disease, dyspnea and fatigue, impaired exercise tolerance
Stage D	Marked symptoms at rest despite maximal medical therapy	Advanced disease requiring hospital-based support, a heart transplant or palliative care

Recently, Harrison et al. suggested a new working hypothesis in which hypertensive stimuli, such as angiotensin II, high salt and ROS (Reactive Oxygen Species) promote sympathetic activity and modest elevation in pressure, further promoting T-cell activation and the initiation of an inflammatory cascade, ultimately causing severe hypertension [13]. This model agrees with the finding that neurohormonal activation, like the renin-angiotensin-aldosterone (RAA) system and sympathetic nervous system (SNS), is implicated already in early stages of HF [14-16]. Initially, these mechanisms have the beneficial goal to maintain adequate blood pressure and peripheral perfusion but excessive activation leads to negative outcome. Intriguingly, several studies found a link between neurohormonal and immune system activation [17-19] and it would be fruitful for further research to recognize autonomic imbalance and inflammation not as separate models but rather related phenomena in the pathogenesis of HF [20, 21].

The transition from stage A to stage B happens when the heart shows structural or functional damage but patients do not yet show symptoms of HF [22-24].

As the heart tries to maintain normal cardiovascular homeostasis, several compensatory mechanisms are activated including the Frank-Starling mechanism, neurohormonal activation and ventricular remodeling, which in the long run worsen the structure and function of the heart [25-27]. The transition from stage A to stage B is not fully understood but it is suggested that persistent low-grade inflammation is an important factor promoting pathophysiological changes [28]. About fifty percent of the stage B patients show left ventricular systolic dysfunction (LVSD) manifested as a low left ventricular ejection fraction (LVEF), the other half has preserved LV function [29]. Reduced LV function comes with high prognosis for developing symptomatic HF [30]. Once the patient establishes HF symptoms he is categorized as stage C. The transition from asymptomatic stage B to even mildly symptomatic stage C is associated with a 5-fold increase in mortality risk in 1-year [31]. Identifying stage B patients at high risk can be accomplished using circulating levels of natriuretic peptides such as B-type natriuretic peptide (BNP) [32]. BNP accurately detects abnormal LV function and predicts risk of future events [33-35]. Currently, biomarker research is one of the most active areas in cardiology and while BNP seems to be one of the favorites, a number of acute phase proteins are in line to become clinically relevant for the diagnosis and prognosis of HF.

Stage C corresponds very closely to NYHA classes II and III. These patients are still comfortable at rest but have marked limitation of physical activity with symptoms like fatigue, palpitation, dyspnea or angina. A defining parameter for symptom severity is the degree of LV dysfunction. Elevated levels of inflammatory cytokines can be found in the circulation and the myocardium [36-40] and have been shown to influence LV function as well as modulate cardiac myocyte hypertrophy, cardiac necrosis and apoptosis and extracellular myocardial remodeling [21, 41, 42]. Interestingly, the same proteins exert cardioprotective effects, at least in the initial phase when they serve as part of compensatory mechanisms [21, 41, 42].

In patients with advanced HF, stage D, the chronic over-activation of inflammatory markers and neurohormones leads to further detrimental damages and precipitates in critical reduction in blood flow to all vital organs. Patients require maximal medical therapy, special interventions like mechanical assist devices and heart transplantations or hospice care. In a last attempt to maximize cardiac output to sufficiently nourish the body's organs the heart is trapped in a cycle of hemodynamic deterioration with a deadly endpoint.

Acute Phase Proteins and HF

As noted in the previous section on HF classifications and pathology, aspects of inflammation and the inflammatory cascade are involved in each stage of HF – from initial risk for development on through the most advanced stages of the disease. In the following pages we will review a number of these key inflammatory mediators with the aim of further understanding their role in the transition from risk to development and advancement of HF (Table 2).

TNF-alpha (Tumor Necrosis Factor-alpha) is the apical cytokine of many inflammatory responses produced by macrophages, lymphocytes, neutrophils and structural cells including cardiac myocytes, fibroblasts and smooth muscle cells.

Table 2. Overview of Biomarkers in Heart Failure

Biomarker	Main Source	Overall Effect in the Organism
TNF-alpha	inflammatory cells, cardiomyocytes, fibroblasts	Transcription of pro-inflammatory mediator genes for cell survival or genes related to apoptosis
IL-6	inflammatory cells, cardiomyocytes, fibroblasts	Induction of inflammatory cascade
CRP	hepatocytes	Pro-inflammatory / Activation of complement pathway
PTX3	endothelial cells, macrophages, neutrophils	Pro-inflammatory / Activation of complement pathway
SAA	hepatocytes	Pro-inflammatory / Cholesterol metabolism
IL-1	inflammatory cells	Pro-inflammatory / Induction of inflammatory cascade
BNP	cardiac myocytes	Relaxation of the myocardium and regulation of sodium homeostasis

Furthermore, adult mammalian myocardial cells are able to produce TNF –alpha after extracellular stimuli such as endotoxin, hypoxia or increased mechanical stress [43]. When released, TNF-alpha acts through two transmembrane receptors TNF-alpha receptor (TNFR) 1 and 2, which can trigger various intracellular signaling pathways. Depending on the stimulus, the cell-type and the local concentration of the cytokine, it can trigger transcription of either pro-inflammatory mediator genes for cell survival or genes related to apoptosis [44]. The central pathway, through which TNF-alpha mitigates its functions, is the famous and complex NFκ-B (Nuclear Factor κ-B) pathway. Curiously, both of the receptors can be cleaved off the cell surface and circulate as soluble TNF receptors (sTNFR), but their biological function is not well defined yet. So far they are believed to act as biologic buffers and neutralize the activities of TNF-alpha [45-47].

Regarding the pathophysiological role of TNF-alpha in HF, both functions - immunity and apoptosis -are feeding into disease development and progression, due to upregulated TNF-alpha expression. Results from the SOLVD (Studies Of Left Ventricular Dysfunction) trial revealed that plasma cytokine levels, among them TNF-alpha, increased proportionally as their functional HF classification progressed [48]. In the first stage of HF, stage A, chronic low-grade inflammation is driving many of the common risk factors and TNF-alpha is involved the symptomatology of many of them, which eventually can lead to the on-set of symptoms of HF. For instance, animal studies on hypertension have identified TNF-alpha as an important contributor in the regulation of blood pressure, although with different hypothesis and mechanisms of how the cytokine is involved [10, 11, 49]. One study, which aims to identify the role of lymphocytes in angiotensin-II induced hypertension, proposes that upregulated renal TNF-alpha in the absence of lymphocytes promotes the induction of NO (Nitric Oxide) by stimulating eNOS (endothelial Nitric Oxide Synthase) activity and COX-2 (cyclooxygenase-2) expression, which in consequence lowers blood pressure [10]. Interestingly, other studies using the TNF-alpha antagonist Etanercept showed decreased blood pressure upon treatment but it remains unclear whether direct inhibition of the cytokine or TNF-alpha-independent mechanisms are responsible for the physiological outcome [11, 49].

Another big source of HF risk, obesity and all associated disorders like type-2 diabetes or sleep apnea, are also characterized by low-grade chronic inflammation and like in hypertension TNF-alpha is one of the usual suspects. In obesity, inflammation and elevated TNF-alpha levels are initiated by excess nutrients in metabolic cells, primarily adipocytes [50]. It has been shown that TNF-alpha and IL-6 interfere with insulin signaling promoting insulin resistance [51, 52]. Fortunately, there is data suggesting that the adverse effects can be reversed with weight loss and accompanied physical exercise [53, 54].

The transition from Stage A to stage B is marked by structural changes in the heart while still asymptomatic in its manifestation. TNF-alpha has been established more than 10 years ago to drive some of these changes. While a short-term expression of the cytokine has beneficial cytoprotective effects as the body's adaption to forms of stress, the long-term expression has deleterious consequences for the heart muscle such as induction of ventricular remodeling and stimulation of cardiomyopathy [55-57]. TNF-alpha impairs myocyte contractility; one possible mechanism is through increasing the levels of inducible nitric oxide synthase (iNOS), an enzyme that enhances nitric oxide production which in turn has negative inotropic effects [58, 59]. Additionally, prolonged overexpression of TNF-alpha leads to myocardial fibrosis and apoptosis [56, 60], which contributes to the left ventricular wall thinning and adverse cardiac remodeling [61, 62]. Transgenic mice which constitutively express TNF-alpha in cardiomyocytes have a phenotype of myocarditis and their hearts show striking similarities to hearts of patients with chronic HF who transition to stage C. At the cellular level, in the murine model as well as in humans, TNF-alpha enhances the activity of extracellular matrix remodeling metalloproteases [62, 63]. Now, in the chronic stage of the disease also skeletal myopathy and endothelial dysfunction can be observed, caused by free radical and nitric oxide overproduction due to TNF-alpha [56, 60].

Because TNF-alpha is so prominent from an early point in HF it became the target for medical therapies, with the premise that TNF-alpha inhibition may be beneficial for disease progression. Etanercept, a drug that binds circulating TNF-alpha, has been used in several trials to assess its impact and efficacy in HF. Initially, results were encouraging. Single dose treatment led to significant improvements of HF symptomatology and the drug was well tolerated by the patients [64]. However, two large studies (RECOVER and RENAISSANCE) that randomized about 2000 patients with HF have been stopped early because the main endpoints did not show a difference between drug and placebo, as the treatment did not hold promise any benefit in terms of symptoms, hospital admissions, or deaths [65, 66]. As a conclusion, high dose anti-TNF-alpha therapy may not be useful in HF patients but the situation in lower doses has not yet been adequately assessed [65].

Interleukin-6 (IL-6) is a prominent cytokine that can activate the immune system by inducing acute phase protein (APP) gene expression but also has regulatory functions in metabolism and regenerative processes [67]. IL-6 is produced by various cell types, including cardiomyocytes, fibroblasts and inflammatory cells. Classically, IL-6 binds to the IL-6 receptor, which exists membrane-bound or soluble; this complex further associates with the central signal transducer subunit gp130 to trigger diverse intracellular pathways. A thorough review of the possible molecular interactions can be found in a review by Scheller et al. [67].

Regarding the cytokine's role in HF, it is on stage from the very beginning. A large community-based multicenter study with over 6000 participants of four ethnicities sought out to reveal the relationships of several risk factors summarized as the metabolic syndrome and HF.

One of the results was that inflammatory markers, among them IL-6, were independently associated with incident HF [68]. In line with this, another study found increased risk of future myocardial stroke associated with elevated levels of IL-6 in apparently healthy men [69]. The results from 2 large population based-cohorts comprising over 2000 patients with a follow-up of up to 20 years give further evidence that long-term IL-6 levels are associated with coronary heart disease risk as strongly as are some other major risk factors [70]. Furthermore, it is now known that adipocytes are a source of elevated IL-6 levels and that the cytokine influences insulin resistance in obese people [71-73].

In stage B patients who have a diagnosis of LV systolic dysfunction, elevated IL-6 levels have been found in the peripheral as well as coronary circulation, pointing to a role of IL-6 in early inflammatory changes in the progression from subclinical LV dysfunction to clinical HF [74]. Parallel to results with TNF-alpha, Torre-Amione et al. saw a similar picture in the SOLVD study, with a significant continuous increase in IL-6 levels during disease progression from healthy subjects to asymptomatic HF patients to symptomatic HF patients [75]. The causality remains uncertain, but it is reinforcing the connection between inflammatory pathways and cardiovascular diseases and within that, puts IL-6 with its central role in mediating immunity, as a potential therapeutic target. Nevertheless, it has to be a careful approach keeping in mind the many regulatory actions of IL-6 within a complex signaling network, including indications that the actual role of IL-6 may well depend on the nature of the inflammatory stimulus [76]. In this regard it has to be mentioned that IL-6 and activation of associated pathways can have beneficial as well as detrimental effects for the syndrome of HF. IL-6 knock-out mice show larger infarct sizes after myocardial infarction with previous coronary occlusion/reperfusion probably through induction of protective genes like inducible NO synthase (iNOS) and COX-2 in cardiomyocytes and through additional anti-apoptotic signaling [77-79]. In gp130 cardiac specific knock-out mice dilated cardiomyopathy can be observed following acute pressure overload and interestingly in the gp130 intact mice a compensatory hypertrophic growth response increased the beneficial role in this setting [80]. On the other hand continuous overexpression of both IL-6 and IL-6R leads to myocardial hypertrophy and thicker LV walls [81]. Another study found that cardiac contractility is decreased after prolonged exposure to IL-6 [82].

Together, the existing inconsistencies in the findings of IL-6 dependent effects on the heart may reflect the complex interactions and that it is not always possible to assign the effects to a single protein, even more so because of the existing redundancy within the IL-6 cytokine family at their convergent signal transducer gp130 [41, 83]. Nevertheless, IL-6 is a strong predictor of morbidity and mortality in patients with HF and it is responsible for mediating expression of several "downstream" inflammatory markers, including C-reactive protein (CRP), another acute phase protein known to contribute to the risk of developing HF [84].

C-reactive protein (CRP), which by the way has the structure of a beautiful pentameric ring, is an acute phase protein whose production by hepatocytes in the liver is triggered by cytokines such as IL-6 in response to most forms of inflammation, infection, and tissue damage [85]. Usually upon stimulation, blood levels of CRP show a rapid increase and decrease after resolution of the condition, so that elevated levels of CRP are a reliable sign of ongoing inflammatory processes in the organism although nonspecific. In general, CRP binds to damaged tissue, to nuclear antigens and to certain pathogenic organisms in a calcium-dependent manner and in consequence activates the classical complement pathway [85].

The stability in plasma and the development of high sensitivity assays for assessing CRP levels made it a prominent candidate to evaluate its potential as a predictor of cardiac events and many studies have indeed shown the association between CRP levels and future cardiac events [86-89]. Additionally, a recent statement from the Centers for Disease Control and Prevention and the American Heart Association concluded that it is reasonable to measure C-reactive protein as an adjunct to the measurement of established risk factors in order to assess the risk of coronary heart disease [90]. However, a large study and following meta-analysis asks for a careful reassessment of the latter recommendation [84]. In this particular study they measured CRP values and other inflammatory markers in approximately 2400 patients with coronary heart disease and approximately 4000 controls nested within the Reykjavik Study, a prospective cohort study with people without a history of myocardial infarction [91]. The results of this study and a following meta-analysis concluded that CRP is only a relatively moderate predictor of coronary heart disease with a lower odds ratio than previously reported and that it added only marginally to the predictive value of established risk factors for coronary heart disease [84].

As Stage A and stage B HF are characterized by ongoing inflammation CRP, which is not only a marker but also acts as an amplifier of inflammation, is a valuable nonspecific marker given that there are studies showing that common risk factors of HF like smoking and obesity are associated with an increase in CRP concentrations [92-94]. Studies on the effects of CRP on endothelial cells in the context of atherosclerosis came to the conclusion that CRP exerts a direct pro-inflammatory effect on endothelial cells by inducing the expression of cell adhesion molecules [95, 96]. However, the mechanism remains to be elucidated. CRP has also been studied looking at the development of hypertension but the contribution and causality remain uncertain to the point that assessing CRP levels in the clinical setting might be helpful for risk stratification but cannot be used as a prognostic tool for high blood pressure [97]. In the case of myocardial infarction CRP levels correlate with the amount of tissue necrosis and there is experimental evidence that the CRP response may contribute to the severity of ischemic myocardial injury [98, 99]. Even though there have been advances to use CRP as a target with statin treatment, a drug originally used to lower cholesterol levels, the clinical value of measuring CRP to guide statin therapy is uncertain [100-102]. Evidence from JUPITER, the Heart Protection Study and the Northern Manhattan Study did not confirm the benefits from statin therapy [103-105]. Thus, CRP concentration is a useful nonspecific biochemical marker of inflammation, its measurement contributes to screening for organic disease but it has to be seen if a direct improvement of cardiovascular outcomes is achieved by specifically inhibiting or reducing the circulating levels of CRP.

Greater levels of CRP have been implicated in the progression into more severe stages of HF [106, 107]. Researchers also found an association of CRP levels and risk for hospitalization [107]. In symptomatic HF CRP appears to be independently related to mortality. However, CRP levels were almost identical in patients with ischemic and non-ischemic HF etiology and high CRP was associated with increased mortality independent of ischemic/non-ischemic etiology as a large study with over 4000 HF patients showed [108]. Patients with higher CRP had lower LVEF, poorer quality of life and worse neurohormonal profile. Causes of higher CRP in symptomatic HF are related to sustained cardiac tissue damage and other organs, probably via induction of IL-6, which activates CRP expression. It is likely that muscle wasting, anemia, and renal dysfunction, common co-morbidities in HF, may be partially caused by inflammatory activation [109, 110].

Pentraxin 3 (PTX3) is a novel emerging marker for inflammation which has a good potential to be adopted clinically but still requires more research to establish the specific frame in which it can be used as a specific biomarker for heart failure. The protein is in the same family as CRP, it is expressed in various cell types including endothelial cells, macrophages and neutrophils and plays a role in innate immunity, tuning inflammation and matrix deposition [111]. The first study to report a specific association with heart failure was by Matsubara et al., who found that pentraxin 3 levels were related to LV diastolic dysfunction and HF with preserved ejection fraction (HFPEF) [112]. The group also claimed that pentraxin 3 is expressed in the coronary sinus, which strengthens the observation that it is involved in cardiac remodeling [113]. Even though these results sound exciting, they have to be taken with a big grain of salt. The relationship that the scientists saw is purely statistical, missing data for possible confounders and the limited size of the study is not enough to clearly discriminate between the associations of pentraxin 3 with HFPEF versus HF with reduced ejection fraction (HFREF). Their finding that pentraxin 3 is expressed in the myocardium supports evidence from another study that it is modulating rather than promoting inflammation in cardiac remodeling [114]. In the latter study, it was demonstrated that mice lacking pentraxin 3 on an apolipoprotein E negative background had greater vascular inflammation and atherosclerotic lesions, pointing to a possible athero-protective function of pentraxin 3 under these circumstances. In another model with pentraxin 3 deficient mice after acute myocardial infarction, increased heart damage was observed when compared to the controls. This phenotype could be reversed when pentraxin 3 was exogenously administered [115].

Regarding HF stages, these results favor the suggestion to measure pentraxin 3 levels already in stages A and B. However, we still do not know whether pentraxin 3 levels can predict the development of HF, help in its clinical diagnosis or carry any prognostic information in the setting of overt HF [116]. Just recently, clinical trials have sought to find out if pentraxin 3 levels are specifically associated with risk and prognosis of cardiovascular events, mortality and incident heart failure [117, 118]. The Heart and Soul Study which included patients with stable coronary heart disease found an association with all-cause mortality, cardiovascular events, and incident HF independently of demographics, traditional CVD risk factors, and systemic inflammation (CRP) [117]. Post-hoc analysis of two trials with patients with chronic HF, namely the Controlled Rosuvastatin Multinational Trial in HF (CORONA) and the GISSI-Heart Failure trial (GISSI-HF) demonstrated that common associates of elevated pentraxin 3 are age, advanced NYHA class, and lower BMI; that changes in pentraxin 3 concentration over time, but not baseline pentraxin 3, can predict fatal outcomes, independently of CRP and of the benchmark prognostic marker in HF, NT-proBNP [118].

Mechanisms of these observed associations remain unknown, calling for further scientific attention to establish pentraxin 3 as a safe and useful new biomarker.

Serum Amyloid-A (SAA) is a highly conserved acute phase protein predominantly produced by the liver. In response to inflammatory signals SAA levels rise fast and substantially up to a 1000-fold and it is a powerful mediator of pro-inflammatory signaling for host defense [119]. Furthermore, SAA plays a role in cholesterol transport and metabolism via binding to high-density lipoprotein (HDL) [120-122]. SAA is also expressed in adipose tissue [123], not in 1000 –fold excess but as a modest elevation, where it is part of chronic inflammatory processes characteristic for obesity.

It was shown that SAA is independently associated with BMI levels and that SAA levels can be beneficially decreased with weight loss interventions [124]. All this evidence made SAA a plausible marker for ongoing inflammation in the body and further research has shown links between SAA levels and risk of developing atherosclerosis and coronary artery disease, however if this link is causal or associative requires further study [125]. Nevertheless, it is used as an indicator for ongoing inflammation in the body [126-128]. There is some evidence that suggests that it may have a direct effect on atherogenesis, that it promotes atherosclerotic plaque destabilization and additionally a strong independent relationship between SAA and future cardiovascular events in women was established [126]. Taken together, SAA is involved in risk factors that can lead to the onset of HF. These risk factors include obesity, atherosclerosis and coronary artery disease with inflammation as a key concept in all of them. It therefore may be useful to assess SAA levels already in the early stages of heart failure (A and B) and follow it over time as the disease develops.

Interleukin-1 (IL-1) is the prototype of cytokines with pro-inflammatory properties, consisting of two distinct ligands IL-1α and IL-1β. IL-1 is expressed by numerous cell types however mostly by innate immune cells including macrophages, monocytes and dendritic cells [129]. The inactive IL-1β precursor gets cleaved by caspase-1, a cysteine protease, to form the active protein [129]. Caspase-1 activity is regulated by a multimeric complex called the inflammasome, which is of major importance in inflammation [130, 131]. There is a naturally occurring IL-1 receptor antagonist (IL-1Ra) which competitively binds to the IL-1 receptor and therefore blocks IL-1 signaling [132]. Thus, the balance of agonist and antagonist is another regulatory factor of IL-1, besides its local concentration, caspase-1 mediated activation and concentration of IL-1 receptor.

Regarding the role of IL-1 in the pathogenesis of heart disease it is central to maladaptive responses in chronic inflammation, inherent to risk factors promoting the development of heat failure. In recent years, research conducted to look at the role of IL-1 in obesity and diabetes found that caspase-1 is upregulated in adipocytes and mediates insulin resistance due to more active IL-1 [133].

These results are supported by another study on type 2 diabetes, in which IL-1 receptor antagonist was used to block IL-1 with the consequence of improved glycemic control and improved function of insulin producing β-cells [134]. Furthermore, IL-1 is involved in several cardiac events. It promotes cardiac myocyte apoptosis leading to loss of viable heart muscle which can then progress into heart failure [135, 136]. It is important in adverse cardiac remodeling of the infarcted heart possibly via several pathways, that are discussed in more detail elsewhere [137].

It also seems to suppress cardiac contractility and induce myocardial hypertrophy, which are mediators in the pathogenesis of heart failure although these results come from mice experimental models and it has to be seen how IL-1 signaling behaves endogenously in patients [138, 139]. There is a high interest in developing treatments that target IL-1 and inhibit its actions for a broad spectrum of diseases [140].

Some studies using anakinra, a recombinant form of IL-1 antagonist, could ameliorate cardiac enlargement and dysfunction after myocardial infarction [135, 136]. This drug is approved by the Food and Drug Administration (FDA) for treatment of rheumatoid arthritis and it holds the potential to be also useful in the treatment of heart disease [141, 142]. More encouragement comes from another trial blocking IL-1 that observed decreased levels of CRP and improvement in exercise tolerance pointing to improved cardiac performance [143].

The results are promising but with drugs targeting a single cytokine in the inflammatory cascade more extensive research is needed to really understand its action and consequences in the pathophysiology of HF.

The most established biomarkers in HF are without doubt natriuretic peptides. Just ten years since their discovery, they are now among the standard care in various settings in cardiology and beyond. Alan Maisel who was among the first investigators to document the importance of BNP as a biomarker has recently summarized the past developments and future questions around BNP [144]. The neurohormone precursor is released into the bloodstream by cardiac monocytes upon volume expansion or pressure overload and initial processing steps result in the biologically active 32-amino acid B-type natriuretic peptide (BNP) and the biologically inactive N-terminus fragment of proBNP (NT-proBNP) [145]. BNP helps with relaxation of the myocardium and exerts an important regulatory role in maintaining sodium homeostasis via interfering with the renin-angiotensin-aldosterone system [146]. The importance of BNP in the diagnosis of HF was first implicated by the Breathing Not Properly Study, where it was found that a BNP cut-off point of 100 pg / mL was 76% specific and 90% sensitive for the diagnosis of HF in patients with dyspnea [33]. Additionally, it was found in other studies that BNP successfully aids in predicting future cardiovascular events in asymptomatic patients without prior heart disease [32, 147]. Other factors that influence BNP levels are age and gender [148, 149]. Therefore "normal" values vary and must be taken into consideration.

One study looked specifically at stage A and B HF patients regarding the prognostic value of their BNP levels and the results indicate that individuals without history of HF with BNP levels >100 pg / mL are at high risk for future cardiovascular events [32]. When compared to stage C/D patients, they had a prognosis just as bad as those with low levels of BNP but history of HF. The risk persisted after adjusting for other common risk factors and it is suggested to be alerted as a physician when confronted with asymptomatic patients but high BNP levels.

Conclusion

Imagine coming back from a Yoga class full of heart opener poses or a good run with a pounding heart, now bursting with joy about a healthy body and a healthy heart - makes one grateful for the gift of health. We, in the scientific community, should always keep in mind that the ultimate goal is to help the patients. HF patients are limited in many areas of their life because of their failing heart. Biomarkers can help detect the first signs of a heart problem prior to any symptoms showing up. And these problems might not even be directly related to the heart yet. Early detection can make all the difference and give patients enough time to find the right treatment and find healthy changes to their lifestyles. Therapies guided by biomarker monitoring have led to better treatment results, which is so urgently needed in HF. A great deal of understanding about the development and progression of HF comes from studying inflammatory and cardiac biomarkers. The challenge now is to integrate the single biomarkers into the larger network of disease pathology and to gain insight how they might be connected and orchestrated with the aim to improve the interpretation of changing levels of these markers and how these biomarker profiles affect the heart.

This scientific knowledge should then be translated into therapies that successfully help the individual and effectively help people with different phenotypes of HF, ideally to support their healing process on many levels.

References

[1] Jessup, M. and Brozena, S. (2003) Heart failure, *N. Engl. J. Med.* 348, 2007-2018.

[2] Roger, V. L., Go, A. S., Lloyd-Jones, D. M., Benjamin, E. J., Berry, J. D., Borden, W. B., Bravata, D. M., Dai, S., Ford, E. S., Fox, C. S., Fullerton, H. J., Gillespie, C., Hailpern, S. M., Heit, J. A., Howard, V. J., Kissela, B. M., Kittner, S. J., Lackland, D. T., Lichtman, J. H., Lisabeth, L. D., Makuc, D. M., Marcus, G. M., Marelli, A., Matchar, D. B., Moy, C. S., Mozaffarian, D., Mussolino, M. E., Nichol, G., Paynter, N. P., Soliman, E. Z., Sorlie, P. D., Sotoodehnia, N., Turan, T. N., Virani, S. S., Wong, N. D., Woo, D., and Turner, M. B. (2012) Heart disease and stroke statistics--2012 update: a report from the American Heart Association, *Circulation* 125, e2-e220.

[3] Hauptman, P. J., Swindle, J., Burroughs, T. E., and Schnitzler, M. A. (2008) Resource utilization in patients hospitalized with heart failure: insights from a contemporary national hospital database, *Am. Heart J.* 155, 978-985.

[4] Dickstein, K., Cohen-Solal, A., Filippatos, G., McMurray, J. J., Ponikowski, P., Poole-Wilson, P. A., Stromberg, A., van Veldhuisen, D. J., Atar, D., Hoes, A. W., Keren, A., Mebazaa, A., Nieminen, M., Priori, S. G., and Swedberg, K. (2008) ESC guidelines for the diagnosis and treatment of acute and chronic heart failure 2008: the Task Force for the diagnosis and treatment of acute and chronic heart failure 2008 of the European Society of Cardiology. Developed in collaboration with the Heart Failure Association of the ESC (HFA) and endorsed by the European Society of Intensive Care Medicine (ESICM), *Eur. J. Heart Fail.* 10, 933-989.

[5] http://www.who.int/mediacentre/factsheets/fs317/en/index.html. 2012. Ref. Type: Online Source

[6] http://www.euro.who.int/en/what-we-do/health-topics/noncommunicable-diseases/cardiovascular-diseases/facts-and-figures. 2013. Ref Type: Online Source

[7] Caccamo, M. A. and Eckman, P. M. (2011) Pharmacologic therapy for New York Heart Association class IV heart failure, *Congest. Heart Fail.* 17, 213-219.

[8] The Criteria Committee of the New York Heart Association. *Nomenclature and Criteria for Diagnosis of Diseases of the Heart and Great Vessels,* 9th ed. Boston, MA: Little, Brown and Co; 1994; 253–256). 9th, 253-256. 1994. Lippincott Williams and Wilkins. LWW Handbooks. Ref Type: Edited Book

[9] Hunt, S. A., Baker, D. W., Chin, M. H., Cinquegrani, M. P., Feldman, A. M., Francis, G. S., Ganiats, T. G., Goldstein, S., Gregoratos, G., Jessup, M. L., Noble, R. J., Packer, M., Silver, M. A., Stevenson, L. W., Gibbons, R. J., Antman, E. M., Alpert, J. S., Faxon, D. P., Fuster, V., Jacobs, A. K., Hiratzka, L. F., Russell, R. O., and Smith, S. C.,

Jr. (2001) ACC/AHA guidelines for the evaluation and management of chronic heart failure in the adult: executive summary. A report of the American College of Cardiology/American Heart Association Task Force on Practice Guidelines (Committee to revise the 1995 Guidelines for the Evaluation and Management of Heart Failure), *J. Am. Coll. Cardiol.* 38, 2101-2113.

[10] Crowley, S. D., Song, Y. S., Lin, E. E., Griffiths, R., Kim, H. S., and Ruiz, P. (2010) Lymphocyte responses exacerbate angiotensin II-dependent hypertension, *Am. J. Physiol. Regul. Integr. Comp. Physiol.* 298, R1089-R1097.

[11] Guzik, T. J., Hoch, N. E., Brown, K. A., McCann, L. A., Rahman, A., Dikalov, S., Goronzy, J., Weyand, C., and Harrison, D. G. (2007) Role of the T cell in the genesis of angiotensin II induced hypertension and vascular dysfunction, *J. Exp. Med.* 204, 2449-2460.

[12] Marvar, P. J., Thabet, S. R., Guzik, T. J., Lob, H. E., McCann, L. A., Weyand, C., Gordon, F. J., and Harrison, D. G. (2010) Central and peripheral mechanisms of T-lymphocyte activation and vascular inflammation produced by angiotensin II-induced hypertension, *Circ. Res.* 107, 263-270.

[13] Harrison, D. G., Guzik, T. J., Lob, H. E., Madhur, M. S., Marvar, P. J., Thabet, S. R., Vinh, A., and Weyand, C. M. (2011) Inflammation, immunity, and hypertension, *Hypertension* 57, 132-140.

[14] Benedict, C. R., Shelton, B., Johnstone, D. E., Francis, G., Greenberg, B., Konstam, M., Probstfield, J. L., and Yusuf, S. (1996) Prognostic significance of plasma norepinephrine in patients with asymptomatic left ventricular dysfunction. SOLVD Investigators, *Circulation* 94, 690-697.

[15] Francis, G. S., Benedict, C., Johnstone, D. E., Kirlin, P. C., Nicklas, J., Liang, C. S., Kubo, S. H., Rudin-Toretsky, E., and Yusuf, S. (1990) Comparison of neuroendocrine activation in patients with left ventricular dysfunction with and without congestive heart failure. A substudy of the Studies of Left Ventricular Dysfunction (SOLVD), *Circulation* 82, 1724-1729.

[16] Parati, G. and Esler, M. (2012) The human sympathetic nervous system: its relevance in hypertension and heart failure, *Eur. Heart J.* 33, 1058-1066.

[17] Brasier, A. R., Recinos, A., III and Eledrisi, M. S. (2002) Vascular inflammation and the renin-angiotensin system, *Arterioscler. Thromb. Vasc. Biol.* 22, 1257-1266.

[18] Prabhu, S. D., Chandrasekar, B., Murray, D. R., and Freeman, G. L. (2000) beta-adrenergic blockade in developing heart failure: effects on myocardial inflammatory cytokines, nitric oxide, and remodeling, *Circulation* 101, 2103-2109.

[19] Wei, G. C., Sirois, M. G., Qu, R., Liu, P., and Rouleau, J. L. (2002) Subacute and chronic effects of quinapril on cardiac cytokine expression, remodeling, and function after myocardial infarction in the rat, *J. Cardiovasc. Pharmacol.* 39, 842-850.

[20] Tracey, K. J. (2009) Reflex control of immunity, *Nat. Rev. Immunol.* 9, 418-428.

[21] Jankowska, E. A., Ponikowski, P., Piepoli, M. F., Banasiak, W., Anker, S. D., and Poole-Wilson, P. A. (2006) Autonomic imbalance and immune activation in chronic heart failure - pathophysiological links, *Cardiovasc. Res.* 70, 434-445.

[22] Goldberg, L. R. and Jessup, M. (2006) Stage B heart failure: management of asymptomatic left ventricular systolic dysfunction, *Circulation* 113, 2851-2860.

[23] Lang, R. M., Bierig, M., Devereux, R. B., Flachskampf, F. A., Foster, E., Pellikka, P. A., Picard, M. H., Roman, M. J., Seward, J., Shanewise, J. S., Solomon, S. D., Spencer,

K. T., Sutton, M. S., and Stewart, W. J. (2005) Recommendations for chamber quantification: a report from the American Society of Echocardiography's Guidelines and Standards Committee and the Chamber Quantification Writing Group, developed in conjunction with the European Association of Echocardiography, a branch of the European Society of Cardiology, *J. Am. Soc. Echocardiogr.* 18, 1440-1463.

[24] Greenberg, B. (2010) Pre-clinical diastolic dysfunction in diabetic patients: where do we go from here?, *J. Am. Coll. Cardiol.* 55, 306-308.

[25] Curry, C. W., Nelson, G. S., Wyman, B. T., Declerck, J., Talbot, M., Berger, R. D., McVeigh, E. R., and Kass, D. A. (2000) Mechanical dyssynchrony in dilated cardiomyopathy with intraventricular conduction delay as depicted by 3D tagged magnetic resonance imaging, *Circulation* 101, E2.

[26] Lee, C. S. and Tkacs, N. C. (2008) Current concepts of neurohormonal activation in heart failure: mediators and mechanisms, *AACN. Adv. Crit. Care* 19, 364-385.

[27] Westerhof, N. and O'Rourke, M. F. (1995) Haemodynamic basis for the development of left ventricular failure in systolic hypertension and for its logical therapy, *J. Hypertens.* 13, 943-952.

[28] Kalogeropoulos, A. P., Georgiopoulou, V. V. and Butler, J. (2012) From risk factors to structural heart disease: the role of inflammation, *Heart Fail. Clin.* 8, 113-123.

[29] Redfield, M. M., Jacobsen, S. J., Burnett, J. C., Jr., Mahoney, D. W., Bailey, K. R., and Rodeheffer, R. J. (2003) Burden of systolic and diastolic ventricular dysfunction in the community: appreciating the scope of the heart failure epidemic, *JAMA* 289, 194-202.

[30] Wang, T. J., Evans, J. C., Benjamin, E. J., Levy, D., LeRoy, E. C., and Vasan, R. S. (2003) Natural history of asymptomatic left ventricular systolic dysfunction in the community, *Circulation* 108, 977-982.

[31] Ammar, K. A., Jacobsen, S. J., Mahoney, D. W., Kors, J. A., Redfield, M. M., Burnett, J. C., Jr., and Rodeheffer, R. J. (2007) Prevalence and prognostic significance of heart failure stages: application of the American College of Cardiology/American Heart Association heart failure staging criteria in the community, *Circulation* 115, 1563-1570.

[32] Daniels, L. B., Clopton, P., Jiang, K., Greenberg, B., and Maisel, A. S. (2010) Prognosis of stage A or B heart failure patients with elevated B-type natriuretic peptide levels, *J. Card Fail.* 16, 93-98.

[33] Maisel, A. S., Krishnaswamy, P., Nowak, R. M., McCord, J., Hollander, J. E., Duc, P., Omland, T., Storrow, A. B., Abraham, W. T., Wu, A. H., Clopton, P., Steg, P. G., Westheim, A., Knudsen, C. W., Perez, A., Kazanegra, R., Herrmann, H. C., and McCullough, P. A. (2002) Rapid measurement of B-type natriuretic peptide in the emergency diagnosis of heart failure, *N. Engl. J. Med.* 347, 161-167.

[34] Miller, W. L., Hartman, K. A., Burritt, M. F., Grill, D. E., Rodeheffer, R. J., Burnett, J. C., Jr., and Jaffe, A. S. (2007) Serial biomarker measurements in ambulatory patients with chronic heart failure: the importance of change over time, *Circulation* 116, 249-257.

[35] Sun, T., Wang, L. and Zhang, Y. (2007) Prognostic value of B-type natriuretic peptide in patients with chronic and advanced heart failure, *Intern. Med. J.* 37, 168-171.

[36] Kalogeropoulos, A., Georgiopoulou, V., Psaty, B. M., Rodondi, N., Smith, A. L., Harrison, D. G., Liu, Y., Hoffmann, U., Bauer, D. C., Newman, A. B., Kritchevsky, S. B., Harris, T. B., and Butler, J. (2010) Inflammatory markers and incident heart failure

risk in older adults: the Health ABC (Health, Aging, and Body Composition) study, *J. Am. Coll. Cardiol.* 55, 2129-2137.

[37] Suzuki, T., Katz, R., Jenny, N. S., Zakai, N. A., LeWinter, M. M., Barzilay, J. I., and Cushman, M. (2008) Metabolic syndrome, inflammation, and incident heart failure in the elderly: the cardiovascular health study, *Circ. Heart Fail.* 1, 242-248.

[38] Bahrami, H., Bluemke, D. A., Kronmal, R., Bertoni, A. G., Lloyd-Jones, D. M., Shahar, E., Szklo, M., and Lima, J. A. (2008) Novel metabolic risk factors for incident heart failure and their relationship with obesity: the MESA (Multi-Ethnic Study of Atherosclerosis) study, *J. Am. Coll. Cardiol.* 51, 1775-1783.

[39] Vasan, R. S., Sullivan, L. M., Roubenoff, R., Dinarello, C. A., Harris, T., Benjamin, E. J., Sawyer, D. B., Levy, D., Wilson, P. W., and D'Agostino, R. B. (2003) Inflammatory markers and risk of heart failure in elderly subjects without prior myocardial infarction: the Framingham Heart Study, *Circulation* 107, 1486-1491.

[40] Hartford, M., Wiklund, O., Hulten, L. M., Persson, A., Karlsson, T., Herlitz, J., Hulthe, J., and Caidahl, K. (2010) Interleukin-18 as a predictor of future events in patients with acute coronary syndromes, *Arterioscler. Thromb. Vasc. Biol.* 30, 2039-2046.

[41] Hedayat, M., Mahmoudi, M. J., Rose, N. R., and Rezaei, N. (2010) Proinflammatory cytokines in heart failure: double-edged swords, *Heart Fail. Rev.* 15, 543-562.

[42] Wilson, E. M., Diwan, A., Spinale, F. G., and Mann, D. L. (2004) Duality of innate stress responses in cardiac injury, repair, and remodeling, *J. Mol. Cell Cardiol.* 37, 801-811.

[43] Kapadia, S. R., Oral, H., Lee, J., Nakano, M., Taffet, G. E., and Mann, D. L. (1997) Hemodynamic regulation of tumor necrosis factor-alpha gene and protein expression in adult feline myocardium, *Circ. Res.* 81, 187-195.

[44] Walczak, H. (2011) TNF and ubiquitin at the crossroads of gene activation, cell death, inflammation, and cancer, *Immunol. Rev.* 244, 9-28.

[45] Bemelmans, M. H., van Tits, L. J. and Buurman, W. A. (1996) Tumor necrosis factor: function, release and clearance, *Crit. Rev. Immunol.* 16, 1-11.

[46] Nophar, Y., Kemper, O., Brakebusch, C., Englemann, H., Zwang, R., Aderka, D., Holtmann, H., and Wallach, D. (1990) Soluble forms of tumor necrosis factor receptors (TNF-Rs). The cDNA for the type I TNF-R, cloned using amino acid sequence data of its soluble form, encodes both the cell surface and a soluble form of the receptor, *EMBO J.* 9, 3269-3278.

[47] Balakumar, P. and Singh, M. (2006) Anti-tumour necrosis factor-alpha therapy in heart failure: future directions, *Basic Clin. Pharmacol. Toxicol.* 99, 391-397.

[48] Torre-Amione, G., Kapadia, S., Benedict, C., Oral, H., Young, J. B., and Mann, D. L. (1996) Proinflammatory cytokine levels in patients with depressed left ventricular ejection fraction: a report from the Studies of Left Ventricular Dysfunction (SOLVD), *J. Am. Coll. Cardiol.* 27, 1201-1206.

[49] Tran, L. T., MacLeod, K. M. and McNeill, J. H. (2009) Chronic etanercept treatment prevents the development of hypertension in fructose-fed rats, *Mol. Cell Biochem.* 330, 219-228.

[50] Gregor, M. F. and Hotamisligil, G. S. (2011) Inflammatory mechanisms in obesity, *Annu. Rev. Immunol.* 29, 415-445.

[51] Alam, I., Lewis, K., Stephens, J. W., and Baxter, J. N. (2007) Obesity, metabolic syndrome and sleep apnoea: all pro-inflammatory states, *Obes. Rev.* 8, 119-127.

[52] Shoelson, S. E., Herrero, L. and Naaz, A. (2007) Obesity, inflammation, and insulin resistance, *Gastroenterology* 132, 2169-2180.

[53] Forsythe, L. K., Wallace, J. M. and Livingstone, M. B. (2008) Obesity and inflammation: the effects of weight loss, *Nutr. Res. Rev.* 21, 117-133.

[54] Kasapis, C. and Thompson, P. D. (2005) The effects of physical activity on serum C-reactive protein and inflammatory markers: a systematic review, *J. Am. Coll. Cardiol.* 45, 1563-1569.

[55] Bristow, M. R. (1998) Tumor necrosis factor-alpha and cardiomyopathy, *Circulation* 97, 1340-1341.

[56] Ferrari, R. (1998) Tumor necrosis factor in CHF: a double facet cytokine, *Cardiovasc. Res.* 37, 554-559.

[57] Melino, G., Bernassola, F., Knight, R. A., Corasaniti, M. T., Nistico, G., and Finazzi-Agro, A. (1997) S-nitrosylation regulates apoptosis, *Nature* 388, 432-433.

[58] De Belder, A. J., Radomski, M. W., Why, H. J., Richardson, P. J., Bucknall, C. A., Salas, E., Martin, J. F., and Moncada, S. (1993) Nitric oxide synthase activities in human myocardium, *Lancet* 341, 84-85.

[59] Habib, F. M., Springall, D. R., Davies, G. J., Oakley, C. M., Yacoub, M. H., and Polak, J. M. (1996) Tumour necrosis factor and inducible nitric oxide synthase in dilated cardiomyopathy, *Lancet* 347, 1151-1155.

[60] Feldman, A. M., Combes, A., Wagner, D., Kadakomi, T., Kubota, T., Li, Y. Y., and McTiernan, C. (2000) The role of tumor necrosis factor in the pathophysiology of heart failure, *J. Am. Coll. Cardiol.* 35, 537-544.

[61] Engel, D., Peshock, R., Armstong, R. C., Sivasubramanian, N., and Mann, D. L. (2004) Cardiac myocyte apoptosis provokes adverse cardiac remodeling in transgenic mice with targeted TNF overexpression, *Am. J. Physiol. Heart Circ. Physiol.* 287, H1303-H1311.

[62] Kubota, T., McTiernan, C. F., Frye, C. S., Slawson, S. E., Lemster, B. H., Koretsky, A. P., Demetris, A. J., and Feldman, A. M. (1997) Dilated cardiomyopathy in transgenic mice with cardiac-specific overexpression of tumor necrosis factor-alpha, *Circ. Res.* 81, 627-635.

[63] Bryant, D., Becker, L., Richardson, J., Shelton, J., Franco, F., Peshock, R., Thompson, M., and Giroir, B. (1998) Cardiac failure in transgenic mice with myocardial expression of tumor necrosis factor-alpha, *Circulation* 97, 1375-1381.

[64] Deswal, A., Bozkurt, B., Seta, Y., Parilti-Eiswirth, S., Hayes, F. A., Blosch, C., and Mann, D. L. (1999) Safety and efficacy of a soluble P75 tumor necrosis factor receptor (Enbrel, etanercept) in patients with advanced heart failure, *Circulation* 99, 3224-3226.

[65] Anker, S. D. and Coats, A. J. (2002) How to RECOVER from RENAISSANCE? The significance of the results of RECOVER, RENAISSANCE, RENEWAL and ATTACH, *Int. J. Cardiol.* 86, 123-130.

[66] Mann, D. L., McMurray, J. J., Packer, M., Swedberg, K., Borer, J. S., Colucci, W. S., Djian, J., Drexler, H., Feldman, A., Kober, L., Krum, H., Liu, P., Nieminen, M., Tavazzi, L., van Veldhuisen, D. J., Waldenstrom, A., Warren, M., Westheim, A., Zannad, F., and Fleming, T. (2004) Targeted anticytokine therapy in patients with chronic heart failure: results of the Randomized Etanercept Worldwide Evaluation (RENEWAL), *Circulation* 109, 1594-1602.

[67] Scheller, J., Chalaris, A., Schmidt-Arras, D., and Rose-John, S. (2011) The pro- and anti-inflammatory properties of the cytokine interleukin-6, *Biochim. Biophys. Acta* 1813, 878-888.

[68] Yan, A. T., Yan, R. T., Cushman, M., Redheuil, A., Tracy, R. P., Arnett, D. K., Rosen, B. D., McClelland, R. L., Bluemke, D. A., and Lima, J. A. (2010) Relationship of interleukin-6 with regional and global left-ventricular function in asymptomatic individuals without clinical cardiovascular disease: insights from the Multi-Ethnic Study of Atherosclerosis, *Eur. Heart J.* 31, 875-882.

[69] Ridker, P. M., Rifai, N., Stampfer, M. J., and Hennekens, C. H. (2000) Plasma concentration of interleukin-6 and the risk of future myocardial infarction among apparently healthy men, *Circulation* 101, 1767-1772.

[70] Danesh, J., Kaptoge, S., Mann, A. G., Sarwar, N., Wood, A., Angleman, S. B., Wensley, F., Higgins, J. P., Lennon, L., Eiriksdottir, G., Rumley, A., Whincup, P. H., Lowe, G. D., and Gudnason, V. (2008) Long-term interleukin-6 levels and subsequent risk of coronary heart disease: two new prospective studies and a systematic review, *PLoS. Med.* 5, e78.

[71] Bastard, J. P., Jardel, C., Bruckert, E., Blondy, P., Capeau, J., Laville, M., Vidal, H., and Hainque, B. (2000) Elevated levels of interleukin 6 are reduced in serum and subcutaneous adipose tissue of obese women after weight loss, *J. Clin. Endocrinol. Metab.* 85, 3338-3342.

[72] Bastard, J. P., Maachi, M., Van Nhieu, J. T., Jardel, C., Bruckert, E., Grimaldi, A., Robert, J. J., Capeau, J., and Hainque, B. (2002) Adipose tissue IL-6 content correlates with resistance to insulin activation of glucose uptake both in vivo and in vitro, *J. Clin. Endocrinol. Metab.* 87, 2084-2089.

[73] Fried, S. K., Bunkin, D. A. and Greenberg, A. S. (1998) Omental and subcutaneous adipose tissues of obese subjects release interleukin-6: depot difference and regulation by glucocorticoid, *J. Clin. Endocrinol. Metab.* 83, 847-850.

[74] Raymond, R. J., Dehmer, G. J., Theoharides, T. C., and Deliargyris, E. N. (2001) Elevated interleukin-6 levels in patients with asymptomatic left ventricular systolic dysfunction, *Am. Heart J.* 141, 435-438.

[75] Torre-Amione, G., Kapadia, S., Benedict, C., Oral, H., Young, J. B., and Mann, D. L. (1996) Proinflammatory cytokine levels in patients with depressed left ventricular ejection fraction: a report from the Studies of Left Ventricular Dysfunction (SOLVD), *J. Am. Coll. Cardiol.* 27, 1201-1206.

[76] Fattori, E., Cappelletti, M., Costa, P., Sellitto, C., Cantoni, L., Carelli, M., Faggioni, R., Fantuzzi, G., Ghezzi, P., and Poli, V. (1994) Defective inflammatory response in interleukin 6-deficient mice, *J. Exp. Med.* 180, 1243-1250.

[77] El-Adawi, H., Deng, L., Tramontano, A., Smith, S., Mascareno, E., Ganguly, K., Castillo, R., and El-Sherif, N. (2003) The functional role of the JAK-STAT pathway in post-infarction remodeling, *Cardiovasc. Res.* 57, 129-138.

[78] Smart, N., Mojet, M. H., Latchman, D. S., Marber, M. S., Duchen, M. R., and Heads, R. J. (2006) IL-6 induces PI 3-kinase and nitric oxide-dependent protection and preserves mitochondrial function in cardiomyocytes, *Cardiovasc. Res.* 69, 164-177.

[79] Yamauchi-Takihara, K. and Kishimoto, T. (2000) Cytokines and their receptors in cardiovascular diseases--role of gp130 signalling pathway in cardiac myocyte growth and maintenance, *Int. J. Exp. Pathol.* 81, 1-16.

[80] Hirota, H., Chen, J., Betz, U. A., Rajewsky, K., Gu, Y., Ross, J., Jr., Muller, W., and Chien, K. R. (1999) Loss of a gp130 cardiac muscle cell survival pathway is a critical event in the onset of heart failure during biomechanical stress, *Cell* 97, 189-198.

[81] Hirota, H., Yoshida, K., Kishimoto, T., and Taga, T. (1995) Continuous activation of gp130, a signal-transducing receptor component for interleukin 6-related cytokines, causes myocardial hypertrophy in mice, *Proc. Natl. Acad. Sci. US* 92, 4862-4866.

[82] Yu, X., Kennedy, R. H. and Liu, S. J. (2003) JAK2/STAT3, not ERK1/2, mediates interleukin-6-induced activation of inducible nitric-oxide synthase and decrease in contractility of adult ventricular myocytes, *J. Biol. Chem.* 278, 16304-16309.

[83] Fischer, P. and Hilfiker-Kleiner, D. (2007) Survival pathways in hypertrophy and heart failure: the gp130-STAT axis, *Basic Res. Cardiol.* 102, 393-411.

[84] Danesh, J., Wheeler, J. G., Hirschfield, G. M., Eda, S., Eiriksdottir, G., Rumley, A., Lowe, G. D., Pepys, M. B., and Gudnason, V. (2004) C-reactive protein and other circulating markers of inflammation in the prediction of coronary heart disease, *N. Engl. J. Med.* 350, 1387-1397.

[85] Pepys, M. B. and Hirschfield, G. M. (2003) C-reactive protein: a critical update, *J. Clin. Invest.* 111, 1805-1812.

[86] Berk, B. C., Weintraub, W. S. and Alexander, R. W. (1990) Elevation of C-reactive protein in "active" coronary artery disease, *Am. J. Cardiol.* 65, 168-172.

[87] Liuzzo, G., Biasucci, L. M., Gallimore, J. R., Grillo, R. L., Rebuzzi, A. G., Pepys, M. B., and Maseri, A. (1994) The prognostic value of C-reactive protein and serum amyloid a protein in severe unstable angina, *N. Engl. J. Med.* 331, 417-424.

[88] Ridker, P. M., Cushman, M., Stampfer, M. J., Tracy, R. P., and Hennekens, C. H. (1997) Inflammation, aspirin, and the risk of cardiovascular disease in apparently healthy men, *N. Engl. J. Med.* 336, 973-979.

[89] Ridker, P. M., Buring, J. E., Shih, J., Matias, M., and Hennekens, C. H. (1998) Prospective study of C-reactive protein and the risk of future cardiovascular events among apparently healthy women, *Circulation* 98, 731-733.

[90] Pearson, T. A., Mensah, G. A., Alexander, R. W., Anderson, J. L., Cannon, R. O., III, Criqui, M., Fadl, Y. Y., Fortmann, S. P., Hong, Y., Myers, G. L., Rifai, N., Smith, S. C., Jr., Taubert, K., Tracy, R. P., and Vinicor, F. (2003) Markers of inflammation and cardiovascular disease: application to clinical and public health practice: A statement for healthcare professionals from the Centers for Disease Control and Prevention and the American Heart Association, *Circulation* 107, 499-511.

[91] Jonsdottir, L. S., Sigfusson, N., Gudnason, V., Sigvaldason, H., and Thorgeirsson, G. (2002) Do lipids, blood pressure, diabetes, and smoking confer equal risk of myocardial infarction in women as in men? The Reykjavik Study, *J. Cardiovasc. Risk* 9, 67-76.

[92] Hak, A. E., Stehouwer, C. D., Bots, M. L., Polderman, K. H., Schalkwijk, C. G., Westendorp, I. C., Hofman, A., and Witteman, J. C. (1999) Associations of C-reactive protein with measures of obesity, insulin resistance, and subclinical atherosclerosis in healthy, middle-aged women, *Arterioscler. Thromb. Vasc. Biol.* 19, 1986-1991.

[93] Tracy, R. P., Psaty, B. M., Macy, E., Bovill, E. G., Cushman, M., Cornell, E. S., and Kuller, L. H. (1997) Lifetime smoking exposure affects the association of C-reactive protein with cardiovascular disease risk factors and subclinical disease in healthy elderly subjects, *Arterioscler. Thromb. Vasc. Biol.* 17, 2167-2176.

[94] Yudkin, J. S., Stehouwer, C. D., Emeis, J. J., and Coppack, S. W. (1999) C-reactive protein in healthy subjects: associations with obesity, insulin resistance, and endothelial dysfunction: a potential role for cytokines originating from adipose tissue?, *Arterioscler. Thromb. Vasc. Biol.* 19, 972-978.

[95] Pasceri, V., Willerson, J. T. and Yeh, E. T. (2000) Direct proinflammatory effect of C-reactive protein on human endothelial cells, *Circulation* 102, 2165-2168.

[96] Pasceri, V., Cheng, J. S., Willerson, J. T., and Yeh, E. T. (2001) Modulation of C-reactive protein-mediated monocyte chemoattractant protein-1 induction in human endothelial cells by anti-atherosclerosis drugs, *Circulation* 103, 2531-2534.

[97] Schillaci, G. and Pirro, M. (2006) C-reactive protein in hypertension: clinical significance and predictive value, *Nutr. Metab. Cardiovasc. Dis.* 16, 500-508.

[98] De Beer, F. C., Hind, C. R., Fox, K. M., Allan, R. M., Maseri, A., and Pepys, M. B. (1982) Measurement of serum C-reactive protein concentration in myocardial ischaemia and infarction, *Br. Heart J.* 47, 239-243.

[99] Griselli, M., Herbert, J., Hutchinson, W. L., Taylor, K. M., Sohail, M., Krausz, T., and Pepys, M. B. (1999) C-reactive protein and complement are important mediators of tissue damage in acute myocardial infarction, *J. Exp. Med.* 190, 1733-1740.

[100] Nissen, S. E., Tuzcu, E. M., Schoenhagen, P., Crowe, T., Sasiela, W. J., Tsai, J., Orazem, J., Magorien, R. D., O'Shaughnessy, C., and Ganz, P. (2005) Statin therapy, LDL cholesterol, C-reactive protein, and coronary artery disease, *N. Engl. J. Med.* 352, 29-38.

[101] Nissen, S. E., Nicholls, S. J., Sipahi, I., Libby, P., Raichlen, J. S., Ballantyne, C. M., Davignon, J., Erbel, R., Fruchart, J. C., Tardif, J. C., Schoenhagen, P., Crowe, T., Cain, V., Wolski, K., Goormastic, M., and Tuzcu, E. M. (2006) Effect of very high-intensity statin therapy on regression of coronary atherosclerosis: the ASTEROID trial, *JAMA* 295, 1556-1565.

[102] Ridker, P. M., Cannon, C. P., Morrow, D., Rifai, N., Rose, L. M., McCabe, C. H., Pfeffer, M. A., and Braunwald, E. (2005) C-reactive protein levels and outcomes after statin therapy, *N. Engl. J. Med.* 352, 20-28.

[103] Elkind, M. S., Luna, J. M., Moon, Y. P., Liu, K. M., Spitalnik, S. L., Paik, M. C., and Sacco, R. L. (2009) High-sensitivity C-reactive protein predicts mortality but not stroke: the Northern Manhattan Study, *Neurology* 73, 1300-1307.

[104] Jonathan, E., Derrick, B., Emma, L., Sarah, P., John, D., Jane, A., and Rory, C. (2011) C-reactive protein concentration and the vascular benefits of statin therapy: an analysis of 20,536 patients in the Heart Protection Study, *Lancet* 377, 469-476.

[105] Ridker, P. M., MacFadyen, J., Libby, P., and Glynn, R. J. (2010) Relation of baseline high-sensitivity C-reactive protein level to cardiovascular outcomes with rosuvastatin in the Justification for Use of statins in Prevention: an Intervention Trial Evaluating Rosuvastatin (JUPITER), *Am. J. Cardiol.* 106, 204-209.

[106] Kaneko, K., Kanda, T., Yamauchi, Y., Hasegawa, A., Iwasaki, T., Arai, M., Suzuki, T., Kobayashi, I., and Nagai, R. (1999) C-Reactive protein in dilated cardiomyopathy, *Cardiology* 91, 215-219.

[107] Alonso-Martinez, J. L., Llorente-Diez, B., Echegaray-Agara, M., Olaz-Preciado, F., Urbieta-Echezarreta, M., and Gonzalez-Arencibia, C. (2002) C-reactive protein as a predictor of improvement and readmission in heart failure, *Eur. J. Heart Fail.* 4, 331-336.

[108] Anand, I. S., Latini, R., Florea, V. G., Kuskowski, M. A., Rector, T., Masson, S., Signorini, S., Mocarelli, P., Hester, A., Glazer, R., and Cohn, J. N. (2005) C-reactive protein in heart failure: prognostic value and the effect of valsartan, *Circulation* 112, 1428-1434.

[109] Anker, S. D. and von, H. S. (2004) Inflammatory mediators in chronic heart failure: an overview, *Heart* 90, 464-470.

[110] Araujo, J. P., Lourenco, P., Azevedo, A., Frioes, F., Rocha-Goncalves, F., Ferreira, A., and Bettencourt, P. (2009) Prognostic value of high-sensitivity C-reactive protein in heart failure: a systematic review, *J. Card Fail.* 15, 256-266.

[111] Deban, L., Jaillon, S., Garlanda, C., Bottazzi, B., and Mantovani, A. (2011) Pentraxins in innate immunity: lessons from PTX3, *Cell Tissue Res.* 343, 237-249.

[112] Matsubara, J., Sugiyama, S., Nozaki, T., Sugamura, K., Konishi, M., Ohba, K., Matsuzawa, Y., Akiyama, E., Yamamoto, E., Sakamoto, K., Nagayoshi, Y., Kaikita, K., Sumida, H., Kim-Mitsuyama, S., and Ogawa, H. (2011) Pentraxin 3 is a new inflammatory marker correlated with left ventricular diastolic dysfunction and heart failure with normal ejection fraction, *J. Am. Coll. Cardiol.* 57, 861-869.

[113] Nebuloni, M., Pasqualini, F., Zerbi, P., Lauri, E., Mantovani, A., Vago, L., and Garlanda, C. (2011) PTX3 expression in the heart tissues of patients with myocardial infarction and infectious myocarditis, *Cardiovasc. Pathol.* 20, e27-e35.

[114] Norata, G. D., Marchesi, P., Pulakazhi Venu, V. K., Pasqualini, F., Anselmo, A., Moalli, F., Pizzitola, I., Garlanda, C., Mantovani, A., and Catapano, A. L. (2009) Deficiency of the long pentraxin PTX3 promotes vascular inflammation and atherosclerosis, *Circulation* 120, 699-708.

[115] Salio, M., Chimenti, S., De, A. N., Molla, F., Maina, V., Nebuloni, M., Pasqualini, F., Latini, R., Garlanda, C., and Mantovani, A. (2008) Cardioprotective function of the long pentraxin PTX3 in acute myocardial infarction, *Circulation* 117, 1055-1064.

[116] Kaess, B. M. and Vasan, R. S. (2011) Heart failure: pentraxin 3-a marker of diastolic dysfunction and HF?, *Nat. Rev. Cardiol.* 8, 246-248.

[117] Dubin, R., Li, Y., Ix, J. H., Shlipak, M. G., Whooley, M., and Peralta, C. A. (2012) Associations of pentraxin-3 with cardiovascular events, incident heart failure, and mortality among persons with coronary heart disease: data from the Heart and Soul Study, *Am. Heart J.* 163, 274-279.

[118] Latini, R., Gullestad, L., Masson, S., Nymo, S. H., Ueland, T., Cuccovillo, I., Vardal, M., Bottazzi, B., Mantovani, A., Lucci, D., Masuda, N., Sudo, Y., Wikstrand, J., Tognoni, G., Aukrust, P., and Tavazzi, L. (2012) Pentraxin-3 in chronic heart failure: the CORONA and GISSI-HF trials, *Eur. J. Heart Fail.* 14, 992-999.

[119] Malle, E. and de Beer, F. C. (1996) Human serum amyloid A (SAA) protein: a prominent acute-phase reactant for clinical practice, *Eur. J. Clin. Invest* 26, 427-435.

[120] Kisilevsky, R. and Subrahmanyan, L. (1992) Serum amyloid A changes high density lipoprotein's cellular affinity. A clue to serum amyloid A's principal function, *Lab. Invest.* 66, 778-785.

[121] Liang, J. S., Schreiber, B. M., Salmona, M., Phillip, G., Gonnerman, W. A., de Beer, F. C., and Sipe, J. D. (1996) Amino terminal region of acute phase, but not constitutive, serum amyloid A (apoSAA) specifically binds and transports cholesterol into aortic smooth muscle and HepG2 cells, *J. Lipid Res.* 37, 2109-2116.

[122] Kisilevsky, R., Tam, S. P. and Ancsin, J. B. (2008) The anti-atherogenic potential of serum amyloid A peptides, *Curr. Opin. Investig. Drugs* 9, 265-273.
[123] Sjoholm, K., Palming, J., Olofsson, L. E., Gummesson, A., Svensson, P. A., Lystig, T. C., Jennische, E., Brandberg, J., Torgerson, J. S., Carlsson, B., and Carlsson, L. M. (2005) A microarray search for genes predominantly expressed in human omental adipocytes: adipose tissue as a major production site of serum amyloid A, *J. Clin. Endocrinol. Metab.* 90, 2233-2239.
[124] Zhao, Y., He, X., Shi, X., Huang, C., Liu, J., Zhou, S., and Heng, C. K. (2010) Association between serum amyloid A and obesity: a meta-analysis and systematic review, *Inflamm. Res.* 59, 323-334.
[125] King, V. L., Thompson, J. and Tannock, L. R. (2011) Serum amyloid A in atherosclerosis, *Curr. Opin. Lipidol.* 22, 302-307.
[126] Johnson, B. D., Kip, K. E., Marroquin, O. C., Ridker, P. M., Kelsey, S. F., Shaw, L. J., Pepine, C. J., Sharaf, B., Bairey Merz, C. N., Sopko, G., Olson, M. B., and Reis, S. E. (2004) Serum amyloid A as a predictor of coronary artery disease and cardiovascular outcome in women: the National Heart, Lung, and Blood Institute-Sponsored Women's Ischemia Syndrome Evaluation (WISE), *Circulation* 109, 726-732.
[127] Kosuge, M., Ebina, T., Ishikawa, T., Hibi, K., Tsukahara, K., Okuda, J., Iwahashi, N., Ozaki, H., Yano, H., Kusama, I., Nakati, T., Umemura, S., and Kimura, K. (2007) Serum amyloid A is a better predictor of clinical outcomes than C-reactive protein in non-ST-segment elevation acute coronary syndromes, *Circ. J.* 71, 186-190.
[128] Ridker, P. M., Hennekens, C. H., Buring, J. E., and Rifai, N. (2000) C-reactive protein and other markers of inflammation in the prediction of cardiovascular disease in women, *N. Engl. J. Med.* 342, 836-843.
[129] Dinarello, C. A. (2009) Immunological and inflammatory functions of the interleukin-1 family, *Annu. Rev. Immunol.* 27, 519-550.
[130] Agostini, L., Martinon, F., Burns, K., McDermott, M. F., Hawkins, P. N., and Tschopp, J. (2004) NALP3 forms an IL-1beta-processing inflammasome with increased activity in Muckle-Wells autoinflammatory disorder, *Immunity.* 20, 319-325.
[131] Martinon, F., Mayor, A. and Tschopp, J. (2009) The inflammasomes: guardians of the body, *Annu. Rev. Immunol.* 27, 229-265.
[132] Dinarello, C. A. (2000) The role of the interleukin-1-receptor antagonist in blocking inflammation mediated by interleukin-1, *N. Engl. J. Med.* 343, 732-734.
[133] Stienstra, R., Joosten, L. A., Koenen, T., van, T. B., van Diepen, J. A., van den Berg, S. A., Rensen, P. C., Voshol, P. J., Fantuzzi, G., Hijmans, A., Kersten, S., Muller, M., van den Berg, W. B., van, R. N., Wabitsch, M., Kullberg, B. J., van der Meer, J. W., Kanneganti, T., Tack, C. J., and Netea, M. G. (2010) The inflammasome-mediated caspase-1 activation controls adipocyte differentiation and insulin sensitivity, *Cell Metab.* 12, 593-605.
[134] Larsen, C. M., Faulenbach, M., Vaag, A., Volund, A., Ehses, J. A., Seifert, B., Mandrup-Poulsen, T., and Donath, M. Y. (2007) Interleukin-1-receptor antagonist in type 2 diabetes mellitus, *N. Engl. J. Med.* 356, 1517-1526.
[135] Abbate, A., Salloum, F. N., Vecile, E., Das, A., Hoke, N. N., Straino, S., Biondi-Zoccai, G. G., Houser, J. E., Qureshi, I. Z., Ownby, E. D., Gustini, E., Biasucci, L. M., Severino, A., Capogrossi, M. C., Vetrovec, G. W., Crea, F., Baldi, A., Kukreja, R. C., and Dobrina, A. (2008) Anakinra, a recombinant human interleukin-1 receptor

antagonist, inhibits apoptosis in experimental acute myocardial infarction, *Circulation* 117, 2670-2683.

[136] Abbate, A., Van Tassell, B. W., Seropian, I. M., Toldo, S., Robati, R., Varma, A., Salloum, F. N., Smithson, L., and Dinarello, C. A. (2010) Interleukin-1beta modulation using a genetically engineered antibody prevents adverse cardiac remodelling following acute myocardial infarction in the mouse, *Eur. J. Heart Fail.* 12, 319-322.

[137] Bujak, M. and Frangogiannis, N. G. (2009) The role of IL-1 in the pathogenesis of eart disease, *Arch. Immunol. Ther. Exp. (Warsz.)* 57, 165-176.

[138] Nishikawa, K., Yoshida, M., Kusuhara, M., Ishigami, N., Isoda, K., Miyazaki, K., and Ohsuzu, F. (2006) Left ventricular hypertrophy in mice with a cardiac-specific overexpression of interleukin-1, *Am. J. Physiol. Heart Circ. Physiol.* 291, H176-H183.

[139] Xia, Y., Lee, K., Li, N., Corbett, D., Mendoza, L., and Frangogiannis, N. G. (2009) Characterization of the inflammatory and fibrotic response in a mouse model of cardiac pressure overload, *Histochem. Cell Biol.* 131, 471-481.

[140] Dinarello, C. A., Simon, A. and van der Meer, J. W. (2012) Treating inflammation by blocking interleukin-1 in a broad spectrum of diseases, *Nat. Rev. Drug Discov.* 11, 633-652.

[141] Fearon, W. F. and Fearon, D. T. (2008) Inflammation and cardiovascular disease: role of the interleukin-1 receptor antagonist, *Circulation* 117, 2577-2579.

[142] Ikonomidis, I., Lekakis, J. P., Nikolaou, M., Paraskevaidis, I., Andreadou, I., Kaplanoglou, T., Katsimbri, P., Skarantavos, G., Soucacos, P. N., and Kremastinos, D. T. (2008) Inhibition of interleukin-1 by anakinra improves vascular and left ventricular function in patients with rheumatoid arthritis, *Circulation* 117, 2662-2669.

[143] Van Tassell, B. W., Arena, R. A., Toldo, S., Mezzaroma, E., Azam, T., Seropian, I. M., Shah, K., Canada, J., Voelkel, N. F., Dinarello, C. A., and Abbate, A. (2012) Enhanced interleukin-1 activity contributes to exercise intolerance in patients with systolic heart failure, *PLoS. One.* 7, e33438.

[144] Maisel, A. S. and Daniels, L. B. (2012) Breathing not properly 10 years later: what we have learned and what we still need to learn, *J. Am. Coll. Cardiol.* 60, 277-282.

[145] Daniels, L. B. and Maisel, A. S. (2007) Natriuretic peptides, *J. Am. Coll. Cardiol.* 50, 2357-2368.

[146] Nakagawa, O., Ogawa, Y., Itoh, H., Suga, S., Komatsu, Y., Kishimoto, I., Nishino, K., Yoshimasa, T., and Nakao, K. (1995) Rapid transcriptional activation and early mRNA turnover of brain natriuretic peptide in cardiocyte hypertrophy. Evidence for brain natriuretic peptide as an "emergency" cardiac hormone against ventricular overload, *J. Clin. Invest.* 96, 1280-1287.

[147] Wang, T. J., Larson, M. G., Levy, D., Benjamin, E. J., Leip, E. P., Omland, T., Wolf, P. A., and Vasan, R. S. (2004) Plasma natriuretic peptide levels and the risk of cardiovascular events and death, *N. Engl. J. Med.* 350, 655-663.

[148] Redfield, M. M., Rodeheffer, R. J., Jacobsen, S. J., Mahoney, D. W., Bailey, K. R., and Burnett, J. C., Jr. (2002) Plasma brain natriuretic peptide concentration: impact of age and gender, *J. Am. Coll. Cardiol.* 40, 976-982.

[149] Wang, T. J., Larson, M. G., Levy, D., Leip, E. P., Benjamin, E. J., Wilson, P. W., Sutherland, P., Omland, T., and Vasan, R. S. (2002) Impact of age and sex on plasma natriuretic peptide levels in healthy adults, *Am. J. Cardiol.* 90, 254-258.

This work was supported by grant HL-073355 from the National Institutes of Health and the Austrian Science Fund (FWF): J3256-B18.

In: Horizons in World Cardiovascular Research. Vol. 6
Editor: Eleanor H. Bennington
ISBN: 978-1-63321-298-5

Chapter 3

Endothelial Dysfunction in Hypertension: From Bench to Bedside and Future Directions

Ify Mordi, MRCP[1], Natalie Sawdon, MRCP[2] and Nikolaos Tzemos*, M.D., MRCP[1]

[1] Institute of Cardiovascular and Medical Sciences, University of Glasgow, Glasgow, UK
[2] Renal Unit, Western Infirmary, Glasgow, UK

Abstract

Introduction: The vascular endothelium plays an important rule in vascular homeostasis, tone and as a consequence, vascular health. Impairment in endothelial function or endothelial dysfunction translates to increased vascular tone and possibly to high blood pressure. Although is still debatable whether endothelial dysfunction remains a cause or consequence of essential hypertension, reversal of this target organ damage undoubtedly leads to improved cardiovascular prognosis. Not unreasonably, reversal of endothelial dysfunction has become therefore an ambitious treatment target. In this article, after exploring and providing evidence for the presence of endothelial dysfunction in hypertension, we also provide a systemic literature search review of endothelial dysfunction reversal in essential hypertension.

Methods: We conducted a MEDLINE, EMBASE etc. search of all of published studies referring to endothelial dysfunction reversal or improvement in hypertension from 1989 to 2012. Studies involving placebo were also included.

Results: We identified several pharmacologic and non-pharmacologic approaches favourably affecting endothelial function. Interestingly, blood pressure reduction per se did not affect vascular function. Modulators of the renin-angiotensin-aldosterone system

* Address for Correspondence: Dr Nikolaos Tzemos, Institute of Cardiovascular and Medical Sciences, University of Glasgow, BHF Glasgow Cardiovascular Research Centre, 126 University Avenue, Glasgow, G12 8TA. Telephone: +44 (0) 141 330 2079; Fax: +44 (0) 141 330 6997. E-mail: niko.tzemos@glasgow.ac.uk

(RAAS) appeared to have a consistent and a powerful effect in ameliorating or even reversing endothelial dysfunction in comparison to other antihypertensive agents for the same blood pressure control.

Conclusions: Reducing blood pressure without specific antihypertensive drugs does not seem to improve endothelial dysfunction. Modulators of the RAAS appear to have a long lasting beneficial effect on endothelial function perhaps providing a mechanistic link to their favourable effects on hypertensive cardiovascular prognosis.

1. The Vascular Endothelium: Anatomy and Physiology

The arterial wall consists of three layers: the adventitia (or tunica externa), the media and the intima, shown in Figure 1. The adventitial layer is made up of loosely tight connective tissue; specifically perivascular fibroblasts and collagen. In addition to the collagen it also contains a rich capillary blood supply and the autonomous nervous system terminals. The collagen gives the artery its stability and anchors it to nearby organs. The media is made up of smooth muscle cells (VSMC) and of a matrix of elastin, collagen and proteoglycans. It is well established that the arterial media layer has a double action: that of container and of damper. A function of container, because gives to the arterial wall its shape and also is responsible for keeping the blood within the vascular system, and a damping function, which is the phasic stress, produced by the elastic properties of the matrix and the tonic contracted or relaxed state of the smooth muscle cells. In addition to the vascular supportive measures, the VSMC also synthesises and matures collagen and the elastin of the extracellular matrix.

The intima is the innermost layer of the blood vessel. It is a single layer of endothelial cells lying on a support basement membrane called the internal elastic lamina. These vascular endothelial cells line every blood vessel in the body as well as the endocardium and are in direct contact with the luminal contents, i.e. blood. The endothelial cell surface in an adult human covers an extensive area and is composed approximately of 1 to 6 X 10^{13} cells and weights approximately 1 kg (Fishman 1982).

Since the pioneering work of Furchgott and Zawadzki [1], who identified that the large blood vessels of rabbits only relaxed in response to acetylcholine if the endothelium was intact, our concept of the endothelium and its functions over the last two decades has radically changed. Hence, rather than being thought of as an inert anatomical shelter, we now understand that the endothelium is actually a metabolically active endocrine, paracrine and autocrine organ with sustainable anti-atherogenic and anti-thrombotic properties. Indeed, one could say that taken altogether, it is the largest organ in the human body, even more so than the skin.

The vascular endothelium has numerous functions, which are summarised in table 1. Regarding hypertension, the most important role of the endothelium is it part in the regulation of vascular tone. The endothelium releases numerous substances with local (paracrine) action. These substances cause vasoconstriction or vasodilatation, and are summarised in table 2. The healthy endothelium is a natural inhibitor in its actions and is thus maintained in a natural state of predominant vasodilatation, and the most important substance for the maintenance of this state is nitric oxide (NO).

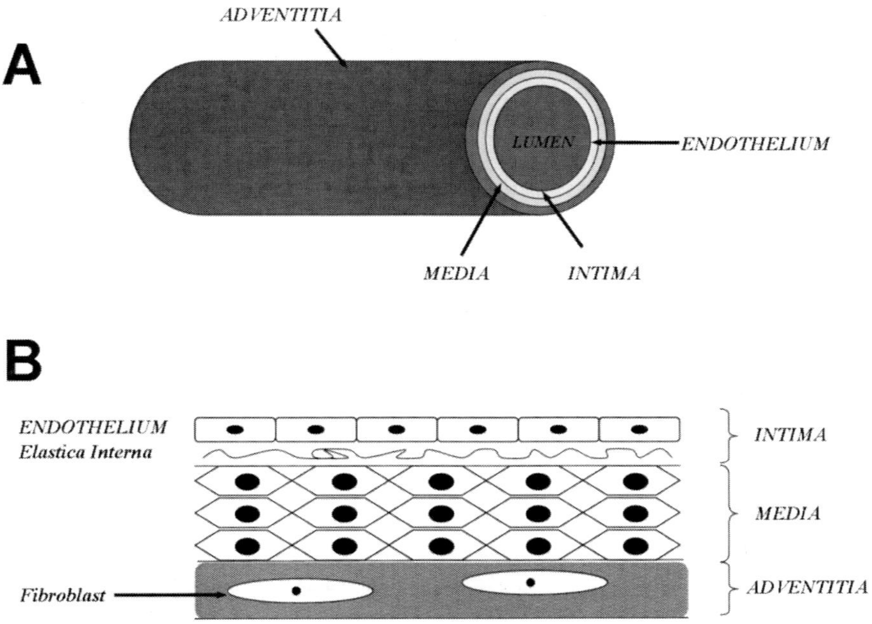

Figure 1. The structure of the human artery.

Table 1. Functions of the human vascular endothelium

Angiogenesis	Numerous growth factors affect the endothelium to cause the repair of old vessels and formation of new ones.
Barrier	The endothelium acts as a semi-selective barrier between the vessel lumen and surrounding tissue, controlling the passage of materials in and out of the bloodstream.
Clotting	The endothelium contains and secretes many pro-thrombotic and antithrombotic factors such as heparin sulphate (antithrombotic). It exists in naturally an antithrombotic state, which allows blood cells to roll along its surface.
Inflammatory	Mediation of inflammatory and immune responses.
Vascular tone	The endothelium contains substances that cause vasoconstriction and vasodilatation.

NO is a lipid and water soluble gas [2], formed by the conversion of the terminal guanidine-nitrogen from L-arginine, a semi-essential amino acid, to L-citrulline by an enzyme called endothelial NO synthase (eNOS), which is constitutive in endothelial cells (summarised in figure 2). There are three distinct isoforms of NO synthase: isoform I or nNOS (present in neuronal cells), isoform II or iNOS (in macrophages) which is calcium independent and cytokine-inducible and isoform III or eNOS originally described in the vascular endothelium but also present in platelets, myocardium and endocardium [3]. The activation of eNOS depends on the intracellular concentration of calcium ions in the endothelial cell, is calmodulin-dependent, and requires nicotinamide-adenine-dinucleotide (NADPH) and 5,6,7,8-tetrahydrobiopterin (BH4) as cofactors. Importantly, the activity of eNOS can be inhibited by endogenous and exogenous analogues of L-arginine such as NG-monomethyl-L-arginine (L-NMMA) and asymmetric dimethyl-arginine (ADMA), respectively [4, 5]. L-NMMA is an analogue of L-arginine that was initially shown to inhibit the generation of nitrite (NO2-) and nitrate (NO3-), which are products of the NO metabolism, in activated macrophages [6]. Subsequently, L-NMMA was also shown to induce contraction of vascular rings in isolated baths, an effect reversed by treatment with L- but not D-arginine [7].

Table 2. Some of the substances involved in maintenance of vascular tone

Endothelium Dependent Relaxing Factors	Endothelium Dependent Contracting Factors
Nitric oxide (NO)	Thromboxane A_2 (TxA_2)
Prostacyclin (PGI_2)	Endothelin
Endothelium derived hyperpolarising factor (EDHF)	Angiotensin II (AII)
C-type naturietic peptide (CNP)	

Once synthesised, part of the NO released diffuses directly to the underlying VSMC and relaxes them by stimulating a cytosolic enzyme, called soluble guanylate synthase. This activation leads to an increase in cyclic 3'-5'-guanisine monophosphate (cGMP) which is the second messenger, and to inhibition of the contractile apparatus, hence to vasodilatation. Apart from its conspicuous vasodilating properties, NO also inhibits VSMC proliferation and migration (hence preventing vascular remodelling) [8-10].

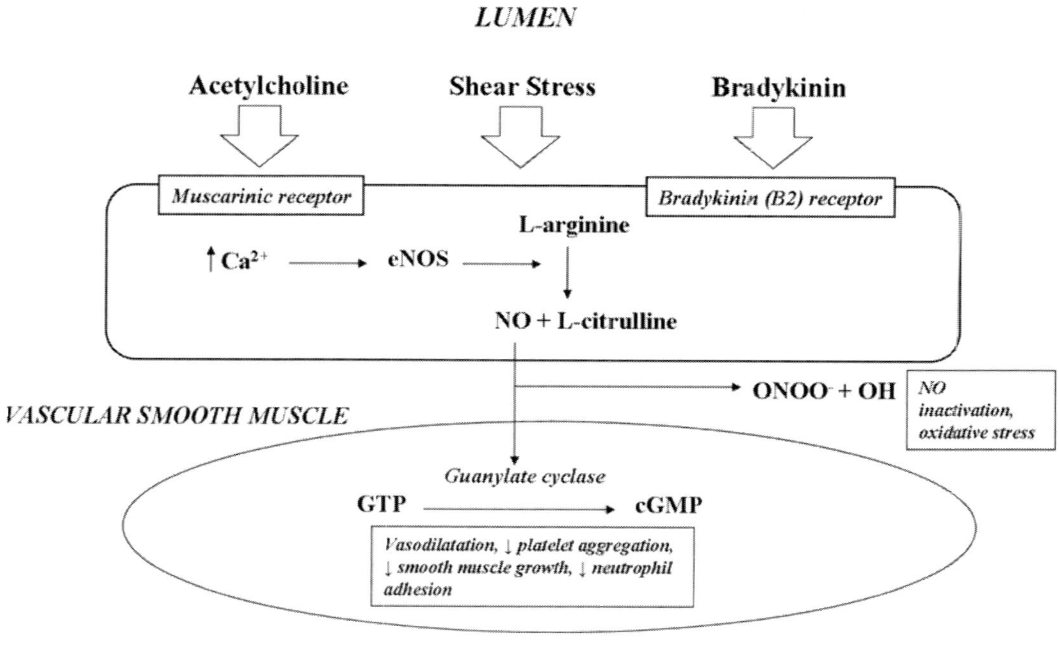

Figure 2. Synthesis of nitric oxide (NO).

In addition, NO relaxes contractile elements in endothelial cells to preserve tight junctions and maintain impermeability [11]. However, the endothelial cells release NO not only abluminally to VSMC but also directly into the lumen. The part of NO released in the lumen interacts with circulating platelets and leukocytes inhibiting their adhesion [12]. Furthermore, NO acting synergistically with prostacyclin inhibits also platelet aggregation. However, nitric oxide has an extremely short half-life of only few seconds. Indeed, after synthesis, NO is rapidly inactivated by locally generated oxygen-derived free radicals (O_2^-) to form peroxynitrite anions ($OONO^-$) which have considerably less vasodilating capacity than NO. Because NO is a free radical itself, the chemical reaction between NO and superoxide anions is extremely fast, faster than that with superoxide dismutase (SODs) or with plasma vitamins which are natural scavengers of superoxide anions. Finally, part of NO released into the lumen is rapidly oxidised to nitrite and then to nitrate by oxygenated haemoglobin, molecular oxygen and superoxide anions and excreted as such in the urine [13].

NO synthesis and release is modulated by physical and humoral stimuli. The endothelial cells, because of their strategic anatomical position between the circulating blood and vascular smooth muscle, are exposed to continuous physical forces as shear stress, hydrostatic pressure and pulsatile stretch, particularly in the arterial circulation. Under resting conditions the interaction between endothelium and blood flow leads to mechanical endothelial changes and to subsequent NO release [14]. Moreover, it has been shown that changes in local flow also acutely increase NO release in vitro and contribute to flow-dependent vasodilatation in vivo [15]. The contribution of this basal NO release in peripheral vascular vasodilation was demonstrated by Vallance et al. [5]. These authors have shown that in healthy subjects intra-arterial brachial administration of L-NMMA (a specific eNOS inhibitor) significantly reduced (up to a total of 40-45% from the basal forearm blood flow) the forearm blood flow in dose-dependent manner. Importantly, because L-NMMA is devoid of intrinsic constrictor activity on vascular smooth muscle cell and does not affect other systems on the arterial wall, its vasoconstrictive action on the arterial wall is endothelium-dependent suggesting that basal or tonic NO release plays a dominant role in the maintenance of peripheral vascular tone. Similarly, it has been shown that systemic L-NMMA infusion in animals and humans induced hypertensive responses predominantly by increasing vascular resistances [16, 17]. These hypertensive responses, although reversible by L-arginine, are not entirely attributed to increased vascular resistance. Indeed, an additional sodium-retaining mechanism might also contribute [18]. In contrast, basal release of NO does not appear to control the resting tone of peripheral veins, although it may have an effect in central veins [19].

Several neurohormonal mediators can cause ‘stimulated’ NO release through activation of specific endothelial receptors. Many substances have been identified as pharmacological NO agonists and few of them have constituted the pharmacological basis of investigating the L-arginine-NO pathway. Muscarinic agents such as acetylcholine, methylcholine and autacoids such as bradykinin and histamine remain the most frequently employed exogenous substances in assessing agonist-evoked endothelium-dependent vasodilation. Similarly, endogenous substances such as circulating hormones (catecholamines, vasopressin) and other mediators released by activated platelets [serotonin, adenosine diphosphate (ADP)] are able to stimulate NO release albeit by different coupling proteins. The endothelium releases other endothelium-dependent vasodilating factors (EDRF) such as prostacyclin [20] and the elusive endothelium-dependent hyperpolarizing factor (EDHF). In contrast, the endothelium also releases endothelium-derived contracting factors (EDCF) such as the peptide endothelin (ET-

1), vasoconstrictor prostanoids (thromboxane A_2, prostaglandin H_2), superoxide anions and angiotensin II (Ang II). Finally, NO is known to be the mediator released in the peripheral nervous system by a complicated network of nerves, previously known as non-adrenergic and non-cholinergic [21, 22]. These nitrergic nerves are known to mediate vasodilation and regulation of blood supply to specific brain regions, by acting on the vascular smooth muscle cells [23]. However, their precise role and contribution in regulating blood pressure is not yet established [22].

Conceivably, the endothelium produces a host of substances clearly favouring those with endothelium-dependent vasodilating properties. The perennial release of NO from the endothelium also ensures additional antiatherogenic, antithrombotic and antiproliferative properties. In health, there is equilibrium between endothelial-derived vasodilating and endothelium-derived vasoconstricting substances favouring those with EDRF properties [24]. However, in several types of vascular disease, including hypertension, the endothelial cells become dysfunctional either structurally or functionally with a consequent impairment in evoking endothelium-dependent relaxations. This alteration is known as endothelial dysfunction and is mainly caused by either a reduction in release and/or increased inactivation and hence bioactivity of EDRF, although an additional excessive and unopposed release of EDCF's may also contribute.

2. Endothelial Dysfunction in Hypertension

The theory for development of hypertension from endothelial dysfunction is clear: we have already seen that dysfunctional endothelium is unable to dilate. We also know that there is a four-fold relationship between lumen diameter and flow. Taking this into consideration, it would be easy to assume that a dysfunctional endothelium would lead to an increase in blood pressure. However, the evidence for this is not entirely definitive; indeed, there is evidence to suggest that hypertension itself may cause hypertension.

Hypertension is a process characterised by elevated arterial blood pressure and its long-term sequelae on target organs leads to a considerably high cardiovascular mortality and morbidity [25]. The changes occurring during the hypertensive process on the wall of the resistant arteries are crucial determining and also perpetuating the hypertensive process itself. Indeed, in response to the increased arterial pressure the vessel structure is actively modified via a process known as vascular remodelling. This vascular process includes an active rearrangement of cellular and non-cellular elements involving elements both in intima and media layers (remodelling) around a smaller lumen [26]. In contrast, the process known as vascular hypertrophy, which involves VSMC proliferation, hypertrophy, and/or poliploidy, is thought to occur throughout the vessel [26, 27]. Therefore, this pressure-induced active restructuring of the arterial wall induces marked changes in luminal vascular dimensions, which along with alteration in endothelial cell shape and dimension results in elevated peripheral vascular resistance. Elevated peripheral vascular resistance, which is the hallmark of hypertension, is not an isolated phenomenon to be found only in macrocirculation but also in microcirculation [28]. Although, the mechanism by which this active remodelling is achieved is not completely understood, the endothelium might have a leading role.

Because of its strategic position within the vascular wall, the endothelium acts both as a 'sensor' detecting signals due to changes in haemo- and humoral factors, and also as a 'transducer' and 'mediator' of these signals. For example, in a condition where an increased flow is achieved (e.g. arterio-venous fistula), the luminal diameter of the artery is increased [29]. In contrast, in conditions with reduced blood flow the lumen diameter is decreased [30]. It is now well established that these vascular homeostatic functions are mediated by the endothelium and in particular via shear stress [31]. However, in hypertension shear stress is only minimally affected whilst in contrast circumferential stretch and/or tension are greatly increased [32]. This increased vascular wall tension promotes the release of vasoconstrictive agents such as EDCFs and PDGF as well as matrix modulators such as collagen [33, 34]. Hence, increased vascular wall stretch and tension will potentially promote vascular hypertrophy and/or formation of myoproliferative lesions, creating a vicious circle. Furthermore, endothelial cells regulate vascular tone, haemostasis, inflammation, cell growth, cell migration and interactions with the extracellular matrix through many receptor-mediated mechanisms. It is now well established that vascular growth factors interacting with specific receptors mediate part of the vascular remodelling in hypertension. In particular, structural changes such as VSMC hypertrophy are mediated partly by an increase of growth factors such as TGF-β1, but also by increased local activation of neurohormones as angiotensin II [35, 36]. In addition, increased matrix proteinases as collegenase and elastase are responsible for the lamellae fragmentation and their consequent replacement by collagen and elastin [37]. Similarly, it has been hypothesised that an increase of VSMC might also amplify the vasoconstrictive response to neurohormones thus further increasing systemic vascular resistance, hence blood pressure [38]. A part from structural changes, it is now accepted that an equal (if not superior) contribution to develop and maintain high peripheral vascular resistances in hypertension is given by functional arterial wall changes.

An impairment of NO bioactivity was initially confirmed in animal models of hypertension in the late 80's. These initial experiments were based on the observation of impaired vascular responses to pharmacological agonists of NO dependent vasodilatation in hypertensive animals [20, 39, 40]. Of particular interest in those initial animal studies was the fact that the degree of impairment of agonist-induced NO release was positively correlated to the level of arterial BP and antihypertensive treatment was able to improve these impaired vascular responses [41-44]. Furthermore, in spontaneous hypertensive rats (SHR) it was shown that the impairment in agonist (ACh) induced vasodilation was secondary to an imbalance between endothelium-dependent vasodilation and vasoconstrictors favouring the latter [45, 46].

In humans, the first demonstration of impaired endothelial dysfunction in hypertensive patients was first reported in the forearm resistance vessels in the early 90's by Panza et al. [47]. Since this first report a plethora of studies by independent researchers also confirmed the presence of endothelial dysfunction in primary and secondary hypertension and also in various vascular territories. Furthermore, it was also confirmed that the abnormality in endothelial-dependent vasodilation was not confined only to the muscarinic receptor level, since acetylcholine was principally deployed as pharmacological NO-agonist, but also extended to other NO evoked agonists [48]. Similarly, the basal NO release assessed by L-NMMA infusion was found also to be blunted in hypertensive patients [49, 50] compared to normotensive controls. In contrast, the endothelium-independent vasoconstricting and vasodilating vascular responses were found to be similar in hypertensive and control groups arguing against an intrinsic alteration of VSMC responsiveness in hypertension [50, 51]. Although, there is overwhelming evidence to suggest the presence of endothelial dysfunction in hypertension, this is not a universal finding. To date only two studies have argued the presence of endothelial dysfunction in hypertension [52, 53]. The discrepancies between those two studies and the rest cannot be clearly explained, suggesting a complex and intriguing mechanism of endothelial dysfunction in hypertension.

The dysfunction of the endothelium is not limited to a reduction in production in NO however. A process called oxidative stress also leads to increased consumption of NO and contributes to an increase in vascular tone. Normal healthy endothelial cells produce dangerous reactive oxygen species (free radicals). The production of these free radicals is normally balanced by their elimination; however, in endothelial dysfunction the production far outweighs their removal [54-56]. Nitric oxide (an anion), after synthesis, is rapidly inactivated by locally (of endothelial and extra-endothelial origin) generated oxygen-derived free radicals ($O^{-}2$) to form peroxynitrite anions ($OONO^{-}$), which have considerably less vasodilating capacity than NO [57, 58]. The chemical reaction between NO and superoxide anions is extremely fast, faster than that with superoxide dismutase (SODs) or with plasma vitamins which are natural scavengers of superoxide anions. An increase in free-radical formation otherwise known as oxidative stress is present in many cardiovascular diseases including hypertension, hyperlipidaemia and heart failure [59-62]. Interestingly, the severity of hypertension appears to correlate with the degree of underlying oxidative stress [63]. Antioxidants, whether endogenous or exogenous in origin are part of an additional scavenging mechanism directed to "overcome" the excess of superoxide anion production. Hypertension has been described as a disease characterised by an excess of oxygen free radicals coupled with an inefficient antioxidant mechanism [61, 64, 65]. There is evidence to suggest that hypertensive patients have significantly lower plasma concentrations of naturally occurring antioxidant factors (thiols, vitamins A, C, E) compared with matched normotensive volunteers [61, 65]. Also, free radical scavengers such as superoxide dismutase (SOD), and glutathione (GSH) are reported to be depressed in hypertensive patients [66, 67]. It appears however, that overall NO is of vital importance to the endothelial dysfunction in hypertension.

3. Clinical Implications of Endothelial Dysfunction in Hypertension

Since there is ample evidence to suggest that NO regulates vascular tone, researchers have focused their interest on the appealing hypothesis of endothelial dysfunction being the promoter of the hypertensive process. Similarly, because NO has vasodilatory and additional anti-atherogenic properties, decreased bioavailability of NO may contribute to the increased peripheral vascular resistance and also provide a link between hypertension and its most important complication, the development of atherosclerosis. This hypothesis was further reinforced by the discovery that systemic administration of the L-arginine analogue L-NMMA induced sustained hypertension both in human and animal models [17], primarily by modulating vascular resistance. Although, it is yet unclear whether endothelial dysfunction is a cause or a consequence of hypertension, there are some intriguing associations between impaired NO bioactivity and hypertension.

The findings of the Framingham study have suggested that hypertensive patients had a twice fold increased risk of cardiovascular death to that of the non-hypertensive population. Since endothelial dysfunction is present before any structural irregularities in the arterial wall [68] it is conceivable that this represents the first vascular target organ damage en route to developing atherosclerosis. Furthermore, the confirmation that endothelial dysfunction was ubiquitous in diverse vascular territories in patients with hypertension led to intriguing speculation on the strong association between hypertension and cardiovascular morbidity and mortality. Brush et al. [69] first showed that hypertensive patients with angina pectoris had a significant reduction in maximal coronary vasodilation (coronary reserve) to pharmacological agents and also myocardial ischaemia without any evidence of atherosclerosis or left ventricular hypertrophy. Therefore, in those patients the 'classical' aetiology of ischaemia by obstructive and/or extrinsic vascular compression of the epicardial arteries by the hypertrophied myocardium was debated. Similarly, Treasure et al. [70] later observed that whilst in normal (morphologically smooth) epicardial coronary arteries the muscarinic agonist acetylcholine (ACh) caused NO release and thus vasodilatation; in subjects with hypertension the same agent caused paradoxical vasoconstriction. Brush et al. [69] also observed a similar 'paradoxical' vasoconstrictive intracoronary response to ACh in hypertensive patients without left ventricular hypertrophy. Importantly, the vascular vasodilatory response to nitroglycerine (a NO donor) in both studies was not different between normotensive and hypertensive group of patients. Treasure et al. showed that the presence of left ventricular hypertrophy in hypertensive patients was strongly associated with coronary endothelial dysfunction and Egashira et al. [71, 72] showed that this abnormal (vasoconstrictive) epicardial response was not limited to the muscarinic agonists but also included substance P. Hence, we can speculate that the presence of impaired endothelial dysfunction at the coronary level in hypertensive patients, even in those without any significant obstructive disease, critically limits the coronary reserve therefore creating a potential source for ischaemia, especially in situations where high metabolic demand is required. Furthermore, the presence of endothelial dysfunction at the coronary level might also explain the discrepancy between angiographically normal coronary arteries and occurrence of cardiac chest pain [73] and/or acute coronary syndromes seen in hypertensive and normotensive patients with cardiovascular risk factors [74].

Ghiadoni et al. [75] have shown that the presence and degree of agonist-evoked endothelium-dependent vasodilation in hypertensives was highly (inversely) correlated to common carotid artery intima-to-media wall ratio. Intima to media wall ratio is a good surrogate marker of atherosclerosis [76] and also correlates (though weakly) to concomitant coronary atherosclerosis [77].

Left ventricular hypertrophy (LVH) is a cardinal manifestation of preclinical cardiovascular disease [78] that strongly predicts future myocardial infarction, stroke, and cardiovascular death in patients with hypertension [79] and also in members of the general population [25, 80]. It has been shown that the risk of death or non-fatal implications, particularly ischaemic vascular events, is increased by to two- to fourfold in the presence of LV hypertrophy, independently of age, gender and other risk factors. Interestingly, although the prognostic significance of hypertensive left ventricular hypertrophy is well established, the mechanism of the adverse association between high LV mass and vascular events has not been well established. The evidence that LVH is associated with an increased systemic arterial wall thickness [81, 82] and more pronounced systemic atherosclerosis [83] has led to the speculation that those changes are also affecting the coronary microcirculation hence limiting coronary reserve. Perticone et al. [84] showed that acetylcholine-evoked endothelium-dependent vasodilation in the forearm microcirculation of never-treated hypertensive patients with echocardiographic left ventricular hypertrophy was inversely related to LV mass and was significantly blunted as compared to normotensive volunteers. Similar results were also obtained by Millgard et al. [85] suggesting a probably significant contribution of endothelial dysfunction in determining LVH, which leads to increased cardiovascular risk.

There is evidence suggesting a significant correlation between the degree of endothelial dysfunction and the severity of high blood pressure in hypertensive patients. Von zur Muhlen *et al* [86] investigated the relationship between ambulatory blood pressure and endothelium-dependent vasodilation in 25 untreated hypertensives. They showed that both 24-hr ambulatory blood pressure and office BP related inversely to the degree of endothelial-dependent vasodilation whilst there was no correlation with endothelium-independent vascular responses. Forte et al. [87] found a strong inverse correlation between mean arterial blood pressure and urinary nitrite and nitrate (index of NO synthesis) in hypertensive patients. Conversely, two independent studies conducted in the normal population found that age, cholesterol, BMI but not BP were significantly related to endothelium-dependent vasodilation [88, 89].

Evidence has now begun to appear confirming the adverse prognostic value of endothelial dysfunction. In several recent studies, the presence of endothelial dysfunction strongly predicted future cardiac outcome [90-92]. The study by Halcox et al. looked at coronary endothelial dysfunction in 308 patients and found that endothelial dysfunction was in fact more predictive of future coronary adverse events than the apparent angiographic severity of any lesion seen. Further studies have also demonstrated the prognostic significance of brachial artery endothelial dysfunction in predicting cardiovascular mortality [93, 94]. These results were mirrored by Yeboah et al. [95] examined FMD in 2792 older patients (age 72-98 years). The authors found that event-free survival was significantly higher in patients with an FMD higher than the median compared to those lower than the median. Again, endothelial dysfunction was an independent predictor of future cardiovascular events. Interestingly, there have also be a couple of studies looking at endothelial dysfunction in patients with risk factors for coronary disease but no prior diagnosis. A study conducted by Perticone et al. [96] examined 225 patients with untreated hypertension looking at brachial artery endothelial function and followed up for cardiovascular events. Endothelial function was measured by looking at arterial response (by forearm blood flow) to acetylcholine infusion. The authors found that the only independent predictors of future cardiovascular events were mean 24-hour blood pressure and endothelial dysfunction as measured by forearm blood flow response. Modena et al. [97] examined 400 women with hypertension and impaired FMD and gave them 6 months of anti-hypertensive therapy. In the group in which there was no change in endothelial dysfunction there were over twice as many adverse cardiovascular events compared to those in who FMD improved, a statistically significant difference. Finally, Anderson et al. [98] in the long-term follow up of the FATE study found that hyperemic velocity was a significant predictor of future cardiovascular events. Hyperemic velocity is a novel measure of blood flow velocity at hyperemia during an FMD examination and has been suggested to be more predictive or future cardiovascular adverse events than FMD alone [99].

It is conceivable that endothelial dysfunction represents a common pathway to all cardiovascular disease whereby, independently of the cause, this leads to atherosclerosis – this hypothesis is being increasingly backed up by the evidence.

4. Reversal of Endothelial Function in Human Hypertension

4.1. Strategies for Improving Endothelial Dysfunction in Hypertension

As we have discussed earlier in the chapter, a functionally and structurally intact endothelium has anti-atherogenic, anti-atherosclerotic and anti-proliferative properties. Thus, in theory an improvement of endothelial dysfunction would further improve cardiac prognosis in hypertensive patients making it an attractive therapeutic target. Hypertension is of course not just about reducing the raw blood pressure figures, but its management should include multiple risk factors intervention, and endothelial dysfunction should also probably be considered as a modifiable risk factor. There is clear evidence suggesting that reducing blood pressure in hypertension is much less effective in lowering coronary events than in lowering cerebral events [100]. This might be because drug treatment that reduces blood pressure might have no impact on the underlying endothelial dysfunction. In other words, although most hypertensives have endothelial dysfunction, most therapies that reduce blood pressure may not improve endothelial dysfunction meaning that, endothelial dysfunction may persist despite adequate control of clinic blood pressure. Because endothelial dysfunction precedes atherosclerosis, ensuring its reversal may well reduce the "coronary shortfall" and hence be a crucial missing link between hypertension and cardiovascular mortality. In this chapter we explore whether this could be true. Firstly, we will discuss non-pharmacological methods to improve endothelial dysfunction.

4.2. Exercise

Exercise is recognised as an effective non-pharmacological measure that reduces BP [101-103]. Regular (at least 3 times/week) aerobic exercise of moderate intensity reduces blood pressure by an average of 4/3mmHg. Exercise is recommended as an integral part of the international guidelines in primary and secondary prevention of hypertension [104]. Kokkinos et al. [102] have previously shown that moderately intense aerobic exercise reduced significantly both systolic (average 7mmHg) and diastolic BP (average 5mmHg) in Afro-Caribbean patients with severe hypertension. In the same study, regression in left ventricular hypertrophy was also achieved. Since basal NO release is facilitated by constant shear stress, it has been postulated that regular exercise increases laminar flow and increases shear stress and hence NO release [105]. The beneficial effects of exercise on endothelial function in hypertensive patients have been confirmed by Higashi *et al* [106]. This group showed that 12 weeks of aerobic exercise, such as walking for 30min, 5 to 7 times per week, improved stimulated (acetylcholine-induced) NO release in previously untreated hypertensives. Interestingly, along with a significant reduction in blood pressure (7/4mmHg), there was also an associated significant reduction in LDL with an increase in HDL. A reduction in circulating LDL might act as a co-factor in improving both endothelial function and reducing BP. Total and LDL cholesterol have been correlated inversely with NO bioactivity both in healthy and in hypertensive subjects [88, 107]. This relationship is probably related to oxidized LDL and its ability to interfere with both NO formation and its inactivation [108, 109].

The results of Hambrecht et al. [110] on the effect of exercise on the coronary vasculature are of particular note. This group showed that regular and programmed exercise improved stimulated NO release (acetylcholine-induced) in patients with established coronary artery disease. This suggests that a simple and moderate exercise program could potentially modify the coronary artery disease process. Indeed, this hypothesis has been recently tested and proven to be correct by Cornelissen et al. [111] who studied endothelial function in 146 patients with stable coronary artery disease who were enrolled in a cardiac rehabilitation program. After twelve weeks there was a mean increase in FMD of 37% (although interestingly there was no improvement in reactive hyperemia index as measured by applanation tonometry). Beyond the effective of exercise on NO, several studies have also suggested an anti-inflammatory effect, reducing the numbers of circulating pro-inflammatory cytokines and CRP. CRP has been shown to have some atherosclerotic properties [112] and elevated levels are a predictor for adverse cardiovascular events [113]. Milani et al. [114] found that an extended cardiopulmonary exercise programme ("cardiac rehabilitation") caused a significant drop in high-sensitivity CRP (42% compared to control). A further study by Vona et al. [115] found that 4 weeks aerobic training provided improvement in endothelial function, either on its own or combined with resistance training. Interestingly, after 1 month of detraining the effect was lost, suggesting that exercise must be continued to have persistent benefit.

There is increasing evidence to suggest that exercise improves markers of endothelial dysfunction. The methods by which it does this are not yet fully understood however, and this remains an interesting area for further research.

4.3. Other Cardiovascular Risk Factors Associated with Hypertension

Endothelial dysfunction in hypertension is worsened by coincidental risk factors with known pro-atherogenic potential such age, total and LDL cholesterol, cigarette smoking, and gender [71, 88, 107, 116]. Taddei et al. [107, 117] found that ageing was associated with progressively impaired NO bioactivity, and in hypertensives, endothelial dysfunction was accelerated with ageing. This group also reported a bimodal relationship between ageing and endothelial dysfunction. In the younger age group (18-30 years) the mechanism of endothelial dysfunction appeared to be related to a relative deficiency of L-arginine (substrate of NO) whereas in later life (>45 years) a cyclooxygenase-dependent mechanism was more apparent. Al-Shaer et al. [118] obtained similar results comparing patients over 60 with atherosclerosis to those over 60 without and young healthy controls using venous occlusion plethysmography. The authors found that there was a significantly higher response in forearm blood flow in the younger group compared to both elderly groups. The group of elderly patients without atherosclerosis were free of all other cardiovascular risk factors, suggesting that age in itself plays a part in endothelial dysfunction. While the process behind which ageing causes endothelial dysfunction is not entirely understood, there is an increasing belief that it is caused by a combination of oxidative stress, reactive oxygen species and an increase in inflammatory cytokines [119]. Furthermore, the endothelium is naturally always in a state of repair and regeneration. As we age, mutations accumulate during the process of mitosis, leading to a slowing of this process. Eventually, the cells become senescent i.e. unable to divide and repair themselves anymore, again contributing to endothelial dysfunction [120]. This of course can be exacerbated by other factors.

Hyperlipidaemia is associated with increased oxidative stress, which adversely affects endothelial NO release [121, 122]. Apart from chronically elevated cholesterol, even a single high-fat meal also transiently impairs stimulated NO release, an effect that can last for up to 6 hours post-prandially [123]. More importantly it has recently been shown that even subjects with normal to high cholesterol levels have endothelial dysfunction [124]. Muiesan et al. [125] looked at the effects of "generic" blood pressure lowering treatment in patients with hypertension and a total cholesterol of >6 mmol/L (mean 6.33). They found that with adequate BP control, irrespective of type of drugs used, forearm reactive hyperaemia was improved after 12 months of treatment. More specifically, Okumura et al. [126] have recently found that small low-density lipoprotein (LDL) cholesterol was an independent predictor of endothelial dysfunction in 120 men. Conversely, low levels of high-density lipoprotein (HDL) cholesterol have been shown to be predictive of adverse cardiovascular risk [127] even if LDL levels are low [128]. Administration of reconstituted HDL cholesterol has been shown to improve endothelial function in several studies [129-131]. This effect has also been reproduced in diabetic patients with natural HDL ([132]). Furthermore, Sorrentino et al. also gave the patients in their study niacin, which incrementally increased the beneficial effects of HDL cholesterol.

Cigarette smoking, whether active or passive causes oxidative stress which is associated with impaired NO release [133-135]. Additionally, smoking also causes a pro-inflammatory state with an increase in leukocytes and inflammatory cytokines, adding to endothelial dysfunction [136, 137]. Gender and race also have important impact on functional integrity of the endothelium [138, 139]. There is the general tendency to exclude pre-menopausal women from vascular endothelial function studies because of the confounding effects of oestrogens on the endothelium pre-menopause [140-142]. Virdis et al. [143] compared the vascular effects of acetylcholine, L-NMMA and vitamin C in healthy women with leiomyoma pre- and post oophorectomy. They found that acute endogenous oestrogen deprivation (oophorectomy) was associated with endothelial dysfunction via a reduction in NO availability and this was restored by oestrogen replacement therapy.

The above-described factors are all capable of initiating and promoting endothelial dysfunction on their own, but their combined vascular effects with high blood pressure have not being investigated. In current management guidelines, patients with coronary artery disease are being treated with a more holistic approach, which address all the concomitant risk factors. This will hopefully lead to improved coronary artery endothelial function. As discussed earlier, there are now long-term data to suggest that endothelial dysfunction of the coronary arteries can predict outcome [90].

4.4. Anti-hypertensive Treatment

Whether endothelial dysfunction is a cause or a consequence of hypertension has long been debated. The evidence that impaired NO bioactivity pre-exists in the normotensive offspring of hypertensive patients, 20-30% of who will later develop hypertension, points towards the probable primary nature of this phenomenon [144-146]. If, however, endothelial dysfunction were the consequence of the hypertensive process then one would expect normalisation of BP should reverse this abnormality, however, this is clearly not the case. Panza et al. [147] showed that adequate BP control with antihypertensive treatment (mainly with beta-blockers/diuretics) did not affect NO bioactivity in the forearm resistance circulation of patients with hypertension. The failure of "first-line" drugs to improve endothelial function supports the notion that endothelial dysfunction is the cause rather than the consequence of hypertension. Alternatively, Millgård and Lind [148] showed that blood pressure rise in itself can impair the endothelial function in that noradrenaline infusion caused both blood pressure rise and impaired stimulated NO release in forearm vasculature of healthy normotensive volunteers. Although the impairment in NO release observed in their study could have been the consequence of complex interaction between norepinephrine and the endothelium rather a pure rise in BP, Paniagua et al. [149] have recently addressed this issue. They obtained similar results on stimulated NO release of small resistance vessels (subcutaneous) in normotensive humans after transient elevation of intravascular hydrostatic pressure. Furthermore, at least in secondary hypertension, removal of the underlying cause (aldosterone-producing adenomas) reverses endothelial dysfunction and also normalises blood pressure [150]. Hence the interaction between endothelial dysfunction and blood pressure might be more complex than simply saying that one must cause the other. In support of this hypothesis, Panza speculated that there are some hypertensive patients where endothelial dysfunction precedes high blood pressure. It could well be that endothelial dysfunction is both a cause and a consequence of hypertension i.e. a vicious circle might exist between endothelial dysfunction and elevated blood pressure.

4.4.1. Beta-blockers and Diuretics

Beta-blockers and thiazide diuretics are commonly prescribed therapies for hypertension. Despite their proven efficacy in improving overall prognosis in hypertension, they appear not to affect the NO-L-arginine pathway [125, 151-153]. One exception is nebivolol, a highly selective β1-blocker that has been shown to improve endothelial dysfunction both in vivo and vitro [154, 155]. Dawes et al. [156] reported that acute intra-arterial administration of nebivolol improved forearm vasculature NO bioactivity in hypertensive patients. Although the mechanism by which nebivolol improves endothelial dysfunction in hypertension is not yet fully elucidated a putative pharmacological cross-reactivity between serotonin and β-receptors might potentially explain these vascular effects [157]. Kakoki et al. [158] showed that 5-HT1 blockade with a specific antagonist almost abolished the vasodilatory response to nebivolol in the rat kidney preparation, suggesting some receptor mediated interaction. Also, a possible antioxidant property of nebivolol has been suggested as an additional factor increasing NO-bioactivity or even a reduction in endothelin (ET-1) release [159, 160]. The beneficial effects of nebivolol on the endothelium were confirmed in humans by Tzemos et al. [161]. In a double-blind crossover trial, 12 hypertensive patients were given 8 weeks of treatment with bendroflumethiazide plus atenolol or nebivolol (and then switched to the other group). With both treatments the blood pressure reduction was the same, however there was a significant increase in both forearm vasodilatory response to acetylcholine and the vasoconstrictor response to L-NMMA, suggesting that there may be a beneficial effect of nebivolol beyond a simple blood pressure reduction. The endothelial effects of nebivolol are unique amongst beta-blockers. For example, carvedilol, which is recommended in heart failure, does not mediate its beneficial effects in that condition by any improvement in endothelial function [162]. Indeed, the tide has recently turned against beta-blockers as first line treatment for hypertension due to poorer outcomes compared with other blood-pressure lowering medications [163-165]. Given the similar anti-hypertensive effects of nebivolol compared with atenolol however [161, 166], it is certainly of interest to investigate outcomes with nebivolol to see if there is an incremental benefit over and above other beta-blockers.

Recently, Sorrentino et al. [167] conducted a study in mice with iatrogenic extensive anterior myocardial infarctions and were randomised to nebivolol, metoprolol or placebo. Although infarct size and heart rate was the same in both groups, left ventricular ejection fraction was significantly higher at 4 weeks in the nebivolol group (32% vs. 17% vs. 19%; $p < 0.05$) and survival was higher in the nebivolol group compared to the placebo group. Furthermore, there was a decrease in left ventricular adverse remodelling in the nebivolol group compared to metoprolol as judged by a more pronounced inhibition of myocyte hypertrophy. The authors felt that this may have been mediated by inhibition of cardiac NADPH oxidase by nebivolol (but not metoprolol), which had also been seen in mouse studies by Doerries and Looi [168, 169]. Nebivolol seems to have beneficial effects on smooth muscle cell proliferation, gene expression and oxidative stress [170, 171].

It seems that there is increasing evidence to support the theory that nebivolol has additional beneficial effects on the endothelium above its anti-hypertensive action. More work needs to be done in this area to ascertain whether these actions are translated to a longer-term prognostic benefit.

4.4.2. Potassium and Spironolactone

Potassium plays an important part in preserving the functional adequacy of the L-arginine-NO pathway. Taddei et al. [172, 173] showed that intra-arterial administration of potassium chloride (KCL) significantly improved stimulated NO release in the forearm vasculature of hypertensive patients. Interestingly, there was no significant effect of KCL on agonist-evoked endothelial dependent vasodilation in the control normotensive group, suggesting an intriguing rule of potassium in NO bioactivity preservation in hypertension. The beneficial effect of potassium in hypertension has previously been highlighted; an analysis of the Syst-EUR trial has shown that hypokalaemia (<3.4mml/L) was associated with a higher incidence of cardiovascular events despite good BP control. Conversely, a high potassium diet appears to prevent deaths due to vascular strokes in hypertensive men, a disease also associated with endothelial dysfunction [174].

Spironolactone, a potassium-sparing diuretic with mineralocorticoid receptor antagonist has received much attention recently. It has been reported to improve NO bioactivity in patients with heart failure [175], consistent with the results of the RALES study in which the use of spironolactone reduced cardiac mortality by a third in subjects with grade III-IV heart failure [176]. The mechanism(s) by which aldosterone impairs endothelial function is unclear. Aldosterone it is known to enhance vascular responsiveness to pressor agents such as norepinephrine and angiotensin II even before the systemic blood pressure begins to increase

[177]. Also, aldosterone can cause direct vascular smooth muscle contraction via a non-genomic pathway that has not yet been characterised. In patients with secondary hypertension due to aldosterone producing adrenal adenomas, surgical excision of these tumours removed the excess circulating aldosterone resulting in a normalised acetylcholine vascular response, i.e. improved endothelial function and BP control [172].

Chronic treatment with aldosterone in rats has been shown to cause impairment of acetylcholine-induced relaxation and increased COX-2 expression in the endothelium of the thoracic aorta in rats [178], perhaps suggesting a mechanism for endothelial dysfunction caused by aldosterone. An interesting study by Garnier et al. [179] examined 62 mice that were genetically modified to over-express aldosterone synthase (and thus over-produce aldosterone) and compared this group to normal mice. The authors found that although there was no difference in myocardial structure or cardiac function by echocardiography, there was a 55% decrease in basal coronary blood flow and vasodilatation to acetylcholine, bradykinin and sodium nitroprusside. Intriguingly, this suggests that there could be both NO-dependent and NO-independent mechanisms by which aldosterone mediates endothelial dysfunction. Given these findings, in theory, spironolactone or eplerenone should improve endothelial dysfunction in hypertensives where excess aldosterone is a factor and evidence has recently been obtained to suggest this.

Kobayashi et al. [180] showed that eplerenone increased eNOS production and reduced oxidative stress and superoxide production in salt-sensitive rats with heart failure. A further study in salt sensitive rats found that the combination of eplerenone and amlodipine enhanced the improvement of vascular endothelial function, cardiac inflammation, fibrosis and diastolic dysfunction compared to that caused by amlodipine alone [181]. The improvement in endothelial function caused by eplerenone has also recently been found in humans [182]. Savoia et al. [183] conducted a randomised controlled trial compared eplerenone to atenolol in 16 patients for 1 year and concluded that eplerenone treatment was associated with reduced arterial stiffness, decreased collagen/elastin ratio, and a reduction in circulating inflammatory mediators. The effects of eplerenone appear to be additive – as well as the combination with amlodipine described earlier, Imanishi et al. [184] found a increased improvement in endothelial function using the combination of enalapril and aldosterone in rabbits.

The recent ESC guidelines for the management of heart failure [185] now place eplerenone and spironolactone as first line therapies – perhaps it is speculation, but the beneficial effects that have been noted in this group may be, at least in part, related to their beneficial effect on endothelial function.

4.4.3. Calcium Channel Blockers

Calcium channel blockers (CCBs) also have outcome data to support their use in hypertension. Two important studies, the NORDIL and INSIGHT trials have shown that diltiazem and long-acting nifedipine (GITS) respectively were as effective as thiazide diuretics in reducing cardiovascular mortality and morbidity in essential hypertension [186-188]. Calcium channel blockers have similarly been shown to have a beneficial effect on nitric oxide bioactivity in coronary, forearm and resistance (subcutaneous) vascular beds. In the forearm microcirculation, Lyons et al. [188] have reported that 6-weeks treatment with amlodipine improved the vasoconstrictive response to L-NMMA (an inhibitor of eNOS) or basal NO release in newly diagnosed hypertensives. In a later study, Perticone et al. [189] showed that oral isradipine also improved both stimulated (ACh-induced) and basal (L-

NMMA induced) NO release in hypertension. However, Taddei et al. demonstrated contrasting effects on the endothelium with acute and chronic administration of a highly lipophilic calcium channel blocker, lacidipine [190]. This group showed that intra-arterial lacidipine did not significantly affect NO bioactivity, but chronic (2 and 8 months) oral treatment with this agent significantly improved stimulated NO release. Interestingly, the improved NO bioactivity persisted after 2-weeks of drug withdrawal, despite returning to hypertensive state. This suggests that BP control in itself may not be sufficient to improve NO release. In the majority of cases, hypertension is treated with combination therapy. Recently, a study by Yamamoto et al. [191] found that azelnidpine in combination with olmesartan had improved endothelial function to a greater extent than olmesartan and hydrochlorothiazide.

Similar beneficial effects of calcium channel blockers on NO bioactivity have also been observed in smaller resistance vessels. The technique required for assessing endothelial function in these vessels involves gluteal subcutaneous tissue biopsy and myography. Schiffrin et al. [192] have observed an improvement in acetylcholine (stimulated NO) response and vascular remodelling in these resistance vessels in hypertensives treated for 1 year with long acting nifedipine.

Of course, reversing endothelial dysfunction in the coronary arteries would be more relevant in hypertension if an improved cardiac outcome were the goal. Freielingsdolf et al. [193] have shown that acute intracoronary administration of either nicardipine or diltiazem in hypertensives reversed endothelial dysfunction in both stenotic and non-stenotic epicardial coronary arteries. Of note, there was no significant effect on the endothelium (NO pathway) of these compounds in normal control subjects. The largest clinical trials looking at CCBs and endothelial function were the ENCORE studies [194, 195]. ENCORE I examined 343 patients undergoing percutaneous coronary intervention and randomised patients to patients were randomized in a double-blind manner to placebo, cerivastatin, nifedipine, or combination therapy for 6 months. In this study the authors demonstrated that nifedipine improved endothelial function at 6 months. In ENCORE II the authors were able to demonstrate that a controlled release preparation of nifedipine was able to improve endothelial function at 2 years.

Calcium channel blockers act directly on voltage dependent L-type calcium channels found on the vascular smooth muscle cells. Blockade of these channels reduces the influx of extracellular calcium into the sarcoplasmic reticulum facilitating vascular smooth muscle cell relaxation. However, endothelial cells are devoid of these receptors for calcium channel blockers to act on. Hence, the mechanism by which calcium channel blockers improve endothelial NO bioavailability is unclear. However, in the coronary microcirculation the addition of a calcium channel blocker appears to indirectly facilitate an increase in intracellular smooth muscle cell cGMP, which is the second messenger of NO and mediates its vasodilation. Therefore, as expected an increase in intracellular cGMP with calcium channel blockers enhances both endothelium dependent and independent vasodilation [193, 196]. This has been confirmed with both dihydropyridine and non-dihydropyridine calcium channel blockers. In contrast, in the forearm microcirculation, calcium channel blockers do not appear to influence the NO-independent pathway whenever exogenous organic sources of NO such as nitrates are present. Two additional mechanisms have been described to explain the effects of calcium channel blocker in the forearm circulation, which might be relevant to the coronary vasculature. The first explanation is that most calcium channel blockers have antioxidant activities [197, 198]. This reduces superoxide anions, which normally inactivate released NO hence reducing NO bioactivity. The second explanation involves a reduction in endothelin release by calcium channel blockers. Endothelin is a potent vasoconstrictor and it is released from the endothelium [199]. Normally, there is a balance between vasoconstrictive and vasodilating substances in the vasculature but in hypertension, the bioavailability of endothelin might be increased in parallel with a reduction in NO bioactivity. Kiowski et al. [200, 201] have shown that calcium channel blockers contributed to improved NO bioactivity by reducing endothelin release. In addition, Cardillo et al. [202] have recently shown that in patients with essential hypertension, the increased endothelin activity is partly responsible for the increased vascular tone [203]. Hence, in a model where vasoconstrictive activity is increased, such as hypertension, a reduction of endothelin release would improve NO bioactivity. Recently, another theory has also been postulated, that CCBs may reduce tissue plasminogen activator activity, thus reducing thrombogenic risk by decreasing platelet activation [204].

4.4.4. Angiotensin Converting Enzyme Inhibitors (ACE-I) and Angiotensin type 2 Receptor Blockers (ARBs)

Since the landmark study on renovascular hypertension by Goldblatt [205], it has been clear that the renin-angiotensin-aldosterone system (RAAS) plays an important role in BP regulation (figure 3). Angiotensin II stimulates angiotensin type 1 receptors (AT1) to mediate arteriolar vasoconstriction and remodelling, superoxide anion production, renal sodium reabsorption, aldosterone secretion and endothelin (ET-1) release [206]. Many of these actions affect the vascular endothelium adversely. On the other hand stimulation of the angiotensin type 2 (AT2) receptor by angiotensin has mainly opposing actions to those of AT1 stimulation and recently has been shown to contribute to endothelial NO release [207]. Hence, AT1 receptor blockade should eventually improve NO bioactivity.

AT2 production can be reduced by angiotensin converting enzyme inhibitors which also increase both tissue and plasma bradykinin by inhibiting kininase II [208]. By stimulating the B2 receptors, bradykinin mediates the release of NO, prostacyclin and the putative endothelial hyperpolarizing factor (EDHF); agents that produce vasodilation [209-211]. Two large studies have investigated the effects of ACE-I and ARBs in the coronary and forearm vasculature (TREND, BANFF) respectively in patients with atherosclerosis [212, 213]. The TREND study showed that quinapril reversed epicardial coronary artery endothelial dysfunction in patients with coronary artery disease. The BANFF study showed an improvement of endothelial dysfunction with quinapril, using reactive hyperaemia, in the forearm vasculature of patients with atherosclerosis. However, such a favourable effect of ACE-I on endothelial dysfunction is less consistent in hypertensives. Two independent long-term studies evaluating respectively the vascular responses to cilazapril and lisinopril on subcutaneous arteries (small resistance vessels) in essential hypertensives showed a considerable improvement in stimulated NO release following prolonged treatment with these agents [214, 215]. Similar results were obtained in the coronary microcirculation of hypertensive patients with ACE-I [216]. Antony et al. showed that intravenous perindoprilat (the active metabolite of perindopril) restored the cold pressure test response and flow-mediated coronary artery vasodilation in 10 patients with untreated (newly diagnosed) essential hypertension.

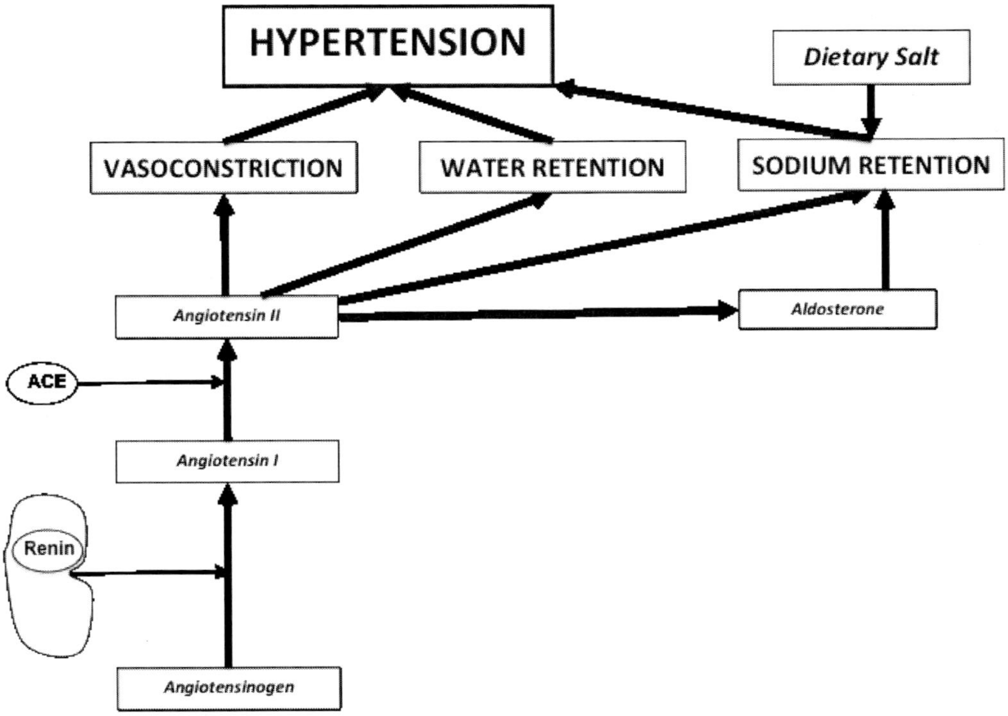

Figure 3. The renin-angiotensin-aldosterone system.

Taddei et al. [217] have reported that 1 year of treatment with lisinopril improved endothelium-dependent and independent vasodilatation in forearm vasculature of hypertensives. However, Kiowski et al. [218] failed to find any improvement on NO bioactivity in the forearm vasculature after 5 months of oral cilazapril treatment despite adequate BP control in a group of hypertensives. Similarly, Creager et al. [219] failed to improve NO bioactivity with 8 weeks treatment with either oral captopril or enalapril. However, two independent studies have shown an improvement of stimulated NO release following a single oral dose of captopril in such patients [220, 221]. Lyons et al. [188] have investigated the effects of ACE-I on basal NO release in hypertensives. They showed that 6 weeks treatment with enalapril improved, but did not normalise, basal NO release in previously untreated hypertensives. Finally, in a large study involving 296 hypertensive patients, Higashi et al. [153] using the technique of forearm reactive hyperaemia (flow-induced NO release) compared the endothelial vascular effects of calcium channel blockers, ACE-I, beta-blockers, and diuretics. They reported that only treatment with ACE-I significantly enhanced the forearm blood flow (an index of endothelium-dependent vasodilation) during reactive hyperaemia whilst the other drug classes had no significant effect although they did equally reduce blood pressure.

There are also reports of the beneficial effects of ARBs on the endothelial function. Schiffrin et al. [152] reported that 1 of year treatment with losartan improved both functional and structural properties of small resistance (subcutaneous) arteries in hypertensive patients. Prasad et al. [222] found the same in patients with atherosclerosis. In contrast, Ghiadoni et al. [223] found that 1 year of treatment with candesartan improved stimulated NO release, but this was accompanied by a concomitant endothelium-independent improvement suggesting an alteration in vascular smooth muscle cell responsiveness. Tzemos et al. [224] also found that valsartan mediated an improvement in endothelial function through both NO-dependent and independent pathways. Interestingly, amlodipine had no effect on nitric oxide. This was similar to the findings of Hirooka et al. in large arteries [225].

In summary, blocking the renin-angiotensin-aldosterone system either at the conversion from Ang I to II or at the Ang II receptor level may favourably affect the NO bioactivity. It is likely that in the forearm microcirculation the tissue renin-angiotensin system is the predominant generator of Ang II hence only ACE-I with high tissue penetration (enough to block the tissue renin-angiotensin system) are likely to be effective [212, 226]. The two large studies, BANFF and TREND, might have obtained positive results because they involved quinalapril, a highly lipophilic ACE-I and this might explain the results. In a sub-analysis of the recent EUROPA study (examining the beneficial effects of ACE-inhibition in patients with stable coronary artery disease), perindopril appeared to increase expression and activity of eNOS by 19% and 27% respectively, as well as a significant reduction in plasma levels of angiotensin II, tumour necrosis factor-α and an increase in bradykinin, nitrate and nitrite [227].

All in all, although there are varying results in studies of ACEIs and ARBs, however the weight of evidence would tend to come down in favour of their beneficial effects. A recent meta-analysis by Miyamoto et al. [228] found 38 studies looking at FMD with these two classes of drugs, and in the majority there was an improvement in endothelial function caused by ACEIs and ARBs. Recent studies have looked at the effects of angiotensin blockade in other subgroups, for example a study by Terashima et al. [229] who found that telmisartan improved coronary endothelial function more than amlodipine in patients with drug eluting stents as measured by response to intracoronary infusion of acetylcholine.

Interestingly, a recent animal study [230] looked at the effects of aliskiren, a direct rennin inhibitor (the initial pathway of the renin-angiotensin-aldosterone axis). In this study, the authors found that aliskiren improved endothelial dysfunction in rat aortas and decreased oxidative stress. The effect of aliskiren was studied in humans by Virdis [231] in a comparative study against ramipril. Aliskiren produced a significantly greater reduction in augmentation index and improved the vasodilatory response to acetylcholine, however blood pressure and pulse wave reduction was the same in both groups. Meanwhile, Cherney et al. suggest that direct renin inhibition using aliskiren might also provide better results than ACE inhibitors in type 2 diabetics [232]. These results may point to a slightly different action of aliskiren, and provide interesting directions for further research.

4.4.5. Endothelin Antagonists

Endothelin 1 (ET-1) acting through the ETA receptor is a potent vasoconstrictor that also promotes vascular smooth muscle cell proliferation [233, 234]. Its gene expression in the vessel wall is promoted by ATII, and its vasoconstrictive effect appears to be enhanced in hypertensives. It may thus play a role in the pathogenesis of hypertension [202, 235, 236]. However, the plasma levels of ET-1 have not been consistently found to be raised in hypertension [237, 238]. Nonetheless, ET-1 is released abluminally rather luminally, hence its plasma levels may not necessarily reflect its activity [239]. Increased ET-1 activity has been found in salt-sensitive hypertension [240, 241]. In animal models of hypertension ET-1 blockade significantly reduces BP and prevents the development of target organ damage [151]. In human hypertension, Cardillo et al. have shown that forearm intrabrachial administration of both selective and non-selective endothelin receptor blockers improved endothelium-dependent vasodilation. The vasodilating properties of endothelin-1 receptor blockers might explain the beneficial effects on BP of bosentan, a non-selective ET-1 receptor blocker. Krum et al. [242] have shown that 4 weeks of treatment with bosentan reduced blood pressure as effectively as enalapril. Moreover, the favourable effect of treatment with bosentan on blood pressure occurred without reflexive neurohormonal activation, which may suggest a more targeted effect of this drug on endothelial ET-1. Coronary endothelial function has also been shown to be improved by atrasentan [243]. A synergistic effect with phosphodiesterase type 5 inhibitors has also been recently found in rats [244].

A recent study has investigated the effects of relaxin on aortic stiffness in rats. Relaxin is a member of the insulin superfamily and has effects on NO production. It also acts as an endothelin receptor antagonist [245, 246]. Acetylcholine mediated endothelial function improved following infusion of relaxin in these rats. The authors noted no difference in eNOS expression but there was increased eNOS activity. Superoxide production was also decreased. Perhaps relaxin may provide a novel target for treatment of endothelial dysfunction.

4.4.6. Vasopeptidase Inhibitors

Vasopeptidase inhibition is a relatively novel concept in blood pressure regulation and in cardiovascular medicine [247]. The actions of this new class of drugs involve the simultaneous inhibition of two different enzymes: angiotensin converting enzyme (ACE) and neutral endopeptidase (NEP). Neutral endopeptidase which degrades natriuretic peptides is widely distributed in endothelial cells, cardiac myocytes, vascular smooth muscle cells and renal epithelial cells [248]. The natriuretic peptides (ANP, BNP, CNP) play a prominent role in cardio-renal blood pressure homeostasis and also in vascular tone and structure [249, 250]. Omapatrilat, a vasopeptidase inhibitor under development, reduces blood pressure more efficiently compared to ACE-I [251]. In theory the dual action of omapatrilat on the NEP/ACE should produce a more substantial vascular response than single enzyme inhibition. This is particularly true in clinical settings where natriuretic peptides are activated, such as salt-sensitive hypertension or in high-renin hypertension. [252, 253]. In 2001, d'Uscio et al. showed that omapatrilat prevented endothelial dysfunction in resistance arteries of salt-sensitive rats. Importantly, in the same study omapatrilat better preserved both structural and functional properties of the arterial wall than captopril. These effects are also seen in the renal vasculature [254]. While there have been several further studies showing a beneficial effect in animals, including in combination with angiotensin blockade [255, 256], there is still yet to be a large study in humans.

4.5. Antioxidants

Impairment in NO bioactivity may be secondary to either decreased synthesis-release and/or increased NO inactivation. Nitric oxide (an anion), after synthesis, is rapidly inactivated by locally (of endothelial and extra-endothelial origin) generated oxygen-derived free radicals ($O^{-}2$) to form peroxynitrite anions ($OONO^{-}$), which have considerably less vasodilating capacity than NO [57, 58]. The chemical reaction between NO and superoxide anions is extremely fast, faster than that with superoxide dismutase (SODs) or with plasma vitamins which are natural scavengers of superoxide anions. An increase in free-radical formation otherwise known as oxidative stress is present in many cardiovascular diseases including hypertension, hyperlipidaemia and heart failure [59-62]. Interestingly, the severity of hypertension appears to correlate with the degree of underlying oxidative stress [63]. Antioxidants, whether endogenous or exogenous in origin are part of an additional scavenging mechanism directed to "overcome" the excess of superoxide anion production. Hypertension has been described as a disease characterised by an excess of oxygen free radicals coupled with an inefficient antioxidant mechanism [61, 64, 65]. There is evidence to suggest that hypertensive patients have significantly lower plasma concentrations of naturally occurring antioxidant factors (thiols, vitamins A, C, E) compared with matched normotensive volunteers. Also free radical scavengers such as superoxide dismutase (SOD), and glutathione (GSH) are reported to be depressed in hypertensive patients [66, 67]. Taddei et al. [257] reported that intra-brachial (forearm) administration of vitamin C, a potent antioxidant, improved both stimulated and basal NO release in hypertensive patients [258] and this has been confirmed by others [61].

Similar effects of vitamin C on NO bioactivity were also obtained in the coronary circulation of hypertensive patients after the intracoronary administration of vitamin C [259]. Also, Jeserich et al. [260], using the cold pressor testing showed an improvement of endothelial dysfunction in the epicardial coronary arteries of patients with hypertension following infusion of vitamin C. Improved endothelial function has also been shown by Engler et al. in children with hyperlipidaemia treated with vitamins C and E [261].

The effect of chronic oral vitamin C on BP lowering has been less consistent. The available data are conflicting with some investigators finding a positive effect whilst others do not [262-265]. The dosages of vitamin C involved in these studies varied widely from 400 to 2000mg daily. Duffy et al. [264] reported that regular vitamin C supplementation (1 gram daily) reduced blood pressure but this was unrelated to endothelial dysfunction. The studies which showed an improvement in endothelial dysfunction in hypertension all used intra-arterially administered vitamin C where it achieved very high or supra-physiological plasma concentrations. Indeed, because of the nature of the pharmacokinetics between NO and superoxide radicals, high plasma levels of any antioxidants would have been necessary to maintain a constant and effective scavenging system. Sherman et al. recently addressed this issue. They showed that, at least in the forearm microcirculation following intra-arterial infusions of vitamin C, its plasma concentration was the main determinant of achieving endothelium-dependent vasodilation and that lower concentrations of vitamin C failed to exert any biological effect. However, recent conflicting evidence has been published suggesting that at least in elderly patients, administration of vitamin C can acute reverse endothelial dysfunction [266]. This effect was not seen in younger patients in this study, and perhaps suggests that the beneficial effects of anti-oxidants and the mechanism by which oxidative stress causes endothelial dysfunction is perhaps age-related.

Not all antioxidants have been shown to be equally effective in reversing endothelial dysfunction. Garcia et al. [267] reported that copper-zinc dismutase, another endothelial superoxide scavenger, did not have a significant effect on acetylcholine-induced endothelial-dependent vasodilation in hypertensive patients. Of note is the fact that in contrast to the high intracellular penetration of vitamin C, copper-zinc dismutase, which is negatively charged, is unable to penetrate the cells. Hence, the use of copper-zinc superoxide dismutase assesses and buffers only the extracellular oxidative environment rather than the intracellular or intimal space. Interestingly, in animal studies the beneficial effects of copper-zinc superoxide dismutase were only obtained after modification of the enzyme to gain access to the endothelial surface [61, 268]. Assessing another antioxidant, Panza et al. [269] failed to show any benefit on the NO pathway by using oxypurinol, an inhibitor of xanthine-oxidase. Although superoxide radicals have been implicated in the genesis and perpetuation of cardiovascular diseases [64], and there is an association between hypertension and increased oxidative stress, the benefits of therapeutic interventions directed to reduce oxidative stress are not evident [270]. Of course, not all anti-oxidants are equal, and so there is still potential for this class of drug to become therapeutically useful.

Conclusion

Endothelial dysfunction is associated with hypertension and its presence correlates with target organ damage. Furthermore, endothelial dysfunction may be both a cause and a consequence of hypertension. In this chapter, we have discussed the pathways by which endothelial dysfunction may occur and the clinical evidence of its utility. Finally, we discussed the evidence looking at reversal of endothelial function, both by antihypertensive medications and therapies more directly targeted at the endothelium. Antihypertensive drug treatment improves and in some cases reverses endothelial dysfunction but this appear to depend very much on drug class and the vascular territories studied. Although calcium channel blockers, ACE-I, and ARBs seem to outperform beta-blockers (with the exception of nebivolol) and diuretics in terms of improving endothelial dysfunction, they do not seem to produce a greater antihypertensive effect. Most importantly, there is still some doubt within the scientific community as to whether the improvement in endothelial function is translated into long-term prognostic benefit. Interestingly the most effective strategy by far to improve endothelial dysfunction is regular aerobic exercise although its antihypertensive effect is only modest and less than most antihypertensive drugs. Recently proposed targets for endothelial dysfunction include oestrogens [271, 272], sirtuins (proteins possessing either histone deacetylase or mono-ribosyltransferase activity) [273] and the effects of coronary stents of endothelial function [274, 275]. Perhaps the most important future direction in this field however is the accumulation of prognostic data regarding endothelial function, especially in various conditions, for example heart failure [276].

Therefore, although endothelial dysfunction is a conceptually attractive therapeutic target in hypertension, at this point in time, we lack convincing data that using endothelial dysfunction to guide our treatment would produce any better outcomes than using blood pressure targets to guide our treatment. This situation may change in the near future as more trials are conducted in this fascinating area.

References

[1] Furchgott, R.F. and J.V. Zawadzki, The obligatory role of endothelial cells in the relaxation of arterial smooth muscle by acetylcholine. *Nature*, 1980. 288(5789): p. 373-6.

[2] Henry, Y., et al., EPR characterization of molecular targets for NO in mammalian cells and organelles. *FASEB J,* 1993. 7(12): p. 1124-34.

[3] Moncada, S. and A. Higgs, The L-arginine-nitric oxide pathway. *N Engl J Med*, 1993. 329(27): p. 2002-12.

[4] Calver, A., J. Collier, and P. Vallance, Nitric oxide and cardiovascular control. *Exp Physiol*, 1993. 78(3): p. 303-26.

[5] Vallance, P., J. Collier, and S. Moncada, Effects of endothelium-derived nitric oxide on peripheral arteriolar tone in man. *Lancet*, 1989. 2(8670): p. 997-1000.

[6] Hibbs, J.B., Jr., R.R. Taintor, and Z. Vavrin, Macrophage cytotoxicity: role for L-arginine deiminase and imino nitrogen oxidation to nitrite. *Science*, 1987. 235(4787): p. 473-6.

[7] Amezcua, J.L., et al., Nitric oxide synthesized from L-arginine regulates vascular tone in the coronary circulation of the rabbit. *Br J Pharmacol*, 1989. 97(4): p. 1119-24.

[8] Furchgott, R.F., Role of endothelium in responses of vascular smooth muscle. *Circ Res*, 1983. 53(5): p. 557-73.

[9] Gorog, P. and I.B. Kovacs, Inhibition of vascular smooth muscle cell migration by intact endothelium is nitric oxide-mediated: interference by oxidised low density lipoproteins. *J Vasc Res*, 1998. 35(3): p. 165-9.

[10] Tare, M., et al., Hyperpolarization and relaxation of arterial smooth muscle caused by nitric oxide derived from the endothelium. *Nature*, 1990. 346(6279): p. 69-71.

[11] Kanwar, S. and P. Kubes, Nitric oxide is an antiadhesive molecule for leukocytes. *New Horiz*, 1995. 3(1): p. 93-104.

[12] Radomski, M.W. and S. Moncada, Regulation of vascular homeostasis by nitric oxide. *Thromb Haemost,* 1993. 70(1): p. 36-41.

[13] Wennmalm, A., et al., Metabolism and excretion of nitric oxide in humans. An experimental and clinical study. Circ Res, 1993. 73(6): p. 1121-7.

[14] Rubanyi, G.M., et al., Mechanoreception by the endothelium: mediators and mechanisms of pressure- and flow-induced vascular responses. *Blood Vessels*, 1990. 27(2-5): p. 246-57.

[15] Pohl, U., et al., Crucial role of endothelium in the vasodilator response to increased flow in vivo. *Hypertension*, 1986. 8(1): p. 37-44.

[16] Rees, D.D., et al., A specific inhibitor of nitric oxide formation from L-arginine attenuates endothelium-dependent relaxation. *Br J Pharmacol*, 1989. 96(2): p. 418-24.

[17] Haynes, W.G., et al., Inhibition of nitric oxide synthesis increases blood pressure in healthy humans. *J Hypertens*, 1993. 11(12): p. 1375-80.

[18] Bech, J.N., et al., Dietary sodium affects systemic and renal hemodynamic response to NO inhibition in healthy humans. *Am J Physiol*, 1998. 274(5 Pt 2): p. F914-23.

[19] Anggard, E., Nitric oxide: mediator, murderer, and medicine. *Lancet*, 1994. 343(8907): p. 1199-206.

[20] Luscher, T.F. and P.M. Vanhoutte, Endothelium-dependent contractions to acetylcholine in the aorta of the spontaneously hypertensive rat. *Hypertension*, 1986. 8(4): p. 344-8.

[21] Rand, M.J., Nitrergic transmission: nitric oxide as a mediator of non-adrenergic, non-cholinergic neuro-effector transmission. *Clin Exp Pharmacol Physiol*, 1992. 19(3): p. 147-69.

[22] Toda, N. and T. Okamura, Role of nitric oxide in neurally induced cerebroarterial relaxation. *J Pharmacol Exp Ther,* 1991. 258(3): p. 1027-32.
[23] Chowdhary, S. and J.N. Townend, Role of nitric oxide in the regulation of cardiovascular autonomic control. *Clin Sci (Lond),* 1999. 97(1): p. 5-17.
[24] Luscher, T.F., Imbalance of endothelium-derived relaxing and contracting factors. A new concept in hypertension? *Am J Hypertens*, 1990. 3(4): p. 317-30.
[25] Levy, D., et al., Prognostic implications of echocardiographically determined left ventricular mass in the Framingham Heart Study. *N Engl J Med,* 1990. 322(22): p. 1561-6.
[26] Heagerty, A.M., et al., Small artery structure in hypertension. Dual processes of remodeling and growth. *Hypertension*, 1993. 21(4): p. 391-7.
[27] Dilley, R.J., et al., Vascular hypertrophy in renal hypertensive spontaneously hypertensive rats. Hypertension, 1994. 24(1): p. 8-15.
[28] Mulvany, M.J., The fourth Sir George Pickering memorial lecture. The structure of the resistance vasculature in essential hypertension. *J Hypertens*, 1987. 5(2): p. 129-36.
[29] Kamiya, A. and T. Togawa, Adaptive regulation of wall shear stress to flow change in the canine carotid artery. *Am J Physiol,* 1980. 239(1): p. H14-21.
[30] Guyton, J.R. and C.J. Hartley, Flow restriction of one carotid artery in juvenile rats inhibits growth of arterial diameter. *Am J Physiol,* 1985. 248(4 Pt 2): p. H540-6.
[31] Langille, B.L. and F. O'Donnell, Reductions in arterial diameter produced by chronic decreases in blood flow are endothelium-dependent. *Science*, 1986. 231(4736): p. 405-7.
[32] Olivetti, G., et al., Morphometry of medial hypertrophy in the rat thoracic aorta. *Lab Invest*, 1980. 42(5): p. 559-65.
[33] Harder, D.R., Pressure-induced myogenic activation of cat cerebral arteries is dependent on intact endothelium. *Circ Res,* 1987. 60(1): p. 102-7.
[34] Iba, T., et al., Stimulation of endothelial secretion of tissue-type plasminogen activator by repetitive stretch. *J Surg Res*, 1991. 50(5): p. 457-60.
[35] Ranieri, G., et al., The effects of diuretic and beta-blocker treatment on cardiac and vascular structural changes in untreated essential hypertensive patients. J *Hypertens Suppl*, 1993. 11(5): p. S368-9.
[36] Morishita, R., et al., Possible role of the vascular renin-angiotensin system in hypertension and vascular hypertrophy. *Hypertension*, 1992. 19(2 Suppl): p. II62-7.
[37] Iwatsuki, K., et al., Hypertension: increase of collagen biosynthesis in arteries but not in veins. *Science*, 1977. 198(4315): p. 403-5.
[38] Dzau, V.J. and G.H. Gibbons, Endothelium and growth factors in vascular remodeling of hypertension. *Hypertension*, 1991. 18(5 Suppl): p. III115-21.
[39] Luscher, T.F., L. Raij, and P.M. Vanhoutte, Endothelium-dependent vascular responses in normotensive and hypertensive Dahl rats. *Hypertension*, 1987. 9(2): p. 157-63.
[40] Raij, L., T.F. Luscher, and P.M. Vanhoutte, High potassium diet augments endothelium-dependent relaxations in the Dahl rat. *Hypertension*, 1988. 12(6): p. 562-7.
[41] Konishi, M. and C. Su, Role of endothelium in dilator responses of spontaneously hypertensive rat arteries. *Hypertension*, 1983. 5(6): p. 881-6.
[42] Winquist, R.J., et al., Decreased endothelium-dependent relaxation in New Zealand genetic hypertensive rats. *J Hypertens,* 1984. 2(5): p. 541-5.

[43] Lockette, W., Y. Otsuka, and O. Carretero, The loss of endothelium-dependent vascular relaxation in hypertension. *Hypertension*, 1986. 8(6 Pt 2): p. II61-6.
[44] Luscher, T.F., P.M. Vanhoutte, and L. Raij, Antihypertensive treatment normalizes decreased endothelium-dependent relaxations in rats with salt-induced hypertension. *Hypertension*, 1987. 9(6 Pt 2): p. III193-7.
[45] Luscher, T.F., Endothelium-derived vasoactive factors and regulation of vascular tone in human blood vessels. *Lung*, 1990. 168 Suppl: p. 27-34.
[46] Luscher, T.F., et al., Endothelium-derived contracting factors. *Hypertension*, 1992. 19(2): p. 117-30.
[47] Panza, J.A., et al., Abnormal endothelium-dependent vascular relaxation in patients with essential hypertension. *N Engl J Med,* 1990. 323(1): p. 22-7.
[48] Panza, J.A., Endothelium-dependent vasodilatation and essential hypertension. *N Engl J Med,* 1994. 331(14): p. 951.
[49] Calver, A., J. Collier, and P. Vallance, Forearm blood flow responses to a nitric oxide synthase inhibitor in patients with treated essential hypertension. *Cardiovasc Res*, 1994. 28(11): p. 1720-5.
[50] Calver, A., et al., Effect of local intra-arterial NG-monomethyl-L-arginine in patients with hypertension: the nitric oxide dilator mechanism appears abnormal. *J Hypertens*, 1992. 10(9): p. 1025-31.
[51] Panza, J.A., et al., Role of endothelium-derived nitric oxide in the abnormal endothelium-dependent vascular relaxation of patients with essential hypertension. *Circulation*, 1993. 87(5): p. 1468-74.
[52] Cockcroft, J.R., et al., Preserved endothelium-dependent vasodilatation in patients with essential hypertension. *N Engl J Med,* 1994. 330(15): p. 1036-40.
[53] Bruning, T.A., et al., In vivo characterization of muscarinic receptor subtypes that mediate vasodilatation in patients with essential hypertension. *Hypertension*, 1995. 26(1): p. 70-7.
[54] Touyz, R.M., Reactive oxygen species, vascular oxidative stress, and redox signaling in hypertension: what is the clinical significance? *Hypertension*, 2004. 44(3): p. 248-52.
[55] Lip, G.Y., et al., Oxidative stress in malignant and non-malignant phase hypertension. *J Hum Hypertens*, 2002. 16(5): p. 333-6.
[56] Higashi, Y., et al., Endothelial function and oxidative stress in renovascular hypertension. *N Engl J Med,* 2002. 346(25): p. 1954-62.
[57] Beckman, J.S., et al., Apparent hydroxyl radical production by peroxynitrite: implications for endothelial injury from nitric oxide and superoxide. *Proc Natl Acad Sci U S A*, 1990. 87(4): p. 1620-4.
[58] Rubanyi, G.M. and P.M. Vanhoutte, Superoxide anions and hyperoxia inactivate endothelium-derived relaxing factor. *Am J Physiol*, 1986. 250(5 Pt 2): p. H822-7.
[59] Laursen, J.B., et al., Role of superoxide in angiotensin II-induced but not catecholamine-induced hypertension. *Circulation*, 1997. 95(3): p. 588-93.
[60] Rajagopalan, S., et al., Angiotensin II-mediated hypertension in the rat increases vascular superoxide production via membrane NADH/NADPH oxidase activation. Contribution to alterations of vasomotor tone. *J Clin Invest,* 1996. 97(8): p. 1916-23.
[61] Sherman, D.L., et al., Pharmacological concentrations of ascorbic acid are required for the beneficial effect on endothelial vasomotor function in hypertension. *Hypertension*, 2000. 35(4): p. 936-41.

[62] Prabha, P.S., et al., Free radical generation, lipid peroxidation and essential fatty acids in uncontrolled essential hypertension. *Prostaglandins Leukot Essent Fatty Acids,* 1990. 41(1): p. 27-33.
[63] Pierdomenico, S.D., et al., Blunted nocturnal fall in blood pressure and oxidative stress in men and women with essential hypertension. *Am J Hypertens*, 1999. 12(4 Pt 1): p. 356-63.
[64] Halliwell, B., Free radicals, antioxidants, and human disease: curiosity, cause, or consequence? *Lancet*, 1994. 344(8924): p. 721-4.
[65] Tse, W.Y., et al., Antioxidant status in controlled and uncontrolled hypertension and its relationship to endothelial damage. *J Hum Hypertens*, 1994. 8(11): p. 843-9.
[66] Sagar, S., et al., Oxygen free radicals in essential hypertension. *Mol Cell Biochem*, 1992. 111(1-2): p. 103-8.
[67] Dhalla, N.S., R.M. Temsah, and T. Netticadan, Role of oxidative stress in cardiovascular diseases. *J Hypertens*, 2000. 18(6): p. 655-73.
[68] Benzuly, K.H., et al., Functional improvement precedes structural regression of atherosclerosis. *Circulation*, 1994. 89(4): p. 1810-8.
[69] Brush, J.E., Jr., et al., Angina due to coronary microvascular disease in hypertensive patients without left ventricular hypertrophy. *N Engl J Med*, 1988. 319(20): p. 1302-7.
[70] Treasure, C.B., et al., Epicardial coronary artery responses to acetylcholine are impaired in hypertensive patients. *Circ Res*, 1992. 71(4): p. 776-81.
[71] Egashira, K., et al., Impaired coronary blood flow response to acetylcholine in patients with coronary risk factors and proximal atherosclerotic lesions. *J Clin Invest*, 1993. 91(1): p. 29-37.
[72] Egashira, K., et al., Impaired endothelium-dependent vasodilation of large epicardial and resistance coronary arteries in patients with essential hypertension. Different responses to acetylcholine and substance P. *Hypertension*, 1995. 25(2): p. 201-6.
[73] Quyyumi, A.A., et al., Endothelial dysfunction in patients with chest pain and normal coronary arteries. *Circulation*, 1992. 86(6): p. 1864-71.
[74] Bhagat, K., Endothelial function and myocardial infarction. *Cardiovasc Res*, 1998. 39(2): p. 312-7.
[75] Ghiadoni, L., et al., Endothelial function and common carotid artery wall thickening in patients with essential hypertension. *Hypertension*, 1998. 32(1): p. 25-32.
[76] Poli, A., et al., Ultrasonographic measurement of the common carotid artery wall thickness in hypercholesterolemic patients. A new model for the quantitation and follow-up of preclinical atherosclerosis in living human subjects. *Atherosclerosis*, 1988. 70(3): p. 253-61.
[77] Salonen, J.T. and R. Salonen, Ultrasonographically assessed carotid morphology and the risk of coronary heart disease. *Arterioscler Thromb*, 1991. 11(5): p. 1245-9.
[78] Devereux, R.B. and M.H. Alderman, Role of preclinical cardiovascular disease in the evolution from risk factor exposure to development of morbid events. *Circulation*, 1993. 88(4 Pt 1): p. 1444-55.
[79] Koren, M.J., et al., Relation of left ventricular mass and geometry to morbidity and mortality in uncomplicated essential hypertension. *Ann Intern Med,* 1991. 114(5): p. 345-52.
[80] Bikkina, M., et al., Left ventricular mass and risk of stroke in an elderly cohort. The Framingham Heart Study. *JAMA*, 1994. 272(1): p. 33-6.

[81] Roman, M.J., et al., Parallel cardiac and vascular adaptation in hypertension. *Circulation*, 1992. 86(6): p. 1909-18.
[82] Roman, M.J., et al., Relation of arterial structure and function to left ventricular geometric patterns in hypertensive adults. *J Am Coll Cardiol*, 1996. 28(3): p. 751-6.
[83] Roman, M.J., et al., Association of carotid atherosclerosis and left ventricular hypertrophy. *J Am Coll Cardiol,* 1995. 25(1): p. 83-90.
[84] Perticone, F., et al., Relationship between left ventricular mass and endothelium-dependent vasodilation in never-treated hypertensive patients. *Circulation*, 1999. 99(15): p. 1991-6.
[85] Millgard, J., et al., Left ventricular hypertrophy is associated with an attenuated endothelium-dependent vasodilation in hypertensive men. *Blood Press,* 2000. 9(6): p. 309-14.
[86] von zur Muhlen, B., et al., Ambulatory blood pressure and endothelium-dependent vasodilation in hypertensive patients. *Blood Press*, 2000. 9(2-3): p. 110-5.
[87] Forte, P., et al., Basal nitric oxide synthesis in essential hypertension. *Lancet*, 1997. 349(9055): p. 837-42.
[88] Gerhard, M., et al., Aging progressively impairs endothelium-dependent vasodilation in forearm resistance vessels of humans. *Hypertension*, 1996. 27(4): p. 849-53.
[89] Celermajer, D.S., et al., Endothelium-dependent dilation in the systemic arteries of asymptomatic subjects relates to coronary risk factors and their interaction. *J Am Coll Cardiol,* 1994. 24(6): p. 1468-74.
[90] Suwaidi, J.A., et al., Long-term follow-up of patients with mild coronary artery disease and endothelial dysfunction. *Circulation*, 2000. 101(9): p. 948-54.
[91] Halcox, J.P., et al., Prognostic value of coronary vascular endothelial dysfunction. *Circulation*, 2002. 106(6): p. 653-8.
[92] Schachinger, V. and A.M. Zeiher, Atherosclerosis-associated endothelial dysfunction. Z Kardiol, 2000. 89 Suppl 9: p. IX/70-4.
[93] Heitzer, T., et al., Endothelial dysfunction, oxidative stress, and risk of cardiovascular events in patients with coronary artery disease. *Circulation*, 2001. 104(22): p. 2673-8.
[94] Neunteufl, T., et al., Late prognostic value of flow-mediated dilation in the brachial artery of patients with chest pain. *Am J Cardiol,* 2000. 86(2): p. 207-10.
[95] Yeboah, J., et al., Brachial flow-mediated dilation predicts incident cardiovascular events in older adults: the Cardiovascular Health Study. *Circulation*, 2007. 115(18): p. 2390-7.
[96] Perticone, F., et al., Prognostic significance of endothelial dysfunction in hypertensive patients. *Circulation*, 2001. 104(2): p. 191-6.
[97] Modena, M.G., et al., Prognostic role of reversible endothelial dysfunction in hypertensive postmenopausal women. *J Am Coll Cardiol*, 2002. 40(3): p. 505-10.
[98] Anderson, T.J., et al., Microvascular function predicts cardiovascular events in primary prevention: long-term results from the Firefighters and Their Endothelium (FATE) study. *Circulation*, 2011. 123(2): p. 163-9.
[99] Philpott, A.C., et al., Comparison of new measures of vascular function to flow mediated dilatation as a measure of cardiovascular risk factors. *Am J Cardiol*, 2009. 103(11): p. 1610-5.
[100] Andersson, O.K., et al., Survival in treated hypertension: follow up study after two decades. *BMJ*, 1998. 317(7152): p. 167-71.

[101] Vallance, P., *Hypertension.* J R Coll Physicians Lond, 1999. 33(2): p. 119-23.

[102] Kokkinos, P.F., et al., Effects of regular exercise on blood pressure and left ventricular hypertrophy in African-American men with severe hypertension. *N Engl J Med*, 1995. 333(22): p. 1462-7.

[103] Duncan, J.J., et al., The effects of aerobic exercise on plasma catecholamines and blood pressure in patients with mild essential hypertension. *JAMA*, 1985. 254(18): p. 2609-13.

[104] Ramsay, L.E., et al., British Hypertension Society guidelines for hypertension management 1999: summary. *BMJ*, 1999. 319(7210): p. 630-5.

[105] Green, D.J., et al., Modification of forearm resistance vessels by exercise training in young men. *J Appl Physiol*, 1994. 77(4): p. 1829-33.

[106] Higashi, Y., et al., Regular aerobic exercise augments endothelium-dependent vascular relaxation in normotensive as well as hypertensive subjects: role of endothelium-derived nitric oxide. *Circulation*, 1999. 100(11): p. 1194-202.

[107] Taddei, S., et al., Aging and endothelial function in normotensive subjects and patients with essential hypertension. *Circulation*, 1995. 91(7): p. 1981-7.

[108] Kugiyama, K., et al., Impairment of endothelium-dependent arterial relaxation by lysolecithin in modified low-density lipoproteins. *Nature*, 1990. 344(6262): p. 160-2.

[109] Chin, J.H., S. Azhar, and B.B. Hoffman, Inactivation of endothelial derived relaxing factor by oxidized lipoproteins. *J Clin Invest*, 1992. 89(1): p. 10-8.

[110] Hambrecht, R., et al., Effect of exercise on coronary endothelial function in patients with coronary artery disease. *N Engl J Med,* 2000. 342(7): p. 454-60.

[111] Cornelissen, V.A., et al., Exercise-based cardiac rehabiliation improves endothelial function assessed by flow-mediated dilation but not by pulse amplitude tonometry. *Eur J Prev Cardiol*, 2012.

[112] Pasceri, V., J.T. Willerson, and E.T. Yeh, Direct proinflammatory effect of C-reactive protein on human endothelial cells. *Circulation*, 2000. 102(18): p. 2165-8.

[113] Ridker, P.M., et al., Comparison of C-reactive protein and low-density lipoprotein cholesterol levels in the prediction of first cardiovascular events. *N Engl J Med*, 2002. 347(20): p. 1557-65.

[114] Milani, R.V., C.J. Lavie, and M.R. Mehra, Reduction in C-reactive protein through cardiac rehabilitation and exercise training. *J Am Coll Cardiol*, 2004. 43(6): p. 1056-61.

[115] Vona, M., et al., Effects of different types of exercise training followed by detraining on endothelium-dependent dilation in patients with recent myocardial infarction. *Circulation*, 2009. 119(12): p. 1601-8.

[116] Vita, J.A., et al., Coronary vasomotor response to acetylcholine relates to risk factors for coronary artery disease. *Circulation*, 1990. 81(2): p. 491-7.

[117] Taddei, S., et al., Hypertension causes premature aging of endothelial function in humans. *Hypertension*, 1997. 29(3): p. 736-43.

[118] Al-Shaer, M.H., et al., Effects of aging and atherosclerosis on endothelial and vascular smooth muscle function in humans. *Int J Cardiol*, 2006. 109(2): p. 201-6.

[119] Herrera, M.D., et al., Endothelial dysfunction and aging: an update. *Ageing Res Rev*, 2010. 9(2): p. 142-52.

[120] Erusalimsky, J.D. and C. Skene, Mechanisms of endothelial senescence. *Exp Physiol*, 2009. 94(3): p. 299-304.

[121] Casino, P.R., et al., The role of nitric oxide in endothelium-dependent vasodilation of hypercholesterolemic patients. *Circulation*, 1993. 88(6): p. 2541-7.

[122] Creager, M.A., et al., Impaired vasodilation of forearm resistance vessels in hypercholesterolemic humans. *J Clin Invest,* 1990. 86(1): p. 228-34.

[123] Vogel, R.A., M.C. Corretti, and G.D. Plotnick, Effect of a single high-fat meal on endothelial function in healthy subjects. *Am J Cardiol*, 1997. 79(3): p. 350-4.

[124] Steinberg, H.O., et al., Endothelial dysfunction is associated with cholesterol levels in the high normal range in humans. *Circulation*, 1997. 96(10): p. 3287-93.

[125] Muiesan, M.L., et al., Effect of treatment on flow-dependent vasodilation of the brachial artery in essential hypertension. Hypertension, 1999. 33(1 Pt 2): p. 575-80.

[126] Okumura, K., et al., Small Low-Density Lipoprotein Cholesterol Concentration is a Determinant of Endothelial Dysfunction by Peripheral Artery Tonometry in Men. J Atheroscler Thromb, 2012.

[127] Ashen, M.D. and R.S. Blumenthal, Clinical practice. Low HDL cholesterol levels. *N Engl J Med*, 2005. 353(12): p. 1252-60.

[128] Barter, P., et al., HDL cholesterol, very low levels of LDL cholesterol, and cardiovascular events. *N Engl J Med*, 2007. 357(13): p. 1301-10.

[129] Bisoendial, R.J., et al., Restoration of endothelial function by increasing high-density lipoprotein in subjects with isolated low high-density lipoprotein. *Circulation*, 2003. 107(23): p. 2944-8.

[130] Spieker, L.E., et al., High-density lipoprotein restores endothelial function in hypercholesterolemic men. *Circulation*, 2002. 105(12): p. 1399-402.

[131] Nicholls, S.J., et al., Reconstituted high-density lipoproteins inhibit the acute pro-oxidant and proinflammatory vascular changes induced by a periarterial collar in normocholesterolemic rabbits. *Circulation*, 2005. 111(12): p. 1543-50.

[132] Sorrentino, S.A., et al., Endothelial-vasoprotective effects of high-density lipoprotein are impaired in patients with type 2 diabetes mellitus but are improved after extended-release niacin therapy. *Circulation*, 2010. 121(1): p. 110-22.

[133] McVeigh, G.E., et al., Effects of long-term cigarette smoking on endothelium-dependent responses in humans. *Am J Cardiol,* 1996. 78(6): p. 668-72.

[134] Celermajer, D.S., et al., Cigarette smoking is associated with dose-related and potentially reversible impairment of endothelium-dependent dilation in healthy young adults. *Circulation*, 1993. 88(5 Pt 1): p. 2149-55.

[135] Toda, N. and H. Toda, Nitric oxide-mediated blood flow regulation as affected by smoking and nicotine. *Eur J Pharmacol,* 2010. 649(1-3): p. 1-13.

[136] Bermudez, E.A., et al., Relation between markers of systemic vascular inflammation and smoking in women. *Am J Cardiol*, 2002. 89(9): p. 1117-9.

[137] Mendall, M.A., et al., Relation of serum cytokine concentrations to cardiovascular risk factors and coronary heart disease. *Heart*, 1997. 78(3): p. 273-7.

[138] Taddei, S., et al., Menopause is associated with endothelial dysfunction in women. *Hypertension*, 1996. 28(4): p. 576-82.

[139] Jones, D.S., N.S. Andrawis, and D.R. Abernethy, Impaired endothelial-dependent forearm vascular relaxation in black Americans. *Clin Pharmacol Ther*, 1999. 65(4): p. 408-12.

[140] Gilligan, D.M., et al., Effects of estrogen replacement therapy on peripheral vasomotor function in postmenopausal women. *Am J Cardiol*, 1995. 75(4): p. 264-8.

[141] Herrington, D.M., et al., Endothelial-dependent coronary vasomotor responsiveness in postmenopausal women with and without estrogen replacement therapy. *Am J Cardiol,* 1994. 73(13): p. 951-2.

[142] Lieberman, E.H., et al., Estrogen improves endothelium-dependent, flow-mediated vasodilation in postmenopausal women. *Ann Intern Med*, 1994. 121(12): p. 936-41.

[143] Virdis, A., et al., Mechanisms responsible for endothelial dysfunction associated with acute estrogen deprivation in normotensive women. *Circulation*, 2000. 101(19): p. 2258-63.

[144] Taddei, S., et al., Endothelium-dependent forearm vasodilation is reduced in normotensive subjects with familial history of hypertension. *J Cardiovasc Pharmacol*, 1992. 20 Suppl 12: p. S193-5.

[145] Taddei, S., et al., Defective L-arginine-nitric oxide pathway in offspring of essential hypertensive patients. *Circulation*, 1996. 94(6): p. 1298-303.

[146] McAllister, A.S., et al., Basal nitric oxide production is impaired in offspring of patients with essential hypertension. *Clin Sci (Lond),* 1999. 97(2): p. 141-7.

[147] Panza, J.A., et al., Effect of antihypertensive treatment on endothelium-dependent vascular relaxation in patients with essential hypertension. *J Am Coll Cardiol,* 1993. 21(5): p. 1145-51.

[148] Millgard, J. and L. Lind, Acute hypertension impairs endothelium-dependent vasodilation. *Clin Sci (Lond),* 1998. 94(6): p. 601-7.

[149] Paniagua, O.A., M.B. Bryant, and J.A. Panza, Transient hypertension directly impairs endothelium-dependent vasodilation of the human microvasculature. *Hypertension*, 2000. 36(6): p. 941-4.

[150] Taddei, S., et al., Vasodilation to acetylcholine in primary and secondary forms of human hypertension. *Hypertension*, 1993. 21(6 Pt 2): p. 929-33.

[151] Schiffrin, E.L., et al., Antihypertensive effect of an endothelin receptor antagonist in DOCA-salt spontaneously hypertensive rats. *Br J Pharmacol*, 1995. 115(8): p. 1377-81.

[152] Schiffrin, E.L., et al., Correction of arterial structure and endothelial dysfunction in human essential hypertension by the angiotensin receptor antagonist losartan. *Circulation*, 2000. 101(14): p. 1653-9.

[153] Higashi, Y., et al., A comparison of angiotensin-converting enzyme inhibitors, calcium antagonists, beta-blockers and diuretic agents on reactive hyperemia in patients with essential hypertension: a multicenter study. *J Am Coll Cardiol,* 2000. 35(2): p. 284-91.

[154] Gao, Y.S., et al., Nebivolol induces endothelium-dependent relaxations of canine coronary arteries. *J Cardiovasc Pharmacol*, 1991. 17(6): p. 964-9.

[155] Cockcroft, J.R., et al., Nebivolol vasodilates human forearm vasculature: evidence for an L-arginine/NO-dependent mechanism. *J Pharmacol Exp Ther*, 1995. 274(3): p. 1067-71.

[156] Dawes, M., et al., The vasodilator action of nebivolol in forearm vasculature of subjects with essential hypertension. *Br J Clin Pharmacol*, 1999. 48(3): p. 460-3.

[157] Fargin, A., et al., The genomic clone G-21 which resembles a beta-adrenergic receptor sequence encodes the 5-HT1A receptor. *Nature*, 1988. 335(6188): p. 358-60.

[158] Kakoki, M., et al., Effects of vasodilatory beta-adrenoceptor antagonists on endothelium-derived nitric oxide release in rat kidney. *Hypertension*, 1999. 33(1 Pt 2): p. 467-71.

[159] Brehm, B.R., et al., Beta-blockers of the third generation inhibit endothelin-1 liberation, mRNA production and proliferation of human coronary smooth muscle and endothelial cells. *J Cardiovasc Pharmacol*, 2000. 36(5 Suppl 1): p. S401-3.

[160] Troost, R., et al., Nebivolol decreases systemic oxidative stress in healthy volunteers. Br J Clin Pharmacol, 2000. 50(4): p. 377-9.

[161] Tzemos, N., P.O. Lim, and T.M. MacDonald, Nebivolol reverses endothelial dysfunction in essential hypertension: a randomized, double-blind, crossover study. *Circulation*, 2001. 104(5): p. 511-4.

[162] Falskov, B., et al., Endothelial function is unaffected by changing between carvedilol and metoprolol in patients with heart failure--a randomized study. *Cardiovasc Diabetol*, 2011. 10: p. 91.

[163] Lindholm, L.H., et al., Cardiovascular morbidity and mortality in patients with diabetes in the Losartan Intervention For Endpoint reduction in hypertension study (LIFE): a randomised trial against atenolol. *Lancet*, 2002. 359(9311): p. 1004-10.

[164] Dahlof, B., et al., Cardiovascular morbidity and mortality in the Losartan Intervention For Endpoint reduction in hypertension study (LIFE): a randomised trial against atenolol. *Lancet*, 2002. 359(9311): p. 995-1003.

[165] Williams, B., et al., Differential impact of blood pressure-lowering drugs on central aortic pressure and clinical outcomes: principal results of the Conduit Artery Function Evaluation (CAFE) study. *Circulation*, 2006. 113(9): p. 1213-25.

[166] Kamp, O., G.T. Sieswerda, and C.A. Visser, Comparison of effects on systolic and diastolic left ventricular function of nebivolol versus atenolol in patients with uncomplicated essential hypertension. *Am J Cardiol*, 2003. 92(3): p. 344-8.

[167] Sorrentino, S.A., et al., Nebivolol exerts beneficial effects on endothelial function, early endothelial progenitor cells, myocardial neovascularization, and left ventricular dysfunction early after myocardial infarction beyond conventional beta1-blockade. *J Am Coll Cardiol*, 2011. 57(5): p. 601-11.

[168] Doerries, C., et al., Critical role of the NAD(P)H oxidase subunit p47phox for left ventricular remodeling/dysfunction and survival after myocardial infarction. *Circ Res*, 2007. 100(6): p. 894-903.

[169] Looi, Y.H., et al., Involvement of Nox2 NADPH oxidase in adverse cardiac remodeling after myocardial infarction. *Hypertension*, 2008. 51(2): p. 319-25.

[170] Brehm, B.R., et al., Effects of nebivolol on proliferation and apoptosis of human coronary artery smooth muscle and endothelial cells. *Cardiovasc Res,* 2001. 49(2): p. 430-9.

[171] Wolf, S.C., et al., Major differences in gene expression in human coronary smooth muscle cells after nebivolol or metoprolol treatment. *Int J Cardiol,* 2008. 125(1): p. 4-10.

[172] Taddei, S., et al., Forearm vasodilation in response to acetylcholine is increased by potassium in essential hypertensive patients. *J Hypertens Suppl,* 1993. 11(5): p. S144-5.

[173] Taddei, S., et al., Effect of potassium on vasodilation to acetylcholine in essential hypertension. *Hypertension*, 1994. 23(4): p. 485-90.

[174] Fang, J., S. Madhavan, and M.H. Alderman, Dietary potassium intake and stroke mortality. *Stroke*, 2000. 31(7): p. 1532-7.

[175] Farquharson, C.A. and A.D. Struthers, Spironolactone increases nitric oxide bioactivity, improves endothelial vasodilator dysfunction, and suppresses vascular angiotensin

I/angiotensin II conversion in patients with chronic heart failure. *Circulation*, 2000. 101(6): p. 594-7.
[176] Pitt, B., et al., The effect of spironolactone on morbidity and mortality in patients with severe heart failure. Randomized Aldactone Evaluation Study Investigators. *N Engl J Med,* 1999. 341(10): p. 709-17.
[177] Ullian, M.E., The role of corticosteriods in the regulation of vascular tone. *Cardiovasc Res*, 1999. 41(1): p. 55-64.
[178] Blanco-Rivero, J., et al., Participation of prostacyclin in endothelial dysfunction induced by aldosterone in normotensive and hypertensive rats. *Hypertension*, 2005. 46(1): p. 107-12.
[179] Garnier, A., et al., Cardiac specific increase in aldosterone production induces coronary dysfunction in aldosterone synthase-transgenic mice. *Circulation*, 2004. 110(13): p. 1819-25.
[180] Kobayashi, N., et al., Cardioprotective mechanisms of eplerenone on cardiac performance and remodeling in failing rat hearts. *Hypertension*, 2006. 47(4): p. 671-9.
[181] Nakamura, T., et al., Eplerenone potentiates protective effects of amlodipine against cardiovascular injury in salt-sensitive hypertensive rats. *Hypertens Res*, 2011. 34(7): p. 817-24.
[182] Fujimura, N., et al., Mineralocorticoid receptor blocker eplerenone improves endothelial function and inhibits Rho-associated kinase activity in patients with hypertension. *Clin Pharmacol Ther*, 2012. 91(2): p. 289-97.
[183] Savoia, C., et al., Selective mineralocorticoid receptor blocker eplerenone reduces resistance artery stiffness in hypertensive patients. *Hypertension*, 2008. 51(2): p. 432-9.
[184] Imanishi, T., et al., Addition of eplerenone to an angiotensin-converting enzyme inhibitor effectively improves nitric oxide bioavailability. *Hypertension*, 2008. 51(3): p. 734-41.
[185] McMurray, J.J., et al., ESC Guidelines for the diagnosis and treatment of acute and chronic heart failure 2012: The Task Force for the Diagnosis and Treatment of Acute and Chronic Heart Failure 2012 of the European Society of Cardiology. Developed in collaboration with the Heart Failure Association (HFA) of the ESC. *Eur Heart J*, 2012. 33(14): p. 1787-847.
[186] Hansson, L., et al., Randomised trial of effects of calcium antagonists compared with diuretics and beta-blockers on cardiovascular morbidity and mortality in hypertension: the Nordic Diltiazem (NORDIL) study. *Lancet*, 2000. 356(9227): p. 359-65.
[187] Brown, M.J., et al., Morbidity and mortality in patients randomised to double-blind treatment with a long-acting calcium-channel blocker or diuretic in the International Nifedipine GITS study: Intervention as a Goal in Hypertension Treatment (INSIGHT). *Lancet*, 2000. 356(9227): p. 366-72.
[188] Lyons, D., J. Webster, and N. Benjamin, The effect of antihypertensive therapy on responsiveness to local intra-arterial NG-monomethyl-L-arginine in patients with essential hypertension. *J Hypertens,* 1994. 12(9): p. 1047-52.
[189] Perticone, F., et al., Calcium antagonist isradipine improves abnormal endothelium-dependent vasodilation in never treated hypertensive patients. *Cardiovasc Res*, 1999. 41(1): p. 299-306.
[190] Taddei, S., et al., Lacidipine restores endothelium-dependent vasodilation in essential hypertensive patients. *Hypertension*, 1997. 30(6): p. 1606-12.

[191] Yamamoto, E., et al., Calcium channel blockers, more than diuretics, enhance vascular protective effects of angiotensin receptor blockers in salt-loaded hypertensive rats. *PLoS One*, 2012. 7(6): p. e39162.

[192] Schiffrin, E.L. and L.Y. Deng, Structure and function of resistance arteries of hypertensive patients treated with a beta-blocker or a calcium channel antagonist. *J Hypertens*, 1996. 14(10): p. 1247-55.

[193] Frielingsdorf, J., et al., Normalization of abnormal coronary vasomotion by calcium antagonists in patients with hypertension. *Circulation*, 1996. 93(7): p. 1380-7.

[194] Effect of nifedipine and cerivastatin on coronary endothelial function in patients with coronary artery disease: the ENCORE I Study (Evaluation of Nifedipine and Cerivastatin On Recovery of coronary Endothelial function). *Circulation*, 2003. 107(3): p. 422-8.

[195] Luscher, T.F., et al., A randomized placebo-controlled study on the effect of nifedipine on coronary endothelial function and plaque formation in patients with coronary artery disease: the ENCORE II study. *Eur Heart J,* 2009. 30(13): p. 1590-7.

[196] Rubanyi, G.M. and P.M. Vanhoutte, Calcium and activation of the release of endothelium-derived relaxing factor. *Ann N Y Acad Sci,* 1988. 522: p. 226-33.

[197] Lupo, E., et al., In vitro antioxidant activity of calcium antagonists against LDL oxidation compared with alpha-tocopherol. *Biochem Biophys Res Commun*, 1994. 203(3): p. 1803-8.

[198] van Amsterdam, F.T., et al., Lacidipine: a dihydropyridine calcium antagonist with antioxidant activity. *Free Radic Biol Med,* 1992. 12(3): p. 183-7.

[199] Haynes, W.G., et al., Pharmacology of endothelin-1 in vivo in humans. *J Cardiovasc Pharmacol*, 1991. 17 Suppl 7: p. S284-6.

[200] Kiowski, W., et al., Endothelin-1-induced vasoconstriction in humans. Reversal by calcium channel blockade but not by nitrovasodilators or endothelium-derived relaxing factor. *Circulation*, 1991. 83(2): p. 469-75.

[201] Kiowski, W. and L. Linder, Reversal of endothelin-1-induced vasoconstriction by nifedipine in human resistance vessels in vivo in healthy subjects. *Am J Cardiol*, 1992. 69(12): p. 1063-6.

[202] Cardillo, C., et al., Role of endothelin in the increased vascular tone of patients with essential hypertension. *Hypertension*, 1999. 33(2): p. 753-8.

[203] Raij, L., Hypertension, endothelium, and cardiovascular risk factors. *Am J Med*, 1991. 90(2A): p. 13S-18S.

[204] Tiryaki, O., et al., Effects of lisinopril, irbesartan, and amlodipine on the thrombogenic variables in the early and late stages of the treatment in hypertensive patients. *Clin Exp Hypertens*, 2012. 34(2): p. 145-52.

[205] Goldblatt, H., et al., Studies on Experimental Hypertension : I. The Production of Persistent Elevation of Systolic Blood Pressure by Means of Renal Ischemia. *J Exp Med*, 1934. 59(3): p. 347-79.

[206] Dzau, V.J., Local expression and pathophysiological role of renin-angiotensin in the blood vessels and heart. *Basic Res Cardiol*, 1993. 88 Suppl 1: p. 1-14.

[207] Siragy, H.M., M. de Gasparo, and R.M. Carey, Angiotensin type 2 receptor mediates valsartan-induced hypotension in conscious rats. *Hypertension*, 2000. 35(5): p. 1074-7.

[208] Erdos, E.G., The angiotensin I converting enzyme. *Fed Proc*, 1977. 36(5): p. 1760-5.

[209] Zhang, X., et al., Role of endothelial kinins in control of coronary nitric oxide production. Hypertension, 1997. 30(5): p. 1105-11.
[210] Vanhoutte, P.M., [Endothelial dysfunction and coronary heart disease. Interaction of endothelium and thrombocytes]. *Schweiz Rundsch Med Prax,* 1993. 82(42): p. 1161-6.
[211] Hornig, B., C. Kohler, and H. Drexler, Role of bradykinin in mediating vascular effects of angiotensin-converting enzyme inhibitors in humans. *Circulation*, 1997. 95(5): p. 1115-8.
[212] Anderson, T.J., et al., Comparative study of ACE-inhibition, angiotensin II antagonism, and calcium channel blockade on flow-mediated vasodilation in patients with coronary disease (BANFF study). *J Am Coll Cardiol*, 2000. 35(1): p. 60-6.
[213] Mancini, G.B., et al., Angiotensin-converting enzyme inhibition with quinapril improves endothelial vasomotor dysfunction in patients with coronary artery disease. The TREND (Trial on Reversing ENdothelial Dysfunction) Study. *Circulation*, 1996. 94(3): p. 258-65.
[214] Schiffrin, E.L., Remodeling of resistance arteries in human hypertension: effects of cilazapril, an angiotensin-I-converting enzyme inhibitor. *Cardiology*, 1995. 86 Suppl 1: p. 16-22.
[215] Rizzoni, D., et al., Effects of long-term antihypertensive treatment with lisinopril on resistance arteries in hypertensive patients with left ventricular hypertrophy. *J Hypertens,* 1997. 15(2): p. 197-204.
[216] Antony, I., G. Lerebours, and A. Nitenberg, Angiotensin-converting enzyme inhibition restores flow-dependent and cold pressor test-induced dilations in coronary arteries of hypertensive patients. *Circulation*, 1996. 94(12): p. 3115-22.
[217] Taddei, S., et al., Effects of angiotensin converting enzyme inhibition on endothelium-dependent vasodilatation in essential hypertensive patients. *J Hypertens*, 1998. 16(4): p. 447-56.
[218] Kiowski, W., et al., Effects of cilazapril on vascular structure and function in essential hypertension. *Hypertension*, 1996. 27(3 Pt 1): p. 371-6.
[219] Creager, M.A. and M.A. Roddy, Effect of captopril and enalapril on endothelial function in hypertensive patients. *Hypertension*, 1994. 24(4): p. 499-505.
[220] Hirooka, Y., et al., Captopril improves impaired endothelium-dependent vasodilation in hypertensive patients. *Hypertension*, 1992. 20(2): p. 175-80.
[221] Millgard, J., et al., Captopril, but not nifedipine, improves endothelium-dependent vasodilation in hypertensive patients. *J Hum Hypertens*, 1998. 12(8): p. 511-6.
[222] Prasad, A., et al., Acute and chronic angiotensin-1 receptor antagonism reverses endothelial dysfunction in atherosclerosis. *Circulation*, 2000. 101(20): p. 2349-54.
[223] Ghiadoni, L., et al., Effect of the angiotensin II type 1 receptor blocker candesartan on endothelial function in patients with essential hypertension. *Hypertension*, 2000. 35(1 Pt 2): p. 501-6.
[224] Tzemos, N., P.O. Lim, and T.M. MacDonald, Valsartan improves endothelial dysfunction in hypertension: a randomized, double-blind study. *Cardiovasc Ther*, 2009. 27(3): p. 151-8.
[225] Hirooka, Y., et al., Effects of valsartan or amlodipine on endothelial function and oxidative stress after one year follow-up in patients with essential hypertension. *Clin Exp Hypertens*, 2008. 30(3): p. 267-76.

[226] Kerth, P.A. and P.M. Vanhoutte, Effects of perindoprilat on endothelium-dependent relaxations and contractions in isolated blood vessels. *Am J Hypertens,* 1991. 4(3 Pt 2): p. 226S-234S.

[227] Ceconi, C., et al., ACE inhibition with perindopril and endothelial function. Results of a substudy of the EUROPA study: PERTINENT. *Cardiovasc Res*, 2007. 73(1): p. 237-46.

[228] Miyamoto, M., et al., The effect of antihypertensive drugs on endothelial function as assessed by flow-mediated vasodilation in hypertensive patients. *Int J Vasc Med,* 2012. 2012: p. 453264.

[229] Terashima, M., et al., Protective effect of telmisartan against endothelial dysfunction after coronary drug-eluting stent implantation in hypertensive patients. *JACC Cardiovasc Interv,* 2012. 5(2): p. 182-90.

[230] Chou, C.L., et al., Direct renin inhibitor prevents and ameliorates insulin resistance, aortic endothelial dysfunction and vascular remodeling in fructose-fed hypertensive rats. *Hypertens Res*, 2012.

[231] Virdis, A., et al., Effect of aliskiren treatment on endothelium-dependent vasodilation and aortic stiffness in essential hypertensive patients. *Eur Heart J*, 2012. 33(12): p. 1530-8.

[232] Cherney, D.Z., et al., The Effect of Direct Renin Inhibition Alone and in Combination With ACE Inhibition on Endothelial Function, Arterial Stiffness, and Renal Function in Type 1 Diabetes. *Diabetes* Care, 2012.

[233] Yanagisawa, M., et al., A novel peptide vasoconstrictor, endothelin, is produced by vascular endothelium and modulates smooth muscle Ca2+ channels. *J Hypertens Suppl*, 1988. 6(4): p. S188-91.

[234] Haynes, W.G., F.E. Strachan, and D.J. Webb, Endothelin ETA and ETB receptors cause vasoconstriction of human resistance and capacitance vessels in vivo. *Circulation*, 1995. 92(3): p. 357-63.

[235] Imai, T., et al., Induction of endothelin-1 gene by angiotensin and vasopressin in endothelial cells. *Hypertension*, 1992. 19(6 Pt 2): p. 753-7.

[236] d'Uscio, L.V., et al., Structure and function of small arteries in salt-induced hypertension: effects of chronic endothelin-subtype-A-receptor blockade. *Hypertension*, 1997. 30(4): p. 905-11.

[237] Kohno, M., et al., Plasma immunoreactive endothelin in essential hypertension. *Am J Med*, 1990. 88(6): p. 614-8.

[238] Russell, F.D., J.N. Skepper, and A.P. Davenport, Endothelin peptide and converting enzymes in human endothelium. *J Cardiovasc Pharmacol*, 1998. 31 Suppl 1: p. S19-21.

[239] Wagner, O.F., et al., Polar secretion of endothelin-1 by cultured endothelial cells. *J Biol Chem*, 1992. 267(23): p. 16066-8.

[240] Schiffrin, E.L., et al., Enhanced expression of endothelin-1 gene in resistance arteries in severe human essential hypertension. *J Hypertens*, 1997. 15(1): p. 57-63.

[241] Ergul, S., et al., Racial differences in plasma endothelin-1 concentrations in individuals with essential hypertension. *Hypertension*, 1996. 28(4): p. 652-5.

[242] Krum, H., et al., The effect of an endothelin-receptor antagonist, bosentan, on blood pressure in patients with essential hypertension. Bosentan Hypertension Investigators. *N Engl J Med*, 1998. 338(12): p. 784-90.

[243] Reriani, M., et al., Long-term administration of endothelin receptor antagonist improves coronary endothelial function in patients with early atherosclerosis. *Circulation*, 2010. 122(10): p. 958-66.

[244] Liang, F., et al., Ambrisentan and tadalafil synergistically relax endothelin-induced contraction of rat pulmonary arteries. *Hypertension*, 2012. 59(3): p. 705-11.

[245] Halls, M.L., R.A. Bathgate, and R.J. Summers, Comparison of signaling pathways activated by the relaxin family peptide receptors, RXFP1 and RXFP2, using reporter genes. *J Pharmacol Exp Ther,* 2007. 320(1): p. 281-90.

[246] Dschietzig, T., et al., Relaxin, a pregnancy hormone, is a functional endothelin-1 antagonist: attenuation of endothelin-1-mediated vasoconstriction by stimulation of endothelin type-B receptor expression via ERK-1/2 and nuclear factor-kappaB. Circ Res, 2003. 92(1): p. 32-40.

[247] Burnett, J.C., Jr., Vasopeptidase inhibition: a new concept in blood pressure management. J Hypertens Suppl, 1999. 17(1): p. S37-43.

[248] Erdos, E.G. and R.A. Skidgel, Neutral endopeptidase 24.11 (enkephalinase) and related regulators of peptide hormones. *FASEB J*, 1989. 3(2): p. 145-51.

[249] Burnett, J.C., Jr., et al., Atrial natriuretic peptide elevation in congestive heart failure in the human. *Science*, 1986. 231(4742): p. 1145-7.

[250] Wei, C.M., et al., Atrial natriuretic peptide and C-type natriuretic peptide in spontaneously hypertensive rats and their vasorelaxing actions in vitro. *Hypertension*, 1994. 23(6 Pt 2): p. 903-7.

[251] Tikkanen, T., et al., Dual inhibition of neutral endopeptidase and angiotensin-converting enzyme in rats with hypertension and diabetes mellitus. *Hypertension*, 1998. 32(4): p. 778-85.

[252] d'Uscio, L.V., et al., Vasopeptidase Inhibition Prevents Endothelial Dysfunction of Resistance Arteries in Salt-Sensitive Hypertension in Comparison With Single ACE Inhibition. *Hypertension*, 2001. 37(1): p. 28-33.

[253] Trippodo, N.C., et al., Effects of omapatrilat in low, normal, and high renin experimental hypertension. *Am J Hypertens*, 1998. 11(3 Pt 1): p. 363-72.

[254] Quaschning, T., et al., Vasopeptidase inhibition restores renovascular endothelial dysfunction in salt-induced hypertension. *J Am Soc Nephrol*, 2001. 12(11): p. 2280-7.

[255] Maniu, C.V., D.M. Meyer, and M.M. Redfield, Hemodynamic and humoral effects of vasopeptidase inhibition in canine hypertension. *Hypertension*, 2002. 40(4): p. 528-34.

[256] Cheng, Z.J., et al., Vascular and renal effects of vasopeptidase inhibition and angiotensin-converting enzyme blockade in spontaneously diabetic Goto-Kakizaki rats. *J Hypertens,* 2005. 23(9): p. 1757-70.

[257] Taddei, S., et al., Vitamin C improves endothelium-dependent vasodilation by restoring nitric oxide activity in essential hypertension. *Circulation*, 1998. 97(22): p. 2222-9.

[258] Frei, B., L. England, and B.N. Ames, Ascorbate is an outstanding antioxidant in human blood plasma. *Proc Natl Acad Sci U S A,* 1989. 86(16): p. 6377-81.

[259] Solzbach, U., et al., Vitamin C improves endothelial dysfunction of epicardial coronary arteries in hypertensive patients. *Circulation*, 1997. 96(5): p. 1513-9.

[260] Jeserich, M., et al., Vitamin C improves endothelial function of epicardial coronary arteries in patients with hypercholesterolaemia or essential hypertension--assessed by cold pressor testing. *Eur Heart J*, 1999. 20(22): p. 1676-80.

[261] Engler, M.M., et al., Antioxidant vitamins C and E improve endothelial function in children with hyperlipidemia: Endothelial Assessment of Risk from Lipids in Youth (EARLY) Trial. *Circulation*, 2003. 108(9): p. 1059-63.

[262] Lovat, L.B., et al., Double-blind trial of vitamin C in elderly hypertensives. *J Hum Hypertens*, 1993. 7(4): p. 403-5.

[263] Ghosh, S.K., et al., A double-blind, placebo-controlled parallel trial of vitamin C treatment in elderly patients with hypertension. *Gerontology*, 1994. 40(5): p. 268-72.

[264] Duffy, S.J., et al., Treatment of hypertension with ascorbic acid. *Lancet*, 1999. 354(9195): p. 2048-9.

[265] Fotherby, M.D., et al., Effect of vitamin C on ambulatory blood pressure and plasma lipids in older persons. *J Hypertens*, 2000. 18(4): p. 411-5.

[266] Wray, D.W., et al., Acute reversal of endothelial dysfunction in the elderly after antioxidant consumption. *Hypertension*, 2012. 59(4): p. 818-24.

[267] Garcia, C.E., et al., Effect of copper-zinc superoxide dismutase on endothelium-dependent vasodilation in patients with essential hypertension. *Hypertension*, 1995. 26(6 Pt 1): p. 863-8.

[268] Nakazono, K., et al., Does superoxide underlie the pathogenesis of hypertension? Proc Natl Acad Sci U S A, 1991. 88(22): p. 10045-8.

[269] Cardillo, C., et al., Xanthine oxidase inhibition with oxypurinol improves endothelial vasodilator function in hypercholesterolemic but not in hypertensive patients. *Hypertension*, 1997. 30(1 Pt 1): p. 57-63.

[270] Kris-Etherton, P.M., et al., Antioxidant vitamin supplements and cardiovascular disease. *Circulation*, 2004. 110(5): p. 637-41.

[271] Traupe, T., et al., Distinct roles of estrogen receptors alpha and beta mediating acute vasodilation of epicardial coronary arteries. *Hypertension*, 2007. 49(6): p. 1364-70.

[272] Meyer, M.R., et al., Deletion of G protein-coupled estrogen receptor increases endothelial vasoconstriction. *Hypertension*, 2012. 59(2): p. 507-12.

[273] Zhou, S., et al., Repression of P66Shc expression by SIRT1 contributes to the prevention of hyperglycemia-induced endothelial dysfunction. *Circ Res*, 2011. 109(6): p. 639-48.

[274] Mitsutake, Y., et al., Coronary endothelial dysfunction distal to stent of first-generation drug-eluting stents. *JACC Cardiovasc Interv*, 2012. 5(9): p. 966-73.

[275] Plass, C.A., et al., Time course of endothelium-dependent and -independent coronary vasomotor response to coronary balloons and stents. Comparison of plain and drug-eluting balloons and stents. *JACC Cardiovasc Interv*, 2012. 5(7): p. 741-51.

[276] Matsue, Y., et al., Endothelial dysfunction measured by peripheral arterial tonometry predicts prognosis in patients with heart failure with preserved ejection fraction. *Int J Cardiol*, 2012.

In: Horizons in World Cardiovascular Research. Vol. 6 ISBN: 978-1-63321-298-5
Editor: Eleanor H. Bennington

Chapter 4

Treatment of Unprotected Left Main Coronary Artery

***Alexandre do Canto Zago*[1,2,3], *Rui Manuel de Sousa de Almeida*[4,5] *and Eduardo Keller Saadi*[1,6,7]**

[1] Federal University of Rio Grande do Sul Medical School (Porto Alegre, RS, Brazil).

[2] Hospital de Clínicas de Porto Alegre and Hospital Mãe de Deus (Porto Alegre, RS, Brazil).

[3] Interventional Cardiology Department at Lutheran University Hospital (Canoas, RS, Brazil).

[4] West Paraná State University Medical School (Cascavel, PR, Brazil)

[5] Cardiovascular Surgery Department at ICCOP (Cascavel, PR, Brazil)

[6]Cardiac Surgery at Hospital de Clínicas de Porto Alegre (Porto Alegre, RS, Brazil)

[7] Cardiovascular Surgery Department at Hospital Mãe de Deus (Porto Alegre, RS, Brazil) and at Lutheran University Hospital (Canoas, RS, Brazil)

1. Introduction

When considering the significance of a left main coronary artery (LMCA) obstruction, one should take into account lesions that obstruct 50% or more of the luminal diameter. The literature shows that, when defined by this criterion, they appear in less than 6% of all patients sent for coronary angiography [1, 2] and 30% of the group submitted to a coronary artery bypass graft surgery (CABG) [3]. Although it is not such a prevalent disease, it is important because of the catastrophic results of LMCA occlusion.

Most of the time LMCA disease occurs in combination with multivessel disease and by itself only in less than 8-18% [4]. Randomized trials comparing percutaneous coronary intervention (PCI) and CABG have shown more favorable results for CABG compared to PCI using only balloon angioplasty or bare metal stents (BMS), especially regarding the target lesion revascularization endpoint.

However, the advent of drug eluting stents (DES) has prompted new studies comparing PCI and CABG due to a significant reduction in target lesion revascularization with DES in relation to BMS.

Another relevant point is that, in the majority of cases, LMCA lesions occur in the distal segment and emerge at the beginning of the left descending anterior (LAD) and circumflex (CX) arteries [5-7]. Therefore, such a compromising branch as LAD and/or CX will require the use of a bifurcation technique, which increases the complexity of the procedure and has an impact on the rate of major adverse cardiovascular events (MACE) [5, 7].

In spite of the anatomic characteristics and challenges discussed above, PCI for LMCA lesions has been increasingly used as an alternative form of treatment.

Thus, the end point of the current discussion is to determine for what kind of anatomical coronary characteristics and for what profile of patients PCI can be indicated with more favorable results or comparable to those of CABG.

2. Bare Metal Stents for Left Main Coronary Artery Disease

Several studies evaluated the use of PCI for treatment of unprotected LMCA disease.

In the balloon angioplasty era, one of the largest studies evaluating the use of PCI for treatment of LMCA analyzed 127 patients. Successful dilatation was achieved in 94% of patients while the 4-year survival rate was only 36% for unprotected LMCA intervention and 90% for protected LMCA intervention. [8] Although the success rate of balloon angioplasty showed to be high, the long-term mortality rate for treatment of unprotected LMCA by this technique was high as well. Therefore, balloon angioplasty for treatment of unprotected LMCA was abandoned and CABG continued to be the gold standard therapy.

In the bare metal stent era, the favorable results of stent over balloon angioplasty for coronary *de novo* lesions prompted several studies to compare both techniques for treatment of unprotected LMCA disease. A registry enrolled 42 patients with unprotected LMCA and normal left ventricule function for PCI with BMS. The procedural success rate was 100%, angiographic restenosis occurred in 22% and the only death occurred 2 days after elective CABG for treatment of in-stent restenosis. [9]

A prospective study with 61 consecutive patients showed an acute procedural success of 100%, symptomatic recurrence of 20% at 6 months, one death before planned angiography and 80% remained asymptomatic during a mean follow-up of 16 months. [10]

A study with 140 consecutive unselected patients included 47 high CABG-risk patients and 93 low-CABG-risk patients. The procedural success rate was 100%. One-month mortality was 9% in the high-CABG-risk group and 0% in the low-CABG-risk group. The restenosis rate was 23% at 6 months while target lesion revascularization was required in 17.4%. [11]

Another study enrolled 92 consecutive patients, surgical revascularization being contraindicated for 39 patients and CABG being feasible for the remaining 53 patients. The group of patients with contraindication for CABG had lower left ventricular ejection fraction, higher surgical risk score and more severe LMCA stenosis. The procedural success rate was 100%. In-hospital mortality was 4% and during the 7 months follow-up the mortality rate was 6.8%, overall mortality being 3.8% in the CABG feasible group and 20.5% in the group of patients with contraindication for CABG. The target lesion revascularization rate was only 6.1% at 7 months. [12]

A study with 67 consecutive patients treated with BMS only (39 patients), rotational atherectomy plus stents (12 patients), directional atherectomy plus stents (13 patients) and directional atherectomy only (3 patients) showed no in-hospital death; however 3% of patients required in-hospital CABG, 3% suffered a Q-wave myocardial infarction, and 4.5% suffered a non-Q-wave myocardial infarction. Follow-up angiography at 5 months revealed 31.4% restenosis and, extending the follow-up to 31 months, the cumulative event rates were 16.4% of deaths (11.9% of them cardiac), 3% of myocardial infarction, and 23.9% of repeat revascularization. Reference vessel size and left ventricular function were found to be the most important predictors of favorable outcomes. [13]

The ULTIMA registry enrolled 279 patients treated with BMS, of these 46% were inoperable or at high surgical risk and 32% were at low risk (age <65 years, left ventricular ejection fraction >30% and without cardiogenic shock). The overall 1-year mortality rate from cardiac cause was 20.2%. There were no periprocedural deaths in the low-risk cohort, the 1-year mortality rate from cardiac cause was only 3.4% and the revascularization rate was 24.5% during the 1-year follow-up. Conversely, in the high-risk cohort the 1-year mortality rate from cardiac cause was 73.7% and the revascularization rate was 67.7%. Excess deaths were observed predominantly in patients initially deemed inoperable and the predictors of cardiac death were severe mitral regurgitation, left ventricular ejection fraction ≤ 30%, myocardial infarction with cardiogenic shock and serum creatinine ≥ 2.0mg/dl. [14]

The series of studies discussed above showed that the use of BMS for treatment of LMCA disease results in excellent procedural success rates as well as low in-hospital mortality and major adverse event rates. Another interesting data is a low mid-term mortality rate, especially among low-risk patients, while high mortality rates were observed predominantly in high-risk patients. However, the high rates of restenosis and target lesion revascularization in overall subgroups of patients were inacceptable when compared to the CABG rates. Therefore, CABG remained as the gold standard treatment, PCI with BMS being recommended only for inoperable or high-risk surgical patients.

3. Recent Advances in CABG

CABG has changed over the last years not only in the morbidity and mortality results over, but also with relation to the profile of patients operated on (older, with more comorbidities, and previously revascularized by PCI or even CABG). For this reason, we would like to stress a few points that have improved results in CABG over the last decades, bringing the overall perioperative mortality to below 2%.

3.1. The Use of Arterial Grafts

The excellent clinical results obtained using the left internal thoracic artery (LITA) and showing superior patency compared to saphenous veins and an improvement in survival of patients led to an increased interest in the use of other arterial grafts.

Therefore, the use of bilateral internal thoracic artery (ITA) has been expanded with the right internal thoracic artery (RITA) directed to revascularize the marginal branches of the CX artery, thus protecting the system from the left coronary artery with two arterial grafts. The use of bilateral ITA both reduced the incidence of a return of angina and myocardial infarction when compared to the use of LITA alone and increased the survival of patients 10 years after surgery [15].

Besides these two arterial grafts, other grafts such as the right gastroepiploic artery (RGEA), which was introduced in the practice of CABG in 1987, and the radial artery initially used as a graft in the 70's are used as well. The RGEA was primarily used to revascularize the right coronary artery and its posterior descending branch.

It gained less popularity among surgeons due to increasing technical difficulties in harvesting and using it [16]. The radial artery was abandoned because of low permeability. In the 90's it was reintroduced due to improvements in techniques, which improved the outcomes. In the literature, the 5-year patency has been reported to be around 80% [17].

The inferior epigastric artery has been used since the late 80's, but its use is limited by its anatomical features and has been directed to revascularize the coronary arteries of lesser importance. [18]

3.2. The Use of Bilateral Internal Thoracic Artery

The use of the LITA to revascularize the LAD allows patency rates to go up 90% at 1 year with more than 90% of grafts still functioning after a 20-year clinical follow-up [19]. The use of bilateral ITA grafts may offer additional benefits to patients, improving survival and lower incidence of cardiovascular events when compared to single ITA grafts. This significant increase in survival occurs when both ITA grafts are attached to the left coronary system, which means the LITA is anastomosed to the LAD and RITA to the branches of the CX (marginal arteries) [20].

The use of bilateral ITA grafts has increased the median survival by 15% in 20 years. Moreover, high-risk patients such as diabetics, the elderly, and those with left ventricular dysfunction also benefit from it. Especially in diabetic patients, the bilateral use of ITAs improves long-term survival and reduces the need for subsequent revasculari-zation procedures [21].

The technique using the RITA routed through the transverse sinus to revascularize the marginal artery was proposed by Puig et al. in the early 80's [22]. More recently, large studies have confirmed that the use of RITA grafts have excellent long-term angiographic patency when compared with that of the LITA to the LAD [20, 21]. The properties of the ITA endothelium contribute to these results. ITA grafts release more nitric oxide than radial artery grafts and saphenous vein do. This turns ITA into a "live conduit" which is able to dilate (adaptation of the flow) and therefore increase blood flow in response to the demand of the coronary and the area of myocardium it supplies. Moreover, the increased production of nitric oxide by the ITA endothelium can reduce and prevent atherosclerosis at the distal bed of the coronary artery revascularized with this graft [23].

3.3. Preservation of Arterial Vascularization of the Sternum

In CABG using bilateral ITA grafting, especially, in diabetic patients, the initial fear was the devascularization of the sternum with increased complications (infection and dehiscence).

The change in the technique of ITA dissection (skeletonization) reduced the incidence of these complications [24]. The skeletonization involves meticulous dissection of the ITA with minimum damage to adjacent tissues and preservation of the vascular trunks that keep sternal irrigation. As a result, it has been shown that there was a reduction in sternal complications (infection and dehiscence), a better preservation of respiratory function and a lower incidence of postoperative pain and dehiscence. Another advantage of this technique is that skeletonized ITA grafts have greater blood flow and allow more coronary artery bypasses when a sequential technique is used [25].

4. Recent Advances in PCI - the DES Era

Interventional cardiology is one of the medical fields in which more progress have been made since its beginning in 1977. It can be divided into 3 stages: (1) balloon angioplasty, (2) BMS, and (3) DES. The procedural success and the restenosis rates significantly improved between the balloon and BMS eras while the most important advance between the BMS and DES eras was a significant reduction in restenosis rates.

4.1. First Generation DES

The first generation of DES comprised sirolimus- and paclitaxel-eluting stents and significantly reduced restenosis rates when compared to BMS in *de novo* coronary lesions, which rekindled enthusiasm for PCI as an alternative to CABG for treatment of LMCA disease. A multicenter and randomized study enrolled 103 patients and compared the efficacy of paclitaxel-eluting stent (PES) to that of BMS for treatment of unprotected LMCA, distal LMCA being compromised in 70% of patients. The rates of death and myocardial infarction were similar, however the PES had lower binary restenosis (6% vs 22%, p=0.021) and target lesion revascularization (2% vs 16%, p=0.014) rates at 6-months follow-up. [26]

A multicenter registry compared clinical outcomes in 238 patients with ostial and shaft lesions after DES or BMS implantation in unprotected LMCA. In this registry, whose population was divided into quintiles according to the propensity score, DES was associated with lower 3-year cardiac mortality (7.8% vs 17.2%, p=0.047); nonetheless no beneficial effect on myocardial infarction (DES= 5.9% vs BMS= 2.1%, p=0.39) and target lesion revascularization (DES= 11.4% vs BMS= 10.7%, p=0.60) was found. [27]

Another multicenter registry enrolled 858 patients and compared clinical outcomes after treatment with sirolimus-eluting stents (SES) or PES at 3 years follow-up. This registry showed similar long-term clinical outcomes in terms of death (9.1% vs 11.0%, p=0.82), myocardial infarction (8.1% vs 8.0%, p=0.47), repeat revascularization (12.1 vs 10.6%, p=0.81) and stent thrombosis (0.6% vs 1.6%, p=0.18) for SES and PES, respectively. [28]

A single center randomized trial named ISAR-LEFT-MAIN compared the safety and efficacy of PES and SES for treatment of unprotected LMCA in 607 patients. The event rate at 1 year for SES and PES were similar: MACE (15.8% vs 13.6%, p=0.44), death (6.6% vs 5.0%, p=0.39), myocardial infarction (4.6% vs 5.0%, p=0.83), binary restenosis (19.4% vs 16.0%, p=0.3), and target lesion revascularization (7.8% vs 6.5%, p=0.49).

At 2 years, the event rates for SES and PES were also similar: MACE (20.6% vs 21.3%, p=0.96), death (8.7% vs 10.4%, p=0.64), myocardial infarction (4.6% vs 5.4%, p=0.69), and target lesion revascularization (10.7% vs 9.2%, p=0.47). Therefore, this study revealed that both SES and PES are safe, effective and provide comparable clinical and angiographic outcomes. [29]

4.2. Second Generation DES

There are several changes and improvements in the second generation of DES when compared to the first generation in terms of its platform, polymers and drugs. Most of the current DES are made of a cobalt-chromium alloy which allows for greater radial strength than stainless steel and thinner struts in the stent design. It is well known that thinner-strut stents cause less vessel wall injury and inflammatory reaction as well as lower restenosis rates. [30] As for polymers, new durable and new bioabsorbable polymers were tested and selected increasing biocompatibility and, consequently, reducing local inflammation. Bioabsorbable polymers are more biocompatible and cause less inflammation since they degrade over time and their degradation products cause less inflammatory reaction than durable polymers [31]. Finally, most of the current DES release sirolimus or analogs instead of paclitaxel or analogs because the limus family drugs are more potent and efficient in the inhibition of neointima hyperplasia [32-34].

A multicenter registry named LEMAX enrolled 173 consecutive patients that received everolimus–eluting stents (EES) for unprotected LMCA. Among them, 140 (81%) had involvement of the distal segment of LMCA, and 129/140 (92%) were treated with provisional side branch T-stenting with a side branch stenting rate of 20%. Angiographic success was achieved in all cases. At 12 months, the cumulative rate of major adverse cardiac or cerebrovascular events (MACCE) was 15%, death rate from any cause was 2.9%, stroke was 2.3%, Q-wave myocardial infarction was 1.2%, non-Q-wave myocardial infarction was 3.5%, target lesion revascularization was 2.9%, and definite or probable stent thrombosis was 0.6%. Therefore, this study revealed that unprotected LMCA stenting using EES and a strategy of provisional side branch T-stenting for distal lesions is safe and effective at midterm follow-up with a relatively low rate of events and reintervention at 1 year. [35]

The PRECOMBAT-2 study assessed 334 consecutive patients who received EES for unprotected LMCA and the results were compared with those of SES from the previous randomized study performed by the same authors. The 18-month incidence rates of MACCE (EES= 8.9% vs SES= 10.8%; 95% CI: 0.51-1.40, p= 0.51), death (EES= 2.1% vs SES= 2.2%; 95% CI: 0.20 to 1.69, p= 0.31), composite end-point of death, myocardial infarction and stroke (EES= 3.3% vs SES= 3.7%; 95% CI: 0.27 to 1.47, p= 0.29), and ischemia driven target vessel revascularization (EES= 6.5% vs SES= 8.2%; 95% CI: 0.63 to 2.06, p= 0.65) did not differ among patients who received EES or SES. However, late loss and restenosis rates in the branch were slightly lower in EES than in SES patients. Furthermore, a focal pattern was predominant in restenotic lesions. This study came to the conclusion that the second generation EES had a similar 18-month clinical outcome as the first generation SES. [7]

When the stenting technique was separated into the single- and 2-stent techniques in the above mentioned study, the kissing stenting technique and crush technique were used the most in SES and EES patients, respectively.

Ischemia-driven target vessel revascularization occurred in 5.3% SES and 5.1% EES patients in the single-stent group (log-rank p= 0.94) and 13.6% SES and 10.4% EES patients in the 2-stent group (log-rank p= 0.51). [7] Therefore, the stenting technique which is related to the coronary anatomy and the involvement of distal LMCA and its branches as well as to the number of stents required for the procedure, is relevant for the PCI outcomes.

4.3. Intravascular Ultrasound-Guided PCI, Thienopyridines and Bioabsorbable DES

The most comprehensive data published to date on the use of intravascular ultrasound (IVUS)-guided PCI in unprotected LMCA stems from a post-hoc analysis from the MAIN-COMPARE registry in which nonrandomized long-term clinical outcomes were evaluated in 201 comparable pairs of patients with balanced baseline differences. Kaplan-Meier incidence curves of log-rank 3-year outcomes revealed a significant lowering of the cumulative mortality rate within the IVUS-guided PCI group receiving DES compared with the angiography-guided group (4.7% vs 16%, p= 0.048). [36, 37].

A study showed that in patients with distal LMCA disease involving bifurcation and requiring 2 stents, a post-intervention ostial CX minimal luminal area (MLA) of $\geq 5.5mm^2$ was associated with a restenosis rate of 15% compared with 67% in those whose ostial CX MLA was $\leq 5.5mm^2$ (p=0.03) [37, 38]. Therefore, if PCI is chosen as the likely mode of LMCA revascularization, IVUS is strongly recommended for the guided PCI and expert consensus also recommends post-dilating the main branch to $> 8.5mm^2$ to reduce target lesion revascularization while aiming for an MLA of $> 5.5mm^2$ for the ostia of each branch [37, 38].

As for the dual antiplatelet therapy, the novel thienopyridines prasugrel and ticagrelor have shown clinical benefit over clopidogrel. The TRITON-TIMI 38 study revealed that prasugrel compared with clopidogrel was associated with significantly reduced rates of MACE (prasugrel= 12.1% vs clopidogrel= 9.9%, p< 0.001), myocardial infarction (7.4% vs 9.7%, p< 0.001), urgent target-vessel revascularization (2.5% vs 3.7%, p< 0.001) and stent thrombosis (1.1% vs 2.4%, p< 0.001) at 15 months; however prasugrel was associated with an increased risk of major bleeding. [39]

The PLATO study trial showed that ticagrelor compared with clopidogrel significantly reduced the rate of MACE (ticagrelor= 9.8% vs clopidogrel= 11.7%, p< 0.001), death from vascular causes (4.0% vs. 5.1%, p= 0.001), myocardial infarction (5.8% vs 6.9%, p= 0.005), and definite stent thrombosis (1.3% vs 1.9%, p= 0.009) without an increase in the rate of overall major bleeding at 12 months. [40]

The bioabsorbable drug eluting stents have shown very promising short- and mid-term results. The ABSORB trial assessed the results of bioabsorbable DES manufactured by Abbott Vascular (US) in 101 patients and revealed no possible, probable or definite thrombosis as well as low rates of ischemic-driven target lesion revascularization (6%) and MACE (9.0%) at 2-years follow-up. [41]

Several advances such as new stent platforms, polymers and drugs as well as new stenting techniques, adjunctive imaging methods, and more efficient and powerful antiplatelet drugs have improved PCI outcomes over the last years, turning PCI into a dynamic and fast-changing revascularization strategy with progressive better results over time.

5. Studies Comparing PCI and CABG

The studies that compared PCI with CABG can be divided into registries, randomized trials and meta-analyses.

5.1. Registries Comparing PCI and CABG

The large multicenter registry MAIN-COMPARE analyzed 2240 patients with unprotected LMCA disease who underwent either PCI or CABG. The majority of patients in this registry were considered to be at low surgical risk and propensity matching was used to define 542 matched pairs of patients in PCI and CABG groups with similar baseline characteristics. In the PCI group, 74.5% of patients received DES while 25.5% received BMS. The majority of patients from the CABG group had LMCA and 3-vessel disease whereas only one-fourth of patients from the PCI group did as well. The results at 3 years showed no difference in the risk of death (PCI= 7.8% vs CABG= 7.9 %, p= 0.45) as well as in the composite outcome of death, myocardial infarction or stroke (PCI= 9.3% vs CABG= 9.2%, p= 0.61). On the other hand, the rate of target vessel revascularization was significantly higher in the PCI group with a hazard ratio of 4.76 (PCI= 12.6% vs CABG= 2.6%; 95% CI: 2.80 to 8.11, p<0.001), which was even higher in the group of patients who received BMS (17.5%) than in the group of patients who underwent DES deployment (9.3%). Despite the markedly smaller rate of target vessel revascularization in patients who received DES compared to those who underwent BMS deployment, CABG continued to be associated with a lower rate of target vessel revascularization at 3 years than DES (PCI= 9.3% vs CABG= 1.6%, p<0.001). [42]

5.2. Randomized Trials Comparing PCI and CABG

The LE MANS was the first randomized trial to compare PCI for unprotected LMCA with CABG [43, 2]. A total of 105 patients were enrolled, of these only 35% of patients from the PCI group received DES and only 72% of patients from the CABG group received internal mammary grafts. The 30-day rate of MACCE was significant lower in the PCI group (PCI= 2% vs CABG= 13%, p= 0.03). At 1 year, there was no significant difference in death or myocardial infarction rates and MACCE was comparable in both groups (PCI= 28.8% vs CABG= 24.5%, p= 0.29), however the increase in the left ventricular ejection fraction was greater in the PCI group than in the CABG group (PCI= 3.3% vs CABG= 0.5%, p= 0.047) whereas repeat revascularization was lower in the CABG group (RR: 1.27; 95% CI: 1.05 to 1.54, p= 0.01). The main limitation of this trial was the small number of patients studied. [43]

The SYNTAX was a multicenter and randomized trial that enrolled 1800 patients to compare the outcomes between PCI with PES and CABG for treatment of LMCA or 3-vessel disease. A subgroup of 705 randomized patients who had LMCA disease out of 1800 patients was analyzed to evaluate the two therapeutic strategies in this setting. The primary end point was the MACCE at 1 year, which included all-cause death, cerebrovascular accident/stroke, myocardial infarction and repeat revascularization.

Out of 705 randomized patients with LMCA disease, approximately 25% had diabetes, 13% had isolated LMCA disease, 20% had LMCA plus 1 vessel, 31% had LMCA plus 2 vessels, and 37% had LMCA plus 3 vessels. Another relevant variable was the involvement of distal LMCA in approximately 61% of patients, which makes PCI more complex and usually requires bifurcation techniques. The overall 1-year results showed no difference in MACCE (PCI= 15.8% vs CABG= 13.6%, p= 0.44), death (PCI= 4.2% vs CABG= 4.4%, p= 0.88) and myocardial infarction (PCI= 4.3% vs CABG= 4.1%, p= 0.97); nevertheless, the cerebrovascular accident/stroke rates were significantly higher in patients who underwent CABG compared to those submitted to PCI (PCI= 0.3% vs CABG= 2.7%, p= 0.009), while the repeat revascularization rates were significantly higher in patients who underwent PCI than in those submitted to CABG (PCI= 12.0% vs CABG= 6.7%, p= 0.02). [5, 44]

SYNTAX outcomes stratified by the extension of vessel involvement showed 1-year MACCE rates higher in the CABG arm than the PCI arm in patients with isolated LMCA or LMCA plus 1 vessel disease, however MACCE rates were higher in the PCI arm than the CABG arm for patients with LMCA plus 2 vessels or LMCA plus 3 vessels disease. There was no significant difference between the groups for the composite safety end point of death, cerebrovascular accident/stroke and myocardial infarction, regardless of the extent of vessel involvement. Revascularization was significantly higher in patients with LMCA plus 2 vessels or LMCA plus 3 vessels disease who underwent PCI compared to those who underwent CABG, but not in patients with isolated LMCA or LMCA plus 1 vessel disease. [5] The SYNTAX 3-year clinical outcomes showed results similar to those of 1-year follow-up. There was no difference in MACCE (PCI= 26.8% vs CABG= 22.3%, p= 0.20), death (PCI= 7.3% vs CABG= 8.4%, p= 0.64) and myocardial infarction (PCI= 6.9% vs CABG= 4.1%, p= 0.14); however, the cerebrovascular accident/stroke rates were significantly higher in patients who underwent CABG compared to those submitted to PCI (PCI= 1.2% vs CABG= 4.0%, p= 0.02), while the repeat revascularization rates were significantly higher in patients who underwent PCI than in those submitted to CABG (PCI= 20.0% vs CABG= 11.7%, p= 0.004). [45] The recent SYNTAX 5-year follow-up results showed no significant difference in MACCE between the PCI and CABG treatment groups (PCI= 36.9% vs CABG= 31.0%, p= 0.12). By contrast, in the LMCA plus 3 vessel disease patients, MACCE rates were more than 50% higher at 5 years in patients assigned to PCI than in those assigned to CABG (PCI= 37.5% vs CABG= 24.2%, p<0.0001). [46]

The PRECOMBAT was a multicenter and randomized trial that assigned 600 patients with unprotected LMCA stenosis to undergo CABG (300 patients) or PCI with SES (300 patients). Isolated LMCA disease was found in only 10% of patients while LMCA plus 3-vessel disease in 41% and bifurcation involvement in 64.5%. The composite primary endpoint of death, myocardial infarction, stroke or ischemia-driven target vessel revascularization showed that PCI was not inferior to CABG at 1 year (PCI= 8.7% vs CABG= 6.7%; 95% CI: -

1.6 to 5.6, p= 0.01 for non-inferiority) and at 2 years (PCI= 12.2% vs CABG= 8.1%; 95% CI: 0.90 to 2.52, p= 0.12). There were no significant between-group differences in ischemia-driven target vessel revascularization at 1 year (PCI= 6.1% vs CABG= 3.4%, p= 0.13), however when the follow-up analysis was extended to 2 years it was lower in the CABG group than in the PCI one (PCI= 9.0% vs CABG= 4.2%, p= 0.022). [6]

The PRECOMBAT-2 study, which was partially discussed above, sought to evaluate the safety and efficacy of EES in 334 consecutive patients with unprotected LMCA stenosis. The results were compared with those of SES and CABG from the PRECOMBAT study; thus the PRECOMBAT 2 can be considered a study complementary to the PRECOMBAT. The second generation EES showed a comparable 18-month composite incidence of death, myocardial infarction, stroke and ischemia-driven target vessel revascularization as SES (EES= 8.9% vs SES= 10.8%; 95% CI: 0.51 to 1.40, p= 0.51) and CABG (6.7%; 95% CI: 0.78 to 2.54, p= 0.26). However, the incidence of ischemia-driven target vessel revascularization in the EES group was higher than in the CABG group (EES= 6.5% vs CABG= 2.6%; 95% CI: 1.17 to 6.58, p= 0.02), but comparable to the SES group (8.2%; 95% CI: 0.64 to 2.06, p= 0.65). [7] (Table 1).

5.3. Meta-Analyses Comparing PCI and CABG

A meta-analysis of 3,773 patients treated with PCI or CABG for unprotected LMCA stenosis of 8 cohort studies and 2 randomized trials showed that composite incidence of death, myocardial infarction and stroke were similar in the PCI- and CABG-treated patients at 1 year (odds ratio [OR]: 0.84; 95% CI: 0.57 to 1.22), 2 years (OR: 1.25; 95% CI: 0.81 to 1.94), and 3 years (OR: 1.16; 95% CI: 0.68 to 1.98). There was no difference in mortality in both patients groups at 1 year (OR: 1.00; 95% CI: 0.70 to 1.41), 2 years (OR: 1.27; 95% CI: 0.83 to 1.94), and 3 years (OR: 1.11; 95% CI: 0.66 to 1.86). Target vessel revascularization was significantly higher in the PCI group at 1 year (OR: 4.36; 95% CI: 2.60 to 7.32), 2 years (OR: 4.2; 95% CI: 2.21 to 7.97), and 3 years (OR: 3.30; 95% CI: 0.96 to 11.33). The interpretation of such results should take into account the usual limitations of a meta-analysis as well as the high rate of BMS (21%) used in PCI. [47]

Another larger meta-analysis with 11,148 subjects from 27 studies compared PCI and CABG in patients with LMCA disease. Patients in the PCI and CABG groups were comparable in terms of cardiovascular comorbidities, including diabetes mellitus, hypertension, chronic renal insufficiency, and prior stroke. However, patients in the CABG arm were older and had a higher proportion of hyperlipidemia, tobbaco smoking, prior myocardial infarction, peripheral arterial disease and history of congestive heart failure. On the other hand, patients in the PCI arm had lower left ventricular ejection fraction and higher proportion of patients with known coronary artery disease and prior PCI. Patients in the CABG arm had a higher proportion of LMCA disease plus 3-vessel involvement (CABG= 55.0% vs PCI= 32.0%, p<0.001), received an internal mammary artery graft in 90.1% of cases, and underwent off-pump CABG in 29.0%.

In the PCI arm, sirolimus- and paclitaxel-eluting stents were the predominant stent type used (58.5% and 27.1%, respectively), however a high proportion of BMS was used in 7 of the 27 studies analyzed.

Table 1. Studies comparing PCI and CABG

Study	N	Design	DES (%)	FU (years)	Death (%)			MI			Stroke			TVR			MACCE		
					PCI	CABG	p	PCI	CABG	p	PCI	CABG	p	PCI	CABG	P	PCI	CABG	P
Main - Compare	1084	Registry	74.5	3	7.8	7.9	0.45	-	-	-	-	-	-	12.6	2.6	<0.001	9.3*	9.2*	0.61
LE MANS	105	Randomized	35	1	1.9	7.5	0.37	1.9	5.7	NS	0	3.8	NS	28.8	9.4	0.01	28.8	24.5	0.29
SYNTAX	705	Randomized	100	1 3 5	4.2 7.3 -	4.4 8.4 -	0.88 0.64 -	4.3 6.9 -	4.1 4.1 -	0.97 0.14 -	0.3 1.2 -	2.7 4.0 -	0.009 0.02 -	12.0 20.0 -	6.7 11.7 -	0.02 0.004 -	15.8 26.8 36.9	13.6 22.3 31.0	0.44 0.20 0.12
PRECOMBAT	600	Randomized	100	1 2	2.0 2.4	2.7 3.4	NS 0.45	1.3 1.7	1.0 1.0	NS 0.49	0 0.4	0.3 .0.7	NS 0.56	6.1 9.0	3.4 4.2	0.13 0.02	8.7 12.2	6.7 8.1	0.01 0.12
PRECOMBAT 2	634	Registry	100	1.5	2.1	3.3	0.57	1.2	1.5	0.95	0.6	0.4	0.84	6.5	2.6	0.02	8.9	6.7	0.26

N: number of patients; DES: drug eluting stent; FU: follow-up; MI: myocardial infarction; TVR: target vessel revascularization; MACCE: major adverse cardiac and cerebrovascular events (all-cause mortality, myocardial infarction, stroke, and repeat revascularization); *data refers to all-cause mortality, myocardial infarction, and stroke; NS: not statistically significant.

The PCI group experienced lower MACCE (OR: 0.57; 95% CI: 0.36 to 0.89) and stroke (OR: 0.22; 95% CI: 0.11 to 0.44) rates in 30 days than the CABG group. At 12 months, PCI was associated with higher rates of repeat revascularization (OR: 3.72; 95% CI: 2.75 to 5.03), but lower rates of stroke (OR: 0.25; 95% CI: 0.14 to 0.44) and all-cause death (OR: 0.69; 95% CI: 0.49 to 0.97). At the longest follow-up of 60 months, PCI was associated with equivalent mortality (OR: 0.87; 95% CI: 0.71 to 1.08) and myocardial infarction (OR: 1.35; 95% CI: 0.99 to 1.85), lower rates of stroke (OR: 0.42; 95% CI: 0.28 to 0.62), and higher rates of repeat revascularization (OR: 3.54; 95% CI: 2.75 to 4.54) and MACCE (OR: 1.30; 95% CI: 1.10 to 1.55). The increased MACCE was driven by the higher repeat revascularization rates of PCI in comparison to CABG. [48]

The results from most of the registries, randomized clinical trials and meta-analyses comparing PCI and CABG for treatment of unprotected LMCA show that major clinical outcomes such as death, myocardial infarction, and composite endpoint of death, myocardial infarction and stroke are similar in both PCI and CABG at 1- to 5-year follow-up; however repeat revascularization rates are higher in patients who underwent PCI, especially, in those patients with LMCA plus 3-vessel disease.

5.4. Future Studies

The EXCEL trial is the major ongoing randomized clinical trial comparing PCI and CABG for treatment of LMCA. The aim of the study is to establish the safety and efficacy of the Xience Prime or Xience V everolimus eluting stents in subjects with unprotected LMCA disease by comparing them to CABG. The estimated enrollment is 2600 patients with unprotected LMCA disease. [49].

The clinical exclusion criteria of the Excel trial are prior PCI of the left main trunk at any time prior to randomization; prior PCI of any other coronary artery lesions within one year prior to randomization; prior CABG at any time prior to randomization; need for any concomitant cardiac surgery other than CABG; any recent myocardial infarction with CK-MB levels still elevated; subjects unable to tolerate, obtain or comply with dual antiplatelet therapy for at least one year; subjects requiring or who may require additional surgery within one year; the presence of any clinical condition(s) which leads the participating interventional cardiologist or participating cardiac surgeon to believe that there is no clinical equipoise; pregnancy or intention to become pregnant; non cardiac co-morbidities with life expectancy less than 3 years; and other investigational drug or device studies that have not reached their primary endpoint. [49]

The angiographic exclusion criteria of the Excel trial are LMCA diameter stenosis $<50\%$; SYNTAX score ≥ 33; left main reference vessel diameter <2.25 mm or >4.25 mm; and the presence of specific coronary lesion characteristics or other cardiac condition(s) which leads the participating interventional cardiologist or the participating cardiac surgeon to believe that there is no clinical equipoise. [49]

The importance of the EXCEL trial is mostly based on the number of subjects enrolled as well as on the characteristics of the drug eluting stents in use for PCI. This trial will be the largest one comparing PCI and CABG for treatment of LMCA, even larger than the SYNTAX trial.

The DES chosen for use in the PCI arm of EXCEL trial comprises a modern platform and a safe and efficacious polymer and drug (everolimus) combination. This second generation EES is superior to the first generation PES used in the SYNTAX trial according to the results of the randomized trials in patients with non-complex coronary artery disease [32, 33]; however there is no trial comparing both EES and PES in patients with LMCA disease. Finally, it should be pointed out that the exclusion of patients with high SYNTAX scores (≥33) in EXCEL trial, which restricts the evaluation to patients with low or intermediate SYNTAX scores, enhances expectation of better outcomes for PCI in the EXCEL trial rather than the ones obtained in SYNTAX trial.

6. Syntax Score

The SYNTAX score is a tool to evaluate the coronary lesion complexity in order to provide guidance to physicians on optimal revascularization strategies for patients with higher risk lesions [44]. Patients were divided into 3 groups according to the coronary and lesions anatomical features as follows: (1) low (Syntax score 0 to 22); (2) intermediate (23 to 32); or (3) high (≥ 33) [5].

The Syntax trial subgroup of patients with LMCA showed comparable MACCE outcomes at 1 year between PCI and CABG with either low (PCI= 7.7% vs CABG= 13.0%, p= 0.19) or intermediate (PCI= 12.6% vs CABG= 15.5%, p= 0.54) baseline Syntax scores. Repeat revascularization rates were also similar in patients who underwent PCI or CABG with either low (PCI= 7.7% vs CABG= 8.1%, p= 0.92) or intermediate (PCI= 9.7% vs CABG= 7.9%, p= 0.65) baseline Syntax scores. The only exception was all-cause death that was significantly higher in patients with intermediate Syntax scores who underwent CABG compared to patients who underwent PCI. On the other hand, in patients with high baseline Syntax scores the group who underwent PCI showed significantly higher MACCE outcomes than those treated by CABG (PCI= 25.3% vs CABG= 12.9%, p= 0.008). These increased MACCE rates in patients with high Syntax scores who underwent PCI were mainly driven by the significantly higher repeat revascularization rates (PCI= 17.2% vs CABG= 4.8%, p< 0.001). It is important to point out that the high Syntax score group of patients showed an increased distribution of LMCA with concurrent 3-vessel disease as well as an increased proportion of distal left main lesions. [5] (Figure 1). The 3-year follow-up showed no significant differences of MACCE in patients with LMCA disease who had low (PCI= 18.0% vs CABG= 23.0%, p= 0.33) or intermediate (PCI= 23.4% vs CABG= 23.4%, p= 0.90) Syntax scores.

However, in patients with LMCA disease and high Syntax scores, MACCE was significantly increased in those treated by PCI (PCI= 37.3% vs CABG= 21.2%, p= 0.003), as was repeat revascularization (PCI= 27.7% vs CABG= 9.2%, p< 0.001). (45) (Figure 2).

At 5 years, the results showed not significant differences of MACCE between PCI and CABG in patients with LMCA disease and low (PCI= 30.4% vs CABG= 31.5%, p= 0.74) or intermediate (PCI= 32.7% vs CABG= 32.3%, p= 0.88) Syntax scores, but, when analyzing patients with LMCA disease and high Syntax scores, the PCI group showed significantly higher MACCE rates than the CABG group (PCI= 46.5% vs CABG= 29.7%, p= 0.003). [46] (Figure 3).

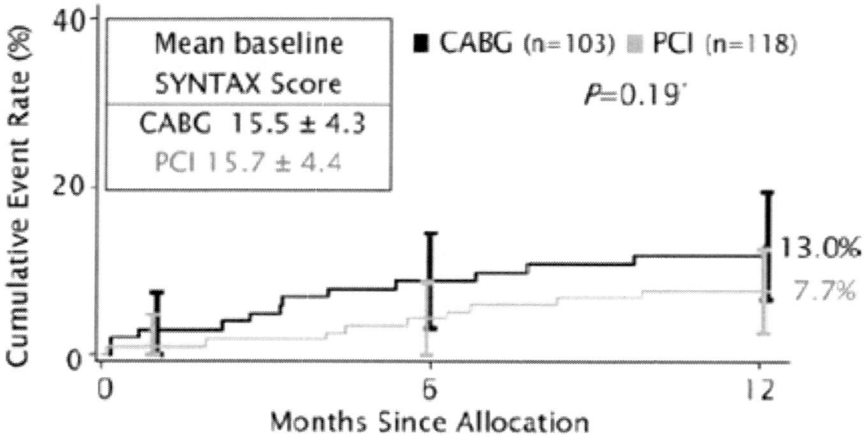

a

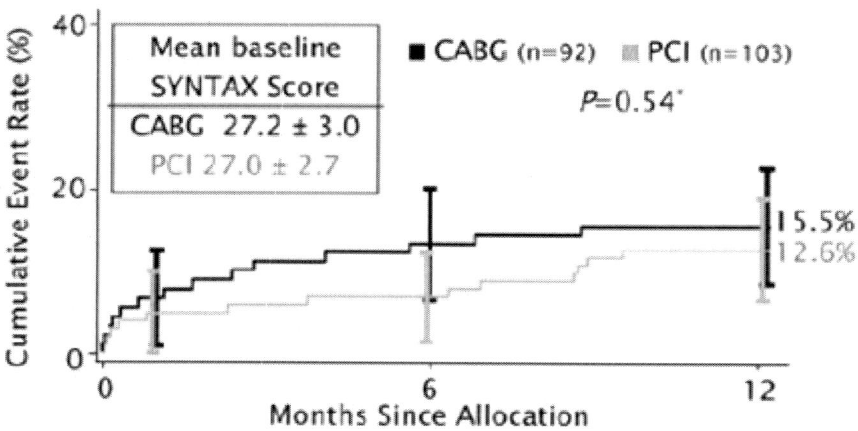

b

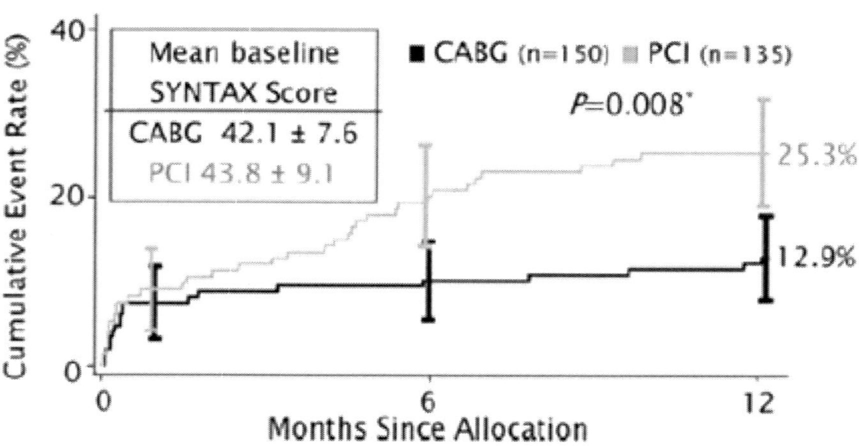

c

Figure 1. Kaplan-Meier estimates of 1-year MACCE by baseline SYNTAX score tercile. A) patients with low baseline SYNTAX score (0-22); B) intermediate baseline SYNTAX score (23-32); and C) high baseline SYNTAX score (≥33). [5]

7. Heart Team

The heart team concept is based on a multidisciplinary team to enable a balanced clinical decision-making according to current available clinical evidence-based data.

This concept allows using the expertise of different professionals to point out the benefits, risks and feasibility of the possible therapeutic strategies for each patient, taking into account the coronary anatomy, coronary artery disease site and severity, and patients' comorbidities.

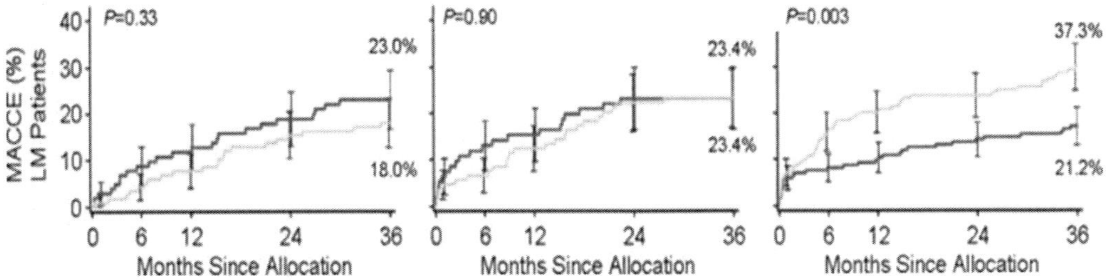

Adapted from Kappetein et al. Eur. H. J. 2011 (32): 2125-34.

Figure 2. MACCE rates in patients with LMCA disease according to the SYNTAX score. Time-to-event curves in the PCI (yellow line) and CABG (blue line) overall cohorts to 3 years according to the Syntax score: A) low (0-22); B) intermediate (23-32); and C) high.

A heart team must comprise at least a clinical cardiologist, an interventional cardiologist, and a cardiac surgeon.

The clinical cardiologist is in charge of searching for patient comorbidities and evaluating cardiac surgery risk. The interventional cardiologist has to evaluate PCI feasibility, estimate procedural risk and success rate, and plan the PCI approach. The cardiac surgeon is in charge of evaluating cardiac surgery risk and planning the CABG approach.

The presence of comorbidities usually requires the participation of additional professionals in the heart team according to the observed comorbidities such as nephrologists, pulmonologist, endocrinologists, neurologists, anesthesiologists, and others. Hence, the combined expertise and experience of different professionals significantly contributes to the most adequate decision-making.

Patients also must participate actively in the therapeutic decision-making process. Information provided to patients ought to be clear, objective, impartial, and based on current clinical evidence-based data, especially in situations in which consensus on the most adequate therapeutic strategy is not achieved. Patients need to understand the risks, benefits, and uncertainties related to their clinical situation and their treatment so that they can form a substantiated opinion and, therefore, help the heart team choose the most appropriate treatment option.

Therefore, the heart team in consonance with the patient's will is the best way to ensure an individualized, non-biased, and adequate decision-making based on a multidisciplinary team consensus as well as on current available clinical evidence-based data. (Figure 4).

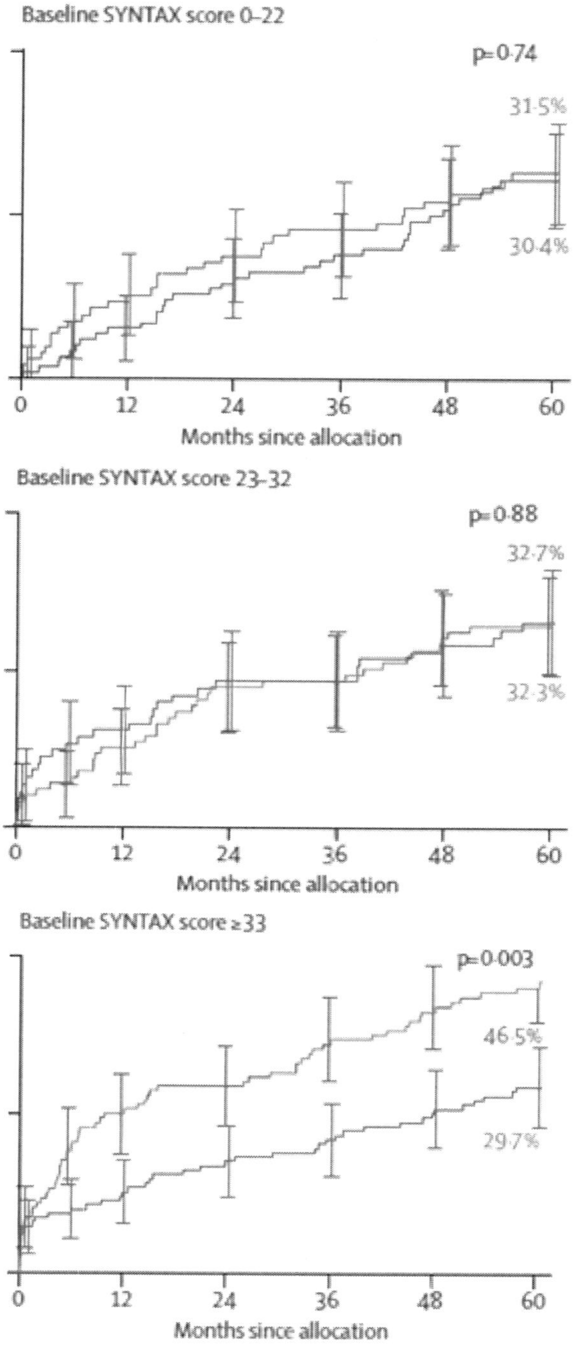

Figure 3. Kaplan-Meier cumulative event curves in patients with LMCA disease according to the SYNTAX score category. Time-to-event curves in the PCI (red line) and CABG (blue line) overall cohorts to 5 years according to the Syntax score: low (0-22), intermediate (23-32), and high [46].

Conclusion

CABG is still the first-choice revascularization strategy for treatment of LMCA disease according to the current guidelines [50, 51], however PCI is nowadays considered as an alternative therapeutic option, especially for high-risk surgical patients and for patients who deny CABG.

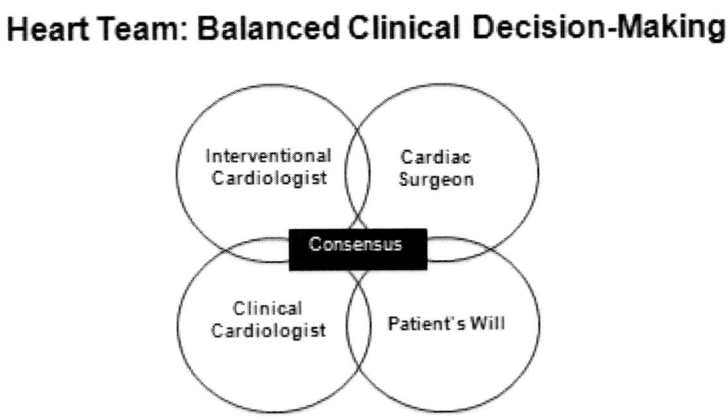

Figure 4. Balanced clinical decision-making based on the heart team consensus in consonance with the patient's will. The heart team is composed of at least an interventional cardiologist, a cardiac surgeon and a clinical cardiologist.

The PCI results change according to anatomical and clinical features and are similar to those of CABG in patients with low or intermediate Syntax scores and inferior to those of CABG in patients with complex LMCA lesions - high Syntax scores. Future randomized trials using second generation DES, IVUS-guided PCI, state-of-art bifurcation techniques and the new thienopyridines are required to define the role of PCI in the LMCA setting. The heart team relevance is already established, thus a multidisciplinary team in consonance with the patient's will is the best way to ensure an individualized, non-biased and adequate decision-making based on current available clinical evidence-based data.

References

[1] Ragosta, M., Dee, S., Sarembock, I. J., Lipson, L. C., Gimple, L. W., Powers, E. R. Prevalence of unfavorable angiographic characteristics for percutaneous intervention in patients with unprotected left main coronary artery disease. *Catheterization and cardiovascular interventions : official journal of the Society for Cardiac Angiography and Interventions*. 2006 Sep.;68(3):357-62. PubMed PMID: 16892431.

[2] Lee, M. S., Faxon, D. P. Revascularization of left main coronary artery disease. *Cardiology in review*. 2011 Jul.-Aug.;19(4):177-83. PubMed PMID: 21646871.

[3] Keogh, B., Kinsman, R. *Fifth National Adult Cardiac Surgical Database Report 2003*. Dendrite Clinical Systems. 2004.

[4] Chaitman, B. R., Bourassa, M. G., Davis, K., Rogers, W. J., Tyras, D. H., Berger, R., et al. Angiographic prevalence of high-risk coronary artery disease in patient subsets (CASS). *Circulation*. 1981 Aug.;64(2):360-7. PubMed PMID: 7249303.

[5] Morice, M. C., Serruys, P. W., Kappetein, A. P., Feldman, T. E., Stahle, E., Colombo, A., et al. Outcomes in patients with de novo left main disease treated with either percutaneous coronary intervention using paclitaxel-eluting stents or coronary artery bypass graft treatment in the Synergy Between Percutaneous Coronary Intervention with TAXUS and Cardiac Surgery (SYNTAX) trial. *Circulation*. 2010 Jun. 22;121(24): 2645-53. PubMed PMID: 20530001.

[6] Park, S. J., Kim, Y. H., Park, D. W., Yun, S. C., Ahn, J. M., Song, H. G., et al. Randomized trial of stents versus bypass surgery for left main coronary artery disease. *The New England journal of medicine*. 2011 May 5;364(18):1718-27. PubMed PMID: 21463149.

[7] Kim, Y. H., Park, D. W., Ahn, J. M., Yun, S. C., Song, H. G., Lee, J. Y., et al. Everolimus-eluting stent implantation for unprotected left main coronary artery stenosis. The PRECOMBAT-2 (Premier of Randomized Comparison of Bypass Surgery versus Angioplasty Using Sirolimus-Eluting Stent in Patients with Left Main Coronary Artery Disease) study. *JACC Cardiovascular interventions*. 2012 Jul.;5(7): 708-17. PubMed PMID: 22814775.

[8] O'Keefe, J. H., Jr., Hartzler, G. O., Rutherford, B. D., McConahay, D. R., Johnson, W. L., Giorgi, L. V., et al. Left main coronary angioplasty: early and late results of 127 acute and elective procedures. *The American journal of cardiology*. 1989 Jul. 15;64 (3): 144-7. PubMed PMID: 2525868.

[9] Park, S. J., Park, S. W., Hong, M. K., Cheong, S. S., Lee, C. W., Kim, J. J., et al. Stenting of unprotected left main coronary artery stenoses: immediate and late outcomes. *Journal of the American College of Cardiology*. 1998 Jan.;31(1):37-42. Pub Med PMID: 9426015.

[10] Wong, P., Wong, V., Tse, K. K., Chan, W., Ko, P., Wong, C. M., et al. A prospective study of elective stenting in unprotected left main coronary disease. *Catheterization and cardiovascular interventions : official journal of the Society for Cardiac Angiography and Interventions*. 1999 Feb.;46(2):153-9. PubMed PMID: 10348534.

[11] Silvestri, M., Barragan, P., Sainsous, J., Bayet, G., Simeoni, J. B., Roquebert, P. O., et al. Unprotected left main coronary artery stenting: immediate and medium-term outcomes of 140 elective procedures. *Journal of the American College of Cardiology*. 2000 May;35(6):1543-50. PubMed PMID: 10807458.

[12] Black, A., Cortina, R., Bossi, I., Choussat, R., Fajadet, J., Marco, J. Unprotected left main coronary artery stenting: correlates of midterm survival and impact of patient selection. *Journal of the American College of Cardiology*. 2001 Mar. 1;37(3):832-8. PubMed PMID: 11693759.

[13] Takagi, T., Stankovic, G., Finci, L., Toutouzas, K., Chieffo, A., Spanos, V., et al. Results and long-term predictors of adverse clinical events after elective percutaneous interventions on unprotected left main coronary artery. *Circulation*. 2002 Aug. 6;106 (6):698-702. PubMed PMID: 12163430.

[14] Tan, W. A., Tamai, H., Park, S. J., Plokker, H. W., Nobuyoshi, M., Suzuki, T., et al. Long-term clinical outcomes after unprotected left main trunk percutaneous

revascularization in 279 patients. *Circulation.* 2001 Oct. 2;104(14):1609-14. PubMed PMID: 11581137.

[15] Kappetein, A. P. Bilateral mammary artery vs. single mammary artery grafting: promising early results: but will the match finish with enough players? *European heart journal.* 2010 Oct.;31(20):2444-6. PubMed PMID: 20852294.

[16] Sasaki, H. The right gastroepiploic artery in coronary artery bypass grafting. *Journal of cardiac surgery.* 2008 Jul.-Aug.;23(4):398-407. PubMed PMID: 18598336.

[17] Kobayashi, J. Radial artery as a graft for coronary artery bypass grafting. *Circulation journal : official journal of the Japanese Circulation Society.* 2009 Jul.;73(7):1178-83. PubMed PMID: 19506319.

[18] Desai, M., Seifalian, A. M., Hamilton, G. Role of prosthetic conduits in coronary artery bypass grafting. *European journal of cardio-thoracic surgery : official journal of the European Association for Cardio-thoracic Surgery.* 2011 Aug.;40(2):394-8. PubMed PMID: 21216613.

[19] Pevni, D., Uretzky, G., Mohr, A., Braunstein, R., Kramer, A., Paz, Y., et al. Routine use of bilateral skeletonized internal thoracic artery grafting: long-term results. *Circulation.* 2008 Aug. 12;118(7):705-12. PubMed PMID: 18663087.

[20] Tatoulis, J., Buxton, B. F., Fuller, J. A. The right internal thoracic artery: the forgotten conduit--5,766 patients and 991 angiograms. *The Annals of thoracic surgery.* 2011 Jul.; 92(1):9-15; discussion -7. PubMed PMID: 21718825.

[21] Gansera, B., Schmidtler, F., Gillrath, G., Angelis, I., Wenke, K., Weingartner, J., et al. Does bilateral ITA grafting increase perioperative complications? Outcome of 4462 patients with bilateral versus 4204 patients with single ITA bypass. *European journal of cardio-thoracic surgery : official journal of the European Association for Cardio-thoracic Surgery.* 2006 Aug.;30(2):318-23. PubMed PMID: 16829096.

[22] Gerola, L. R., Puig, L. B., Moreira, L. F., Cividanes, G. V., Gemha, G. P., Souto, R. C., et al. Right internal thoracic artery through the transverse sinus in myocardial revascularization. *The Annals of thoracic surgery.* 1996 Jun.;61(6):1708-12; discussion 12-3. PubMed PMID: 8651771.

[23] Bayram, Z., Golbasi, I., Ozdem, S. S. The role of nitric oxide and potassium channels in the effect of adrenomedullin in human internal thoracic arteries. *Regulatory peptides.* 2010 Apr. 9;161(1-3):92-6. PubMed PMID: 20079376.

[24] Choo, S. J., Lee, S. K., Chung, S. W., Kim, J. W., Sung, S. C., Kim, Y. D., et al. Does bilateral pedicle internal thoracic artery harvest increase the risk of mediastinitis? *Yonsei medical journal.* 2009 Feb. 28;50(1):78-82. PubMed PMID: 19259352. Pubmed Central PMCID: 2649852.

[25] Une, D., Shimizu, S., Kamiya, A., Kawada, T., Shishido, T., Sugimachi, M. Both skeletonized and pedicled internal thoracic arteries supply adequate graft flow after coronary artery bypass grafting even during intense sympathoexcitation. *The journal of physiological sciences : JPS.* 2010 Nov.;60(6):407-13. PubMed PMID: 20839081.

[26] Erglis, A., Narbute, I., Kumsars, I., Jegere, S., Mintale, I., Zakke, I., et al. A randomized comparison of paclitaxel-eluting stents versus bare-metal stents for treatment of unprotected left main coronary artery stenosis. *Journal of the American College of Cardiology.* 2007 Aug. 7;50(6):491-7. PubMed PMID: 17678730.

[27] Tamburino, C., Di Salvo, M. E., Capodanno, D., Marzocchi, A., Sheiban, I., Margheri, M., et al. Are drug-eluting stents superior to bare-metal stents in patients with

unprotected non-bifurcational left main disease? Insights from a multicentre registry. *European heart journal*. 2009 May;30(10):1171-9. PubMed PMID: 19276194.

[28] Lee, J. Y., Park, D. W., Yun, S. C., Lee, S. W., Kim, Y. H., Lee, C. W., et al. Long-term clinical outcomes of sirolimus- versus paclitaxel-eluting stents for patients with unprotected left main coronary artery disease: analysis of the MAIN-COMPARE (revascularization for unprotected left main coronary artery stenosis: comparison of percutaneous coronary angioplasty versus surgical revascularization) registry. *Journal of the American College of Cardiology*. 2009 Aug. 25;54(9):853-9. PubMed PMID: 196 95467.

[29] Mehilli, J., Kastrati, A., Byrne, R. A., Bruskina, O., Iijima, R., Schulz, S., et al. Paclitaxel- versus sirolimus-eluting stents for unprotected left main coronary artery disease. *Journal of the American College of Cardiology*. 2009 May 12;53(19):1760-8. PubMed PMID: 19422982.

[30] Pache, J., Kastrati, A., Mehilli, J., Schuhlen, H., Dotzer, F., Hausleiter, J., et al. Intracoronary stenting and angiographic results: strut thickness effect on restenosis outcome (ISAR-STEREO-2) trial. *Journal of the American College of Cardiology*. 2003 Apr. 16;41(8):1283-8. PubMed PMID: 12706922.

[31] Pendyala, L. K., Matsumoto, D., Shinke, T., Iwasaki, T., Sugimoto, R., Hou, D., et al. Nobori stent shows less vascular inflammation and early recovery of endothelial function compared with Cypher stent. *JACC Cardiovascular interventions*. 2012 Apr.; 5(4):436-44. PubMed PMID: 22516402.

[32] Onuma, Y., Miquel-Hebert, K., Serruys, P. W., Investigators. S. I. Five-year long-term clinical follow-up of the XIENCE V everolimus-eluting coronary stent system in the treatment of patients with de novo coronary artery disease: the SPIRIT II trial. *EuroIntervention : journal of EuroPCR in collaboration with the Working Group on Interventional Cardiology of the European Society of Cardiology*. 2013 Jan. 22;8(9): 1047-51. PubMed PMID: 23339811.

[33] Yamasaki, M., Tsujino, I., Lima-Filho, M. O., Ako, J., Shimohama, T., Hasegawa, T., et al. Comparison of vascular response to the everolimus-eluting stent versus the paclitaxel-eluting stent: intravascular ultrasound results from the SPIRIT III trial. *EuroIntervention : journal of EuroPCR in collaboration with the Working Group on Interventional Cardiology of the European Society of Cardiology*. 2012 Oct.;8(6):724-31. PubMed PMID: 23086791.

[34] Silber, S., Windecker, S., Vranckx, P., Serruys, P. W., investigators RAC. Unrestricted randomised use of two new generation drug-eluting coronary stents: 2-year patient-related versus stent-related outcomes from the RESOLUTE All Comers trial. *Lancet*. 2011 Apr. 9;377(9773):1241-7. PubMed PMID: 21459430.

[35] Salvatella, N., Morice, M. C., Darremont, O., Tafflet, M., Garot, P., Leymarie, J. L., et al. Unprotected left main stenting with a second-generation drug-eluting stent: one-year outcomes of the LEMAX Pilot study. *EuroIntervention : journal of EuroPCR in collaboration with the Working Group on Interventional Cardiology of the European Society of Cardiology*. 2011 Oct. 30;7(6):689-96. PubMed PMID: 21986327.

[36] Park, S. J., Kim, Y. H., Park, D. W., Lee, S. W., Kim, W. J., Suh, J., et al. Impact of intravascular ultrasound guidance on long-term mortality in stenting for unprotected left main coronary artery stenosis. *Circulation Cardiovascular interventions*. 2009 Jun.;2 (3):167-77. PubMed PMID: 20031713.

[37] Puri, R., Kapadia, S. R., Nicholls, S. J., Harvey, J. E., Kataoka, Y., Tuzcu, E. M. Optimizing outcomes during left main percutaneous coronary intervention with intravascular ultrasound and fractional flow reserve: the current state of evidence. *JACC Cardiovascular interventions*. 2012 Jul.;5(7):697-707. PubMed PMID: 228147 74.

[38] Leon, M. B. *How to improve upon the left main cohort results from SYNTAX*. New York, NY2011.

[39] Wiviott, S. D., Braunwald, E., McCabe, C. H., Montalescot, G., Ruzyllo, W., Gottlieb, S., et al. Prasugrel versus clopidogrel in patients with acute coronary syndromes. *The New England journal of medicine*. 2007 Nov. 15;357(20):2001-15. PubMed PMID: 179 82182.

[40] Wallentin, L., Becker, R. C., Budaj, A., Cannon, C. P., Emanuelsson, H., Held, C., et al. Ticagrelor versus clopidogrel in patients with acute coronary syndromes. *The New England journal of medicine*. 2009 Sep. 10;361(11):1045-57. PubMed PMID: 197178 46.

[41] Ormiston, J. A., Serruys, P. W., Onuma, Y., van Geuns, R. J., de Bruyne, B., Dudek, D., et al. First serial assessment at 6 months and 2 years of the second generation of absorb everolimus-eluting bioresorbable vascular scaffold: a multi-imaging modality study. *Circulation Cardiovascular interventions*. 2012 Oct.;5(5):620-32. PubMed PMID: 23048057.

[42] Seung, K. B., Park, D. W., Kim, Y. H., Lee, S. W., Lee, C. W., Hong, M. K., et al. Stents versus coronary-artery bypass grafting for left main coronary artery disease. *The New England journal of medicine*. 2008 Apr. 24;358(17):1781-92. PubMed PMID: 183 78517.

[43] Buszman, P. E., Kiesz, S. R., Bochenek, A., Peszek-Przybyla, E., Szkrobka, I., Debinski, M., et al. Acute and late outcomes of unprotected left main stenting in comparison with surgical revascularization. *Journal of the American College of Cardiology*. 2008 Feb. 5;51(5):538-45. PubMed PMID: 18237682.

[44] Ong, A. T., Serruys, P. W., Mohr, F. W., Morice, M. C., Kappetein, A. P., Holmes, D. R., Jr., et al. The SYNergy between percutaneous coronary intervention with TAXus and cardiac surgery (SYNTAX) study: design, rationale, and run-in phase. *American heart journal*. 2006 Jun.;151(6):1194-204. PubMed PMID: 16781219.

[45] Kappetein, A. P., Feldman, T. E., Mack, M. J., Morice, M. C., Holmes, D. R., Stahle, E., et al. Comparison of coronary bypass surgery with drug-eluting stenting for the treatment of left main and/or three-vessel disease: 3-year follow-up of the SYNTAX trial. *European heart journal*. 2011 Sep.;32(17):2125-34. PubMed PMID: 21697170.

[46] Mohr, F. W., Morice, M. C., Kappetein, A. P., Feldman, T. E., Stahle, E., Colombo, A., et al. Coronary artery bypass graft surgery versus percutaneous coronary intervention in patients with three-vessel disease and left main coronary disease: 5-year follow-up of the randomised, clinical SYNTAX trial. *Lancet*. 2013 Feb. 23;381(9867):629-38. Pub Med PMID: 23439102.

[47] Naik, H., White, A. J., Chakravarty, T., Forrester, J., Fontana, G., Kar, S., et al. A meta-analysis of 3,773 patients treated with percutaneous coronary intervention or surgery for unprotected left main coronary artery stenosis. *JACC Cardiovascular interventions*. 2009 Aug.;2(8):739-47. PubMed PMID: 19695542.

[48] Alam, M., Huang, H. D., Shahzad, S. A., Kar, B., Virani, S. S., Rogers, P. A., et al. Percutaneous coronary intervention vs. coronary artery bypass graft surgery for unprotected left main coronary artery disease in the drug-eluting stents era--an aggregate data meta-analysis of 11,148 patients. *Circulation journal : official journal of the Japanese Circulation Society*. 2013;77(2):372-82. PubMed PMID: 23123552.

[49] Stone, G. W. S., P. W.; Sabik, J., Kappetein, A. P., et al. Evaluation of XIENCE PRIME Everolimus Eluting Stent System (EECSS) or XIENCE V EECSS Versus Coronary Bypass Surgery for Effectiveness of Left Main Revascularization. [Clinical Trial]. In press 2012.

[50] Fihn, S. D., Gardin, J. M., Abrams, J., Berra, K., Blankenship, J. C., Dallas, A. P., et al. 2012 ACCF/AHA/ACP/AATS/PCNA/SCAI/STS guideline for the diagnosis and management of patients with stable ischemic heart disease: a report of the American College of Cardiology Foundation/American Heart Association task force on practice guidelines, and the American College of Physicians, American Association for Thoracic Surgery, Preventive Cardiovascular Nurses Association, Society for Cardiovascular Angiography and Interventions, and Society of Thoracic Surgeons. *Circulation*. 2012 Dec. 18;126(25):e354-471. PubMed PMID: 23166211.

[51] Task Force on Myocardial Revascularization of the European Society of C, the European Association for Cardio-Thoracic S, European Association for Percutaneous Cardiovascular I, Wijns, W., Kolh, P., Danchin, N., et al. Guidelines on myocardial revascularization. *European heart journal*. 2010 Oct.;31(20):2501-55. PubMed PMID: 20802248.

In: Horizons in World Cardiovascular Research. Vol. 6
Editor: Eleanor H. Bennington
ISBN: 978-1-63321-298-5

Chapter 5

Does Cholesterol Drive Coronary Atherosclerosis?

William R. Ware*
University of Western Ontario, Canada

Introduction

The hypothesis that total cholesterol or LDL cholesterol is a risk factor or causative factor for coronary atherosclerosis was advanced without supporting evidence but rather was based on what appeared to be an association between serum cholesterol and acute coronary events. This observation was then extrapolated backwards since it was assumed that atherosclerosis was a prerequisite precursor of myocardial infarction or unstable angina. But this ignored several autopsy studies that showed no correlation between coronary atherosclerosis and circulating cholesterol in healthy accident victims, studies that were prior to or contemporary with the early evolution of the cholesterol-atherosclerosis hypothesis [1-3]. Atherosclerosis frequently starts at a relatively young age and progresses to eventually generate plaque, atheromas and stenosis with an impact on coronary circulation, and this pathology increases dramatically with age. To study the cholesterol-atherosclerosis hypothesis, it seems reasonable that one must actually observe the associated arterial manifestations and progression and how they relate to cholesterol levels, rather than focus on acute coronary events or one or two selected atheromas. However, for a considerable period, this was not or could not be done, but the cholesterol-atherosclerosis hypothesis still evolved to become a dogma as did the cholesterol-heart disease hypothesis.

In a review published in 2008, Paul Rosch describes and documents the early history of the cholesterol-heart disease hypothesis which was originally also called the heart-diet hypothesis [4]. In 1856 Virchow found cholesterol in human atheroma and thought it arose from an inflammatory process that injured the intimal lining of the arteries. This notion was

* Emeritus Professor, Faculty of Science; 14 Metamora Cres. London, Ontario, Canada N6G 1R3. E-mail: warewr@rogers.com. Tel: 519-472-2359.

reinforced in a studies where rabbits were fed large amounts of meat, eggs and milk. In 1909 Ignatowski reported this produced lesions similar to those seen in human atherosclerosis and Windaus subsequently found that such intimal atheromatous deposits contained enhanced cholesterol compared to normal arterial walls. These observations were quickly followed by experiments where rabbits were fed purified cholesterol and this also produced lipid-laden lesions. However, evidence of inflammation characteristic of obstructive plaque in humans was absent in rabbits. It is also well known that rabbits do not normally consume meat, eggs or cholesterol, and similar experiments on carnivores were a failure.

Rosch also points out that few physicians in the U.S. were aware of this early research and there was little interest in coronary heart disease. It was not a major problem since it caused less than 10% of all deaths in the 1920s. The dormant period lasted until the 1950s when Ancel Keys became interested in the increasing rate of heart disease in the US which was not seen in Italy. His approach involved ecological studies in a limited number of countries which produced remarkable correlations between mortality from heart disease and either fat intake or serum cholesterol levels. However, when others examined the data from 22 countries actually available at the time Keys published his early work involving 6 countries, the correlation was poor [5]. The cholesterol-heart disease hypothesis was nevertheless successfully launched and Keys' early research labelled "landmark." However, twenty years after the Keys' studies, Rosch quotes him as admitting on the basis of his feeding experiments that cholesterol in the diet does not matter unless you are a chicken or rabbit [4]. A recent review of the literature confirmed this, finding that the risk CVD associated with dietary cholesterol is at best very low and that dietary cholesterol has negligible clinical implications [6]. It is thus interesting that limiting dietary cholesterol is still a pillar of modern guidelines.

The cholesterol-heart disease hypothesis was then examined in the famous and still ongoing Framingham study, based on a long follow-up of the population of a small city in Massachusetts. Framingham is widely viewed as providing solid evidence that high cholesterol levels are associated with elevated risk of heart attack. Cholesterol was described as a powerful predictor in spite of the observation that half of heart attacks occurred in individuals with normal or low cholesterol [7]. Framingham also found that those with a decline in serum cholesterol over a 30-year period had a *greater* risk of heart-disease related mortality. With each 1% drop in cholesterol resulted in an 11% increase in coronary mortality [8]. In 1992 in a paper on Framingham results, William Castelli, the director of the study at the time, stated that "the more saturated fat one ate, the more cholesterol one ate, the more calories one ate, the lower the person's serum cholesterol" [9].

The next significant study was the *Multiple Risk Factor Intervention Trial* (MRFIT). The results of one part of the MRFIT trial which involved following 300,000 so-called screenees for 6 years were presented as definitive by pointing to the result that the risk of dying from a heart attack (MI) with total cholesterol (TC) above 265 mg/dL was an impressive 4.3 times higher than if it was below 170 mg/dL [10]. However, the absolute percentage difference between the number of deaths from heart attack when these two groups were compared was only 1% (1.3% vs. 0.3%). Thus as a risk factor, elevated cholesterol did not seem to make much difference to almost all of the subjects studied. This is an example where relative risk can be very misleading, but the practice of emphasizing relative risk continues to this day. Nevertheless, cholesterol was accepted as a major risk factor for heart disease and even cardiovascular disease in general, and dietary cholesterol, while having a significant influence on serum levels in only a very small fraction of individuals, was demonized and this became a significant food-marketing tool.

The large number of lipid lowering trials that followed after the development of statin drugs provided the icing on the cake. Very small absolute differences in benefit were found for true primary prevention and somewhat larger but still small benefits observed for secondary prevention, but the large relative risk reductions of 20-30% were extremely persuasive. Only the critics kept harping on absolute risk reduction. The decrease in events associated with statin therapy was believed to be due to the lowering of LDL cholesterol, a fallacy in formal logic commonly termed *post hoc ergo propter hoc*. Attempts to establish a causative relationship have been plagued by the ever increasing number of pleiotropic effects (non-lipid lowering effects) associated with statins [11-13]. Furthermore, a series of recent negative lipid lowering trials have unsettled some who held the cholesterol-heart disease hypothesis as proven [14].

Over the years since the cholesterol-heart disease hypothesis was put forward and accepted, there have been numerous studies which have exposed inconsistencies and contradictions. For example, a further examination of the Framingham data revealed that once men reached 47, it did not matter if cholesterol was high or low if survival was the issue [8]. For sudden cardiac death, which is the case in about 50% of acute cardiac event-related deaths, the risk has been found in all studies to be completely independent of cholesterol levels [15]. Many other examples could be cited, but in the overall picture that emerged, it became evident that there were many factors at play including age, gender, country of residence and its culture, diet, exercise, smoking, hypertension, lipid sub-fractions such as lipoprotein(a) and apolipoproteins A and B, C-reactive protein, diabetes, obesity, the dyslipidemia of the metabolic syndrome, poor dental hygiene, homocysteine and psychological stress [16, 17]. In the context examining hypotheses concerning coronary atherosclerosis and the primary prevention of coronary heart disease, the formation, prevalence and progression of coronary plaque should now be primary endpoints in studies that evaluate the significance of this collection of risk factors, especially since plaque can be quantified by non-invasive CT scans. To some extent, this is ongoing, but it may take decades for a real evidence base to be developed and observational studies will remain essential. As will be discussed and documented below, non-invasive CT scans have provided a serious obstacle to the cholesterol-atherosclerosis hypothesis by failing to find any association between cholesterol levels and the prevalence or progression of calcified coronary plaque, which incidentally is in agreement with the early autopsy studies.

Since the cholesterol-heart disease hypothesis was advanced, critics wrote books, commentary in journals and letters-to-the-editor of journals detailing and documenting the problems with the hypothesis in an attempt to provide perspective, but these were ignored or ridiculed or simply not published. The authors of three of the books summarizing the critics' evidence are medical doctors [18-20]. These books, while written for a mixed audience, are a good source of citations for studies in the earlier peer reviewed literature that over the years have raised concerns. A very comprehensive and thoroughly documented book dealing with all the essential aspects of the heart-diet-cholesterol subject also recently appeared [21].

Unrecognized heart disease and in particular silent atherosclerosis is very common. When an "inside view" from a CT scan is lacking, clinicians attempt to non-invasively quantify the risk of developing symptomatic coronary or cardiovascular disease and clinically relevant events by using factors such as blood pressure, total and HDL cholesterol, smoking, age, gender and the presence or absence of diabetes, the latter being generally regarded as a risk equivalent to established heart disease. The end result is a score such as the Framingham Risk Score from which is derived an estimated 10-year risk of an acute coronary event and patient stratification into low, intermediate and high risk categories [22]. Such an approach is common but not without its critics or its defects, especially since age plays a central role. A man can be 74 with no risk factors and still be at intermediate risk. The Framingham Risk Score also has variable validity outside of the North America. The results of risk assessment influence medication decisions and treatment targets. So called "novel" or "emerging" risk factors such as homocysteine, triglycerides, C-reactive protein, apopolyprotein B, lipoprotein (a) and fibrinogen are also on occasion considered in treatment decisions since they can be quantified [23, 24], but evidence of the actual benefits of intervention to influence these emerging risk factors is sparse, inconsistent or non-existent.

Intermediate risk according to the Framingham Risk Score (10-20%) involves a huge grey area. Thus one school of thought believes that a more effective approach should employ the non-invasive measurement of coronary plaque by CT scanning in order to confirm the assignment of intermediate risk of acute events. When this approach has been tested, it is always found that some individuals change risk categories, both up and down, and such changes have a significant impact on treatment recommendations [25]. However, the use of CT screening for large populations has encountered considerable opposition from those concerned with overdiagnosis and overtreatment, and also from those who believe the cancer risk of the radiation exposure is significant. Incidentally, the magnitude of the risk associated with low-level radiation is considerably more debatable than generally recognized, and the field of so-called radiation hormesis is attracting increased attention [26-29]. Given the discovery of significant coronary plaque, there remains the question of an appropriate and in particular an effective intervention and, as will be discussed below, the typical response to a significant plaque burden often entails aggressive management of all traditional risk factors.

It is not the purpose in this review to examine in detail the all the issues outlined above. Rather, the focus is on subclinical atherosclerosis in both non-diabetic and diabetic individuals and its association with circulating cholesterol. Related aspects include primary prevention intervention based on cholesterol levels in populations free of symptomatic cardiovascular disease at baseline. Coronary atherosclerosis is, for almost all individuals, a prerequisite precursor of acute coronary events. Evaluating coronary atherosclerosis advanced rapidly after the introduction of electron beam computed tomography (EBCT) and the Agatston method of generating a convenient measure (calcium score) of the extent of calcified coronary artery plaque. The coronary artery calcium score provides significant improvement in risk assessment of coronary atherosclerosis in asymptomatic individuals, both non-diabetics [25] diabetics [30], as compared to using traditional risk factors. EBCT also represents an improvement over ultrasonic carotid artery assessment extrapolated to coronary atherosclerosis since there is very poor correlation between carotid and coronary atherosclerotic burden [31]. EBCT or variations of this non-invasive technique also offer an attractive adjunct to studies using acute coronary events as endpoints and allows examination of risk factor correlations that are relevant to the arterial process that preceded these events.

In the past 15 years a number of studies have examined the prevalence or progression of coronary plaque for both non-diabetic and non-diabetic individuals viewed as free of symptomatic coronary heart disease or cardiovascular disease. In these studies there was also extensive risk factor information collected, including blood lipid levels. In addition, the results of pharmaceutical intervention to halt or reverse progression of coronary atherosclerosis have been reported in a number of studies. Thus the information needed for a critical evaluation of the cholesterol-atherosclerosis hypothesis now exists. The focus in this review will be on the association between serum cholesterol and silent or so-called subclinical atherosclerosis, as manifest by calcified plaque.

Individuals Free of Coronary Heart Disease and Diabetes

Cholesterol and in particular LDL has been called *the driving force of atherosclerosis* [32]. But this widely held view is merely a hypothesis based almost entirely on studies with cardiac event endpoints rather than direct measurement of coronary plaque burden and progression. But as briefly discussed above, cholesterol and LDL are rather weak predictors of CHD events and statin drugs produce very small absolute risk reduction in the context of primary prevention.

As will be discussed at length below, extensive data continues to accumulate indicating that serum total cholesterol (TC) and LDL cholesterol in individuals asymptomatic of CHD are not associated with either the extent or progression of coronary plaque [33]. The vast majority of the data relevant to the issues addressed in this review are based on EBCT scans. Most radiologists use the Agatston Score protocol to quantify plaque burden. This score ranges from zero to several thousand and provides the basis for inter-study comparisons and the development of generalized risk-score relationships. This non-invasive imaging can prevent unnecessary concern or lead to therapy [34]. A zero calcium score is particularly significant for the individual involved. Eight studies involving over 27,000 asymptomatic patients found that those with zero calcium score had an extremely low average annual coronary event rate (6.6 per 10,000), even though individuals with a zero calcium score may still have non-calcified plaque or stenosis [35]. Furthermore, the risk of adverse coronary events strongly increases with calcified plaque burden [34].

Some Inconvenient Questions

Those who believe the conventional wisdom that cholesterol in general and LDL in particular drives coronary atherosclerosis must address the following inconvenient questions which are based on the measurement mostly of calcified but also non-calcified coronary plaque as surrogates for coronary atherosclerosis. It is important to note that this approach avoids the use of carotid artery intima thickness as a surrogate for coronary atherosclerosis, a popular approach which suffers from being indirect and, as mentioned above, from a very poor correlation. It is also important to note that the correlation between carotid artery intima-media thickness and coronary atherosclerosis, the earlier traditional method of judging atherosclerosis, is modest, especially in asymptomatic individuals or those merely suspected of CHD, where correlation coefficients range mostly between 0.2 and 0.3 [31]. Results based on carotid intima-media studies, still a popular approach especially in studies of progression-regression, should be extrapolated to coronary artery atherosclerosis only with reservations.

If the hypothesis is true, then:

- Why have autopsy studies of the correlation between the extent of coronary atherosclerosis and serum cholesterol yielded null results [1-3]? The objection that the blood samples, mostly from accident or suicide victims, were obtained too long after death has been discredited [3]. These studies, incidentally, looked all types of plaque.
- Why was it found by Hecht et al. [36] that total cholesterol (TC) and LDL cholesterol did not correlate with either the extent or prematurely of coronary artery calcium (CAC) burden in 1105 consecutive, asymptomatic individuals self-referred for EBCT? Why did these same researchers [37] fail to find a correlation between LDL or TC and the CAC percentile (correlation coefficient 0.06 with a scatter plot showing no visible correlation) for 304 asymptomatic women?
- Why did Johnson et al. [38] find when 1653 men and women without a history of CHD were subjected to coronary CT angiography using contrast media that there was there no correlation between total plaque burden (calcified, mixed and non-calcified) and total serum cholesterol with Spearman's rho = -0.04?
- Why in a study of the impact of psychosocial factors on coronary calcification in 780 male and female asymptomatic individuals, did Kop *et al* find that there was no correlation between TC or LDL and CAC score with Spearman correlation coefficients near zero? Multivariate analysis gave an odds ratio of 1.005 for LDL [39].
- Why in the St. Francis Heart Study [40] was no correlation found between LDL levels and CAC scores in 4,903 asymptomatic individuals?
- Why for adults with familial hypercholesterolemia, were age-adjusted CAC scores not associated with cholesterol levels, according to a study by Jensen et al. [41]?
- Why in a study by Kornmal et al. [42] of approximately 2900 individuals was the relative risk of incident CAC associated with LDL only 1.03 per 10 mg/dL and barely reached statistical significance (lower CI 1.01)?
- Why did Sung et al. [43] in a recent study of CAC and coronary risk find negligible correlation between LDL or TC and calcium scores in 1653 asymptomatic individuals judged free of CHD (Spearman's coefficients = 0.07 and 0.08 respectively)?
- Why in a study by Ramadan et al. [44] of 177 asymptomatic patients of intermediate risk of CHD was a null result found for the odds of a positive association between CAC and LDL in a multivariate model (OR = 1.022, $p = 0.361$)?
- Why when 100 asymptomatic individuals underwent EBCT were Takamiya *et al* [45] unable to find any association whatsoever between LDL and CAC when using three multiple logistic regression models?
- Why did a study by Lee et al. [46] find that while insulin resistance positively correlated with CAC progression in a community based group of about 900 healthy adults, they failed to find in multivariate regression any correlation with TC or LDL.
- Why in a study by Budoff et al. [47] of CAC progression and all-cause mortality, was a strong association found for subjects with calcium score (CACS) ≥ 30, and this relationship was not changed by adjustment for hypercholesterolemia?

- Why in a study by Park et al. [48] of 5239 asymptomatic patients free from known coronary artery disease did multivariate analysis of factors significant for a CACS > 100 not include TC or LDL?
- Why did a recent study from Korea by Lee et al. [49] of the relationship between CAC and bone mineral density fail to find in either univariate of multivariate analysis any correlation between the CACS and LDL?
- Why in a study by Jeon et al. [50] of the association between estradiol and CAC in postmenopausal women did a univariate analysis of factors associated with a calcium score ≥ 100 fail to find LDL significant ($p = 0.49$). Age, time since menopause and hypertension were the strongest risk factors.
- Why in a study by Rondanelli et al. [51] of progression in a group initially having CACS of zero, was it found in univariate analysis that dyslipidemia was insignificant and thus omitted from multivariate analysis? Diabetes, hypertension and age > 40 remained significant.
- Why in a study by Coylewright et al. [52] was neither TC or LDL significant in a multivariate analysis when one compared the risk of having high (400-999) or very high (≥ 1000) calcium scores. This also found that while high coronary calcium was associated with the risk of CHD death and myocardial infarct, very high values were more predictive of angina.
- Finally and perhaps the most important question, why is there no association between TC or LDL and the progression of CAC? At least 10 studies in addition to those mentioned above have directly addressed this issue and all cited involved EBCT [42,53-61].

One study Turner *et al* [62] recently appeared which appears to contradict the above picture. As part of the Multi-Ethnic Study of Atherosclerosis (MESA), the association of CAC with a combination of lipid parameters with was examined. For CAC, the question was zero or > zero. The lipid parameters were hypercholesterolemia (LDL ≥ 160 mg/dL, TGs < 150mg/dL) and no restriction on HDL. Combined hyperlipidemia changed the TGs to ≥ 150 mg/dL. The analysis treated the variables as dichotomous and found a small but statistically significant risk of CAC > 0 when hypercholesterolemia or hyperlipidemia was present. The association with LDL became progressively weaker with increasing age. While elevated TGs have been implicated in some studies, the finding for just hypercholesterolemia is surprising and may reflect the design of the study since the result is contrary to all of the above cited studies as well as those discussed below that concern diabetics.

A noteworthy exception to the above picture was reported in 2010. The results were part of the ongoing Coronary Artery Risk Development in Young Adults study (CARDIA) and indicated that non-optimal levels of LDL and HDL during the early years of adulthood were independently associated with coronary atherosclerosis two decades later, but at this later time, the plaque burden was no longer dependent on lipid levels [63]. The investigators calculated time-averaged cumulative exposures to blood lipids between ages 20 and 35 and then examined CAC burden later in life at mean age of 45. This implies LDL as a factor in the initiation of atherosclerosis at a young age, but as has been discussed above and confirmed in this study, in older persons the correlation disappears.

One explanation for this apparent inconsistency is psychological stress which elevates LDL cholesterol in this age group [64-66]. The cited studies apply to the age group studied in CARDIA, the stress was mostly of academic origin, and the LDL elevations similar when compared to the CARDIA data. In this view, LDL is simply a marker for psychological stress. When the stress was continuous, as it was in one study, the elevation of LDL levels persisted [64]. Psychological stress might then operate to produce atherosclerosis through a blood pressure mechanism, and this has been documented in another CARDIA study of young adults where blood pressure reactivity to psychological stress was a positive factor in predicting CAC 13 years later [67].

Hypotheses are not proven but exist until falsified (to paraphrase Karl Popper). One is reminded of the famous black swan example. Here we seem to have a significant number of black swans! The obvious answer to the questions raised is that the hypothesis is false. Twenty-eight studies, all clearly relevant, contradict the hypothesis that TC or LDL drives atherosclerosis, either when plaque burden or progression is at issue, and this observation does not include twelve studies cited below that focus entirely or type 2 diabetic populations and reach the same conclusion. These questions directly address coronary plaque and thus do not involve arguments based on studies concerning other vascular beds. The results are consistent over a wide range of age and nationality for both genders. In many of the studies presented as evidence, the lack of an association was based on multivariate analysis. It seems justified to regard this as compelling evidence.

It might be argued that total plaque rather than calcified plaque should be the basis for judging the hypothesis, but in general, non-calcified plaque represents a small fraction of the total plaque burden. One study cited in the above set of questions [38] did indeed look at total plaque including non-calcified, calcified and mixed and found no correlation with TC. In addition, another study [68] found progression of non-calcified plaque volume in coronary arteries to be independent of whether patients had high or low LDL. Also, the autopsy studies looked at total plaque. The issue of different plaque types will be discussed in more detail below.

Implications and Related Cholesterol Issues

LDL as a Surrogate Endpoint for CHD Risk

The above results do not support the widely held view that a diet high in saturated fat is atherogenic and increases the risk of CHD because it modestly raises LDL which in turn, so it is argued, stimulates atherosclerosis. This role of saturated fat in CHD was already conclusively challenged two decades ago [69]. Since then three studies and a meta-analysis all reached the same negative conclusion [70-73]. Also, increased saturated fat intake leads to a beneficial *decrease* in small dense LDL, and greater intake in saturated fat was found to *reduce* progression of coronary arthrosclerosis [74]. Nevertheless, reduction of saturated fat intake has for a long time been central to preventive and treatment guidelines. A general discussion of the use surrogates in the context of CHD has recently appeared [75].

Determinants of Plaque Progression

In the ten coronary plaque progression studies cited above, the prior existence of calcified plaque and hypertension were the most frequently found statistically significant positive risk factors, followed by diabetes, lipoprotein(a), triglycerides, smoking, the Framingham risk score, and HDL (negative association), but these latter factors were not consistently identified. In terms of modifiable factors, the only strong association consistently found was with hypertension. This association was also found in a study of individuals having a zero calcium score at baseline [57]. However, insulin resistance also appears very important not only in progression but also in plaque burden [46, 76]. Diet and exercise can influence insulin resistance, HDL and triglyceride levels, and patients are presumably always advised to stop smoking.

Plaques and Lipid Lowering

The null results from the large number of trials cited above suggest that lowering LDL should have no impact on the prevalence or progression of coronary plaque and calls into question the proposed approach which targets LDL for asymptomatic persons of intermediate traditional risk of CHD who exhibit elevated coronary calcium [77, 78]. Several randomized clinical trials employing statins and enrolling asymptomatic individuals support this inference. Randomized, placebo controlled studies found that statin therapy had no effect on the progression of coronary calcification as measured by the calcium score [79-81].

In trials comparing doses or different statins, atherosclerosis progression as measured by calcified plaque showed no relationship with on-treatment LDL levels and intensive therapy was unable to attenuate coronary artery calcium progression [80, 82, 83]. A recent randomized trial also failed to support the hypothesis that baseline CRP levels modify the vascular benefits of statin therapy [84]. However, one study found statin therapy reduced plaque burden for non-calcified plaque but not CAC score or total plaque burden [85]. This is inconsistent with the studies discussed above and only 11% of the patients had non-calcified plaque.

Lipid-Lowering Trials in Primary Prevention

The failure of statins to influence prevalence or progression of atherosclerosis prompts questions regarding statins for primary prevention of CHD. Michel de Lorgeril has discussed nine CHD-related negative cholesterol lowering trials done since the Vioxx affair of 2005 resulted in tightening of rules and regulations concerning conduct and reporting of trials [14]. This paper extends earlier related observations from de Lorgeril and colleagues [86, 87]. These recent results challenge the cholesterol hypothesis as did the observation that half of a large serial cohort admitted to a hospital for heart attack (MI) had low or very low LDL [88]. In addition, a recent meta-analysis that recalculated primary prevention trial results after excluding all subjects with CHD found no impact on all-cause mortality [89]. It is interesting in view of the recent JUPITER lipid and CRP lowering trial [90], that three recent studies directly examined the correlation between the coronary calcium score and high-sensitivity CRP levels and found that there was no association [54, 91, 92]. This was confirmed in the JUPITER cohort where obesity was the important factor associated with atherosclerosis [93]. JUPITER has also been criticized as flawed [94]. It may also have been confounded by the fact that rosuvastatin appears unique among statins in that it strongly elevates vitamin D levels and it is well known that low vitamin D status is a risk factor for CHD and also for coronary atherosclerosis [95].

A recent study reported a meta-analyses of statin intervention RTCs restricted to pure primary prevention (11 studies) and selected studies after eliminating 4 trials because of suspected high risk of bias according to the Cochrane Risk of Bias Tool. It was found for the restricted set that there was no statistically significant risk associated with overall mortality, an absolute risk reduction of 1.3% in major CHD events with an a number needed NNT to treat over the period of the study (typically 4-5 years) of 77 to prevent one event. For 11 studies the absolute risk reduction for major CHD events was 1% with a resultant NNT of 100 [96]. Of the seven RTCs, AFCAPS, ALLHAT-LLT, ASPEN, PROSPER, WOSCOP carried most of the weight with HYRIM, and PREVEND-IT contributing less than 2%.

Cholesterol as a Risk Factor for CHD

This association is based mostly on studies of the risk of CHD events and not on directly observed coronary atherosclerosis identified by calcified plaque. A recent review [97] summarizes six disturbing facts including the evidence that for women, men over 47 and in general the elderly, hypercholesteremia is a very weak risk factor for CHD, or in most cases, not a risk factor at all. Studies of familial hypercholesteremia (FH) also fail to support the hypothesis if one considers that in young people, where most of the excess mortality is seen, FH includes well known abnormalities in the coagulation system which constitute a strong CHD risk factor. In young men, the observed association may be confounded by the connection between cholesterol levels and stress-induced exaggerated blood pressure response [98]. The major studies frequently cited to support the hypothesis that cholesterol causes coronary heart disease continue to come under attack [99]. If one uses the prevalence and progression of coronary atherosclerosis as criteria instead of events, the association disappears completely.

Diabetic Individuals Free of Coronary Heart Disease

Individuals with diabetes represent a special case since they are at enhanced risk of cardiovascular mortality and morbidity. Current estimates indicate that 1 in 3 individuals in the US will develop diabetes in their lifetime with concomitant lifespan reduction of 10--15 years. Furthermore, more than half of diabetics will die as the result of cardiovascular disease [100]. In the INTERHEART Study, a large case-control study of incident acute MI, diabetes was among the strongest risk factors identified. The combination of diabetes and hypertension was found to be particularly dangerous [16].

This review will focus on cholesterol and atherosclerosis in type 2 diabetics since they represent the vast majority of those with this disorder. While type 2 diabetes is generally characterized by much later onset, current trends in obesity and the metabolic syndrome among young people will no doubt alter this natural history dramatically over the next few decades with the associated comorbidities occurring much earlier.

In 2011, the American Diabetes Association (ADA) published their view of the standard of medical care for diabetes [101]. Under prevention and management of complications, they discuss hypertension, blood lipids, antiplatelet therapy and smoking cessation. Central to the lipid management recommendation is the focus on LDL cholesterol and the recommendation of statin use by many diabetics. Thus, it is of interest to examine the evidence for the central role given LDL and the magnitude of the benefits associated with statin use in diabetic patients, especially those without cardiovascular or coronary heart disease but with type 2 diabetes.

There are a number of studies including randomized, placebo controlled trials and observational studies published over the past 8 years that are of interest. In addition, it is clearly important to examine the factors associated with the prevalence and progression of subclinical coronary atherosclerosis in diabetics using non-invasive imaging.

Coronary Artery Calcification Prevalence Studies in Diabetics

A number of studies have been published recently that find LDL is not a factor in the prevalence of coronary artery calcium (CAC) in diabetics as measured by electron beam computed tomography (EBCT) or coronary computed tomography angiography.

- Mazzone et al. (CHICAGO study) examined the prevalence of CAC in type 2 diabetics [102]. They excluded type 1 diabetics and anyone with coronary artery disease (CAD), cerebrovascular or peripheral vascular disease, heart failure, very high triglycerides (TGs) or BMI >45. Lipoprotein determinants of the CACS were HDL, TGs, ApoB, and cholesterol components called triglyceride rich lipoproteins (TRLs). Significant factors on multivariate analysis were age, systolic blood pressure, gender, race, and TRLs. Neither LDL nor statin use (50%) was significant in the multivariate analysis.
- Anand et al. examined factors associated with CHD event-free survival over about 2 years and the prevalence of CAC in Type 2 diabetics [103]. They excluded subjects with documented CAD, atypical angina, abnormal ECGs, cerebrovascular or peripheral artery disease, or renal impairment. Multivariate analysis predictors of CAC were age, male gender, ethnicity, hypertension, duration of diabetes, statin use (positive) and UKPDS risk score (weak association). The input data included hyperlipidemia which was not significant in multivariate analysis. This study also examined cardiovascular event-free survival over about 2 years. LDL was not a significant predictor and statin use did not enter into the analysis.
- Elkeles et al. studied the association between CAC and conventional risk factors in individuals with type 2 diabetes [104]. Subjects had no known coronary heart disease

(CHD). Multivariate analysis yielded waist-hip ratio, systolic blood pressure, male gender and statin use as positive risk factors. Factors not appearing as significant in multivariate analysis included non-HDL cholesterol, LDL, the cholesterol ratio TC/HDL, TGs and HbA1c.

- Wolfe et al. examined the association between CAC and traditional risk factors [105]. They found in a study of 71 diabetics with no evidence of CHD that the extent of CAC was independent of LDL levels in an adjusted model. Age, male gender and BMI were the only significant factors.
- A study by Martin et al. (Penn Diabetes Heart Study) examined factors associated with CAC in type 2 diabetics with no clinical evidence of CHD [106]. Only white individuals were enrolled. Analysis found only ApoB as a significant factor and in particular, LDL was not significantly associated with CAC after adjustment for age, sex, hypertension, smoking, alcohol, exercise, family history of premature cardiovascular disease (CVD), C-reactive protein, medications (including statins) and the metabolic syndrome. However, ApoB and LDL are correlated. Also, ApoB is a measure of LDL particle number and total the particle number viewed as atherogenic. In this study, there was a large difference between statin use in diabetics (57%) and non-diabetics (14%), but ApoB predicted CAC even after controlling for differences in statin use and in subgroup analysis of non-statin users. This study also found a weak but positive association with LDL and CAC in non-diabetics, an association which, as discussed above, is almost universally absent in numerous other studies.
- The PREDICT study reported in 2006 on the results of a study involving 573 subject with type 2 diabetes [107]. Excluded were those with past or present heart disease and uncontrolled hypertension. It was found in a multivariate analysis that age was the major factor influencing the CACS with weaker contributions from waist-to-hip ratio and duration of diabetes. Other traditional or novel risk factors were found to have insignificant positive effect, including TC, HDL,TGs and the use of statins (34-45% of subjects).
- A Japanese study examined the association of the prevalence and extent of CAC with insulin resistance in chronic kidney disease patients free of symptomatic CVD or any history of previous MI [108]. It was found that CAC becomes more prevalent and severe with an increase in the severity of kidney disease. In a univariate analysis, all the classical lipid parameters as well as statin use failed to achieve significant association with the CACS, with LDL the weakest ($p = 0.59$). In a multivariate analysis for factors associated with the CACS, only the common measure of insulin resistance (HOMA-IR) exhibited a significant association. Of the 111 subjects, 38 (34%) had type 2 diabetes although none used insulin.

In all but the study by Wolfe et al., a significant percentage of subjects were taking statin drugs (range 34% to 51% with most studies around 40%). Thus the mean LDL levels were, with the exception of Wolfe et al., about 108mg/dL, but there was in general a large enough range to make the LDL level a meaningful variable to examine. When the association with statin use was examined, two studies found the prevalence of CAC increased with statin use, while for remainder there was either no association or in Wolfe *et al* it was not noted in the baseline data. Based on the conventional wisdom, one might have expected an inverse correlation with statin use, i.e. statin use yields lower LDL which lowers the prevalence of CAC. This was not observed even though there were significant statin users, but rather, the opposite was found in two of the studies. This anomalous positive association with statin use persists in studies of progression of CAC, and a potential explanation will be discussed below.

Coronary Artery Calcification Progression Studies in Diabetics

What factors impact the progression of CAC in diabetics with no symptoms of heart disease? There are several relevant studies.

- A substudy of the Veterans Affairs Diabetes Trial examined the progression of CAC in 189 type 2 diabetics [109]. Individuals were excluded who had experienced stroke, MI, or revascularization in the past 6 months or who had congestive heart failure or significant angina. CAC progression was found in > 75% of subjects but was not influenced by standard risk factors. Univariable predictors of CAC progression were ethnicity, lipoprotein-associated phospholipase (Lp-PLA2) and the albumin to creatinine ratio. Lipids were not significant. The albumin to creatinine ratio and LP-PLA2 predicted progression independent of adjustment for age or other traditional risk factors. Treatment assignment to standard or aggressive glycemic control did not influence progression, irrespective of baseline CACS. LP-PLA2 has also been associated with the progression of subclinical atherosclerosis in a study involving individuals either with or without type 1 diabetes [110].
- Anand *et al* have reported the results of a study of the determinants of progression of CAC in type 2 diabetics without prior CHD or peripheral vascular disease, intermittent claudication, stroke, transient ischemic attack or renal impairment [111]. In the final multivariate analysis, odds ratios for independent factors for progression of CAC were baseline CAC > 400 mm^3 (OR = 6.38), HbA1c > 7 (OR =1.95), and statin use (OR = 2.27), but not hyperlipidemia or smoking status. It is noteworthy that the researchers found that statin therapy failed to inhibit progression of CAC but rather accelerated it.
- Progression of atherosclerosis measured by CAC in type 2 diabetics without previous clinical CVD was also addressed as part of the PREDICT study [112]. CAC was measured at baseline and after 4 years follow-up. The rate of change was strongly related to baseline CACS and also correlated positively with waist to hip ratio, male gender, the use of antihypertensive drugs or statins and the albumin to creatinine ratio. The majority of subjects showed progression. There was no relationship with traditional lipid risk factors. Independent of baseline CACS, blood pressure, central adiposity and microalbuminuria were found significant in the context of progression and the authors suggest these as areas for risk factor modification especially relevant to type 2 diabetics.

- It is well know that depression is a comorbid condition associated with diabetes [113]. The nature and details of the interaction are not clear. This is relevant to the present discussion since depressive symptoms are a risk factor for CHD and it has now been shown that depressive symptoms are a risk factor for the progression of coronary calcification. A recent report documented this in midlife women in the SWAN Heart Study, where depressive symptoms were independently associated with progression as measured by CAC [114]. In a multivariate analysis, the only other predictors of significance for progression of CAC were systolic blood pressure, and a low level of education. Lipids did not qualify statistically for inclusion in the analysis, and statin use, which was included, turned out to be insignificant.
- In a CAC progression study based on the Kaiser Permanente of Northern California database, Lee et al. [46] examined a sample of about 900 healthy adults age 60-72 initially free of clinical CAD. They included measures of insulin resistance, noted the presence of diabetes in the group, and then examined associations via univariate and multivariate analysis. In the univariate analysis, TC, LDL, HDL and TG were not even close to being significantly associated with progression of CAC over 2 years. However, dyslipidemia was a factor, but the authors fail to provide their working definition. In the context of the study this probably means the dyslipidemia associated with prediabetes and diabetes which involves elevated TGs and low HDL. In multivariate analysis, progression was associated with age, female gender, African American, diabetes, fasting insulin, dyslipidemia, hypertension, diastolic BP and pulse pressure but not lipid lowering medication.

In some of these studies, 30-50% of the subjects were on statin therapy at baseline. It is thus curious that statin use turns up in multivariate analysis in some of these studies to be a positive risk factor. Elkeles in his 2010 review of coronary calcium and CVD in diabetics suggests that the positive associations may have been caused by some study cohorts including individuals who had been given statins because they were perceived to be at the greatest risk [115]. Not all of the studies of prevalence or progression examined the same set of baseline factors but all included the traditional blood lipids and blood pressure. For prevalence, systolic blood pressure and the waist to hip ratio were most frequently found on multivariate analysis. For progression, the albumin to creatinine ratio, blood pressure and statin use were the most common positive factors. The strength in these studies appears to be the consistent finding of no association between total cholesterol or LDL cholesterol and the extent or progression of subclinical coronary atherosclerosis, a result consistent with studies on non-diabetic cohorts discussed above. Nevertheless, statins are recommended for most diabetics. This raises the question of the comparative effectiveness of lipid lowering in the context of acute events in diabetics as compared to non-diabetics.

Primary and Secondary Prevention of Diabetic CHD/CVD Events with Statins

Individuals with diabetes have enhanced risk of coronary heart disease and vascular disease in general. As discussed above, in the context of true primary prevention in non-diabetics, statins provide only a small (approximately 1%) absolute benefit in terms of acute coronary events and no impact on mortality. Thus it is of interest to examine this therapy in diabetics. If one examines the 2011 ADA standard of care [101], three primary prevention lipid lowering studies are cited where it is possible to stratify both by diabetes and the presence or absence of baseline CHD, thus obtaining information on the role of statins in risk reduction in the context of primary prevention of acute CHD events in type 2 diabetes. Their Table 11 indicates endpoint restriction to fatal CHD and non-fatal heart attack, but it is extrapolated to 10-year risk. It is thus of interest to look at the individual primary prevention trials. The results were as follows for absolute percent risk reduction, (ARR) the numbers needed to treat to prevent one event (NNT), the relative risk reduction (RRR) and the untreated event rate (UTER) for the endpoint of fatal and non-fatal heart attack over 4-5 years (calculated from reported events over the study period).

The HPS (MRC/BHF) trial [119], which the ADA included, is omitted because for the endpoint in question, the study included in the diabetic group individuals with arterial disease, including 33% with previous heart attack or other CHD and 18% with other occlusive artery disease. HPS only stratified diabetics by prior CHD when the endpoint includes coronary events, all strokes, and coronary and non-coronary revascularization, which inflates the benefit. Its inclusion with the data presented in the ADA table is inconsistent with the other primary prevention studies cited.

The very small absolute risk reduction (average 1.1%) with large NNT seen in the above table was also found in studies of cohorts where diabetes is present in only in a small fraction or absent. In this essentially non-diabetic population, when meta-analyses were rigorously restricted to primary prevention statin trials [96], absolute risk reduction for major CHD events was 1.0% (11 studies) and the NNT 100. Thus it is interesting that in the context of primary prevention, there is little difference between diabetics and non-diabetics. In addition, the above results call into question the use of statin therapy for diabetics free of CHD/CVD.

The largest meta-analysis of statin trials where both diabetes and primary vs. secondary prevention were stratified is the Cholesterol Treatment Trialists' Collaborators (CCT) study. The results are summarized below for the composite endpoint of MI, coronary deaths, stroke, or coronary revascularization over 4-5 years, calculated from reported event numbers [120]. Most participants in these trials were at elevated risk of adverse CVD events.

These results illustrate the greater impact of statins in secondary prevention. The result for diabetics with no vascular disease is somewhat higher than in CARDS, ASPEN and ASCOT discussed above, presumably because of the expanded endpoint which increases event rates. The results for no diabetes and no vascular disease are slightly higher than those reported above [96], again probably for the same reason.

Table 1. Primary prevention trials of statins among patients with diabetes

Trial	ARR	NNT	RRR	UTER
ASCOT [116]	0.6%	166	16%	1.4%
ASPEN [117]	0.7%	142	27%	3.6%
CARDS [118]	1.9%	53	36%	3.6%

Table 2. Summary of outcomes from the Cholesterol Treatment Trialists' Collaborators study

Category	ARR	NNT	RRR	UTER
Diabetes and no vascular disease	2.6%	39	27%	11.8%
Diabetes with vascular disease	5.3%	19	20%	31.6%
No diabetes and no vascular disease	1.6%	63	22%	8.3%
No diabetes with vascular disease	5.0%	20	21%	23.5%

The recent Cochrane meta-analysis [121] of primary prevention trials which included up to 10% subjects with heart disease and significant numbers with diabetes and hypertension presented data that yielded a 1.9% AAR (27% RRR) for CHD [75], which, given the cohorts, compares well with the CCT value of 1.6%.

The CCT results tabulated above which include the NNT should be viewed with some caution since the combined studies average over somewhat different populations. The NNT, as it is being used to illustrate clinical utility, can only be rigorously applied for comparisons when the baseline absolute risks are similar. Also, the NNT decreases dramatically with the duration of studies [122-124]. In the CCT results, duration probably does not confuse the issue. Nevertheless, for primary prevention when 60-80 individuals without diabetes and about 40 with diabetes must be treated to prevent one acute event, the treatment appears to be without benefit for too many individuals receiving the drug to make it attractive, given that there are potentially serious side effects. These results, instead of justifying the use of the therapy, should prompt a search for something better.

There is growing suspicion that a significant and perhaps major part of the action of statin drugs involves non-lipid lowering (pleiotropic) effects, of which there is a long and impressive list containing actions that can influence acute events, but have nothing to do with lower circulating cholesterol [11-13]. This may explain the higher absolute risk reduction in secondary prevention trials seen in Table 2. Pleiotropic effects significantly impact the use of LDL lowering trials to prove that LDL is a causative factor. Some might argue that for secondary prevention it does not matter what the mechanism is as long as there is a modest (5%) absolute benefit.

However, there are the statin adverse effects. For liver dysfunction, cataracts and myopathy, the number needed to treat to harm one patient with statin therapy has been estimated for men at 142, 52 and 81 and for women 136, 33 and 259, respectively [125]. It is doubtful that cataracts disappear if statin therapy is terminated. It is also strongly suspected that adverse events are significantly under-reported, downplayed or prevalence data suppressed. The point at which the ARR is large enough and the adverse side effects small enough to justify treatment is of course debatable, and the attitudes of both patients and physicians highly variable. Conservative clinicians might conclude that the treatment is not justified in general for very small ARRs, especially in the absence of symptomatic heart disease [96].

A side effect of statin treatment which is receiving increasing attention involves the enhanced risk of incident diabetes. In fact, at the 2011 annual meeting of the European Association for the Study of Diabetes held in Lisbon, Portugal in September, a special symposium was devoted to this topic. Diabetes incidence has been examined as a side effect in studies that were controlled by a placebo and studies where two doses of statin were compared.

Sattar *et al* [126] have performed a meta-analysis on a large number of randomized statin trials. When diabetes incidence was not in the published report, they obtained the data from the authors. A total of 13 trials were used involving over 91,000 participants. Statin therapy was associated with a statistically significant 9% relative risk increase. In absolute terms, this represented one new case per 255 statin users or an absolute risk enhancement of about 0.4% over 4 years of therapy.

Waters *et al* [127] has reviewed three studies not included in the above analysis that employed atorvastatin. Only the SPARCL study compared the drug with a placebo. This study involved 80 mg /day, a dose considered high. A 37% increase in the risk of new-onset diabetes was found (2.7% absolute increase). The diabetes risk factors were fasting glucose ≥ 220 mg/dL, triglycerides ≥ 150 mg/dL, BMI ≥ 30 and history of hypertension (yes/no). Individuals with none of these risk factors had a hazard ratio (HR) or 1.37 whereas when all for factors were present, the HR jumped to 2.44. The other two trials reviewed involved comparison of 80 mg and with 10 mg (TNT trial) or 20 mg (IDEAL trial) of atorvastatin. For the TNT trial, the HR for new-onset diabetes for all statin users was 1.10 but not significant. For the IDEAL trial, the HR was 1.19, also not significant. While the SPARCL result indicated higher risk, the upper confidence limit overlapped that in the meta-analysis of Sattar et al. discussed above.

The general conclusion seems to be that there is a small absolute enhanced risk of diabetes associated with statin treatment which becomes stronger with the presence of all the identified risk factors, but that the absolute risk increase may be smaller than the absolute risk reduction for incident CVD. These studies involved mostly cohorts at high risk of CVD or were CVD secondary prevention trials.

Fibrate Therapy

A class of drug called fibrates has also been tested for reducing CVD/CHD events in diabetics. Fibrates are interesting in the context of diabetes because diabetic dyslipidemia is characterized by elevated TGs and low HDL and fibrates are very effective in lowering TGs (30-50%). When combined with a statin, they dramatically reduce TGs and modestly elevate HDL. The most extensive testing has occurred with fenofibrate. In the FIELD randomized controlled study [128] which reported in 2005, fenofibrate did not significantly reduce the risk of CHD death or non-fatal MI, but there was a significant (about 14%) relative risk reduction in total cardiovascular events, driven in part by revascularizations which represent a soft endpoint due to prevalence influenced by physician recommendations (and persuasive ability??). Additional analysis of the outcomes in the FIELD study has revealed beneficial effects on the need for laser therapy for patients with or without known baseline diabetic retinopathy and fenofibrate treatment was also associated with slower progression of kidney disease and reduced risk of diabetes-related amputation [129].

The FIELD trial was followed by the ACCORD-DIAB-FENO trial [130] which compared type 2 diabetics taking simvastatin to those where fenofibrate was added for a combined therapy. This combined therapy did not reduce the rate of fatal cardiovascular events, non-fatal MIs, or non-fatal stroke (the combined primary endpoint) as compared to the statin alone. However, there was evidence of benefit in a reduction in the rate for the primary endpoint in individuals with significantly elevated TGs (≥ 204 mg/dL) and low HDL (≤ 34 mg/dL) where approximately a 30% decrease in relative rate was found, but the result was only close to statistical significance.

In 2011, the FDA has issued a warning regarding fenofibric acid, stating that the drug may not lower the risk of major cardiovascular events, which is the rationale for its use. This was prompted by the ACCORD trial. Furthermore, women receiving the combination may have an increase in risk of a major cardiac event compared to the statin treatment alone. Fenofibrate was approved in 2008 to be used with a statin to reduce triglycerides and increase HDL in diabetics with dyslipidemia and coronary heart disease or at risk of coronary heart disease who were already at their "official" LDL target.

A Paradox?

The above studies, viewed together, suggest a paradox. Acute coronary events, aside from those associated with "electrical problems," almost always require atherosclerosis. The more CAC the more coronary plaque and the higher risk of acute events with very low risk associated with zero plaque [131]. The prevalence and progression of coronary plaque as measured by EBCT is independent of serum LDL and TC levels over a very wide range of calcium score, age, gender, ethnic background and the presence of diabetes. But it is almost universally believed that the risk of CHD as manifest by acute ischemic events is strongly and continuously associated with LDL levels and thus LDL lowering targets form one of the pillars of modern preventive medicine in asymptomatic individuals with and without diabetes and as well in secondary prevention. This has the earmarks of a paradox.

The belief that the risk of coronary heart disease (CHD) events is strongly and continuously associated with LDL levels has resulted in LDL lowering targets which can generally only be attained with drugs. These targets are strongly dependent on meta-analyses of intervention studies which involve mostly secondary prevention. Cholesterol, we are also told, is related in observational studies to the risk of acute CHD evens which mostly require atherosclerosis, and at the same time, the evidence is compelling that neither TC nor LDL is driving atherosclerosis in men or women.

This apparent paradox can be resolved merely by assuming that the pathophysiology of acute events is different from that involved in the natural history of atherosclerosis. This gives LDL the role of an event trigger. However, this seems inconsistent with the apparent absence of a dose relationship since as pointed out above, it has been observed that half of a large cohort presenting with MI had low or very low LDL. Nevertheless, this explanation may have some merit.

There is an alternative. A way to resolve this paradox is to take the view that the association between TC and LDL and acute coronary events is in fact very weak, clinically insignificant, and for some segments of the population, nonexistent, a view that goes strongly against the conventional wisdom and guidelines from a number of professional organization. This has already been briefly discussed above. The literature supporting this contrary view is extensive, spans almost three decades, is in general ignored and has had negligible impact on those who believe in the cholesterol-heart disease hypothesis.

Put another way, the critical question is simply, does elevated TC and LDL increase the risk of heart disease related acute coronary events to an extent which is clinically significant? The conventional wisdom is that this question is already answered, and that the science clear with vast and robust evidence, even if the mechanism is far from clear or at least far from proven. If the notion that cholesterol increases the risk of symptomatic heart disease is viewed as a hypothesis, then careful consideration must be given to evidence that falsifies it, since as mentioned above, hypotheses are not proven, they survive until falsified.

The several meta-analyses cited above involving primary prevention of healthy individuals and yielding large numbers needed to treat with lipid lowering to prevent one acute CHD event would appear to support the notion of only a very weak association between cholesterol and CHD even after significant LDL lowering and up to 4-5 years follow-up.

A dispassionate examination of this contrarian evidence is thus important and It turns out to be informative to examine this question with stratification by age and gender.

Women

A pooled analysis involving 15 observational studies and about 125,000 women examined the question of total cholesterol and all-cause, cardiovascular, and coronary heart disease mortality [132]. Only events that occurred ≥ 5 years after the study baseline were considered and the reference was 160-199 mg/dL. Hazard ratios adjusted for age, diastolic blood pressure, BMI, and alcohol and smoking were derived. For total cardiovascular mortality, there was no significant association at any cholesterol level from < 160 to ≥ 240 mg/dL. For coronary heart disease mortality, the association became significant at levels ≥ 240 mg/dL but this may have included individuals with familial hypercholesterolemia which confuses the issue because of the non-lipid related triggers for acute coronary events associated with this disorder.

In 2004, Walsh and Pignone reported on pooled analysis of 6 lipid lowering trials involving women with endpoints of CHD and total mortality and CHD events [133]. Follow-up was from 3 to 5 years and 5 of the 6 studies used statins. For women without cardiovascular disease, lipid lowering was not associated with total or CHD mortality. For CHD events, the data was insufficient to permit a conclusive result. A more recent meta-analysis found that for women without prior cardiovascular disease, statin therapy did not reduce CHD events nor the risk of total mortality [134]. A similar conclusion was reached in a study motivated by legal aspects of drug company claims of efficacy which was also based on meta-analysis [135]. It is unusual to see a study on this subject in a legal journal, although one of the two authors was a professor of medicine at Harvard.

The famous JUPITER trial was the first to find benefit of lipid lowering for women. This study enrolled subjects with relatively low LDL (<130 mg/dL, mean 108 mg/dL) with C-reactive protein levels > 2 mg/L [136]. While described as healthy, 42% of the cohort had the metabolic syndrome and most were overweight and some obese. The study was prematurely terminated at a median follow-up about 2 years with maximum follow-up of 5 years, even though the number of events was very small. Using the tabulated events during the study, the absolute risk reduction for any heart attack was 0.41% and for combined heart attack, stroke or death from cardiovascular causes, it was 0.83%. Since these results span a considerable range of follow-up times of up to 5 years, the small absolutes risk reductions appear more meaningful than approximate numbers needed to treat which one might calculate. Women and men had similar relative risks, and thus the absolute risk reductions for women were also very small, although the relative risk reductions were very large. What is generally not recognized about this trial is that Crestor is unique in its very strong influence on vitamin D levels. The increase in vitamin D levels could easily account for the small absolute cardiovascular benefits [95]. Until this potential confounding is taken into account, JUPITER should be viewed with reservations. Serious problems with JUPITER have also been discussed by de Logeril [137]. Put simply, some of the numbers do not make any sense clinically.

Thus from the above studies one may reasonably conclude that TC or LDL are only very weak or non-existent factors for acute coronary events for women. This of course accounts for the interest from the legal profession. It is important to recognize that women younger than 50 years have such low risk of CHD that studies of events are difficult due to the very large number of participants needed to obtain useful data. It is no doubt also the reason why, historically, women were under-represented in studies conducted to justify drug therapy.

The Elderly

There have been a number of studies addressing the association between cholesterol and CHD or CVD events and related mortality in the elderly.

- Framingham looked at an elderly subgroup and the data for those 60 to 74 years of age assessed statistically and discussed by Larson [138]. For women, the rate ratio for cardiovascular disease was J shaped and showed *enhanced* risk at levels below about 200 mg/dL and then no risk until there was a modest increase above 300 mg/dL, which is both very high and in the FH range. For men, the curve was U shaped, with small *enhanced* risk below about 160 mg/dL and a modest increase in risk with a threshold of about 250 mg/L.
- Nissinen *et al* [139] found no association between cholesterol and CVD or CHD in a group aged 65-75. Systolic blood pressure was the most significant factor, and smoking declined in importance with age.
- Siegel *et al* [140] found for men and women with a mean age of 72 that when the data was adjusted for covariables, cholesterol was not associated with the risk of first cardiovascular event.
- Krumholz *et al* [141] studied the association between cholesterol and CHD mortality and morbidity in persons older than 70. They state that their results failed to support the hypothesis that hypercholesterolemia was an important factor for CHD mortality, or hospitalization for MI or unstable angina.
- Simons *et al* [142] found cholesterol and other lipids predicted CHD in the elderly, but only in those below 70 years of age. However, for the 60-69 age group, a hazard ratio > 1.0 was found only for the 5th quintile of TC which for women was 274 and men 294 mg/dl.

- The most frequently cited study in the context of primary prevention with a statin in an elderly population is the PROSPER trial which reported in 2002. This was a combined primary and secondary prevention trial which involved 5800 men and 3000 women aged 70-82 treated with a statin drug. For the primary prevention arm, no statistically significant treatment benefit was observed for CHD death, non-fatal MI or fatal and non-fatal stroke [143]. PROSPER is frequently cited supporting the opposite result, but this is incorrect in the context of primary prevention.

In a review published in 2011, Long *et al* attempt to convince readers that in fact statin intervention is important in the elderly for primary prevention [144]. If one ignores JUPITER because of issues discussed above, then the review is based on 5 primary prevention studies, AFCAPS, ASCOT, MEGA, PROSPER AND WOSCOP which included the elderly as a fraction or all of the study cohort. The researchers only cite stroke results for PROSPER. If one examines the data from these studies for the endpoint of major coronary events, the relative risk reductions range from 23% to 36%. The authors then claim that in studies where subgroup analysis was done, age did not influence the results. However, aside from PROSPER, the studies covered a range of age from 40 to 76, and thus did not provide an ideal design to examine the impact of old age. Absolute risk reductions were not mentioned. However, if one calculates the overall pooled absolute risk reduction it is only 1% yielding a NNT of 100 over the average duration of the studies. As discussed above, the PROSPER study, which was specifically targeted at the elderly, found no association with the incidence of major cardiac events from statin intervention. Thus for those who are impressed by relative risk reduction, the elderly definitely benefit from statins. However, if one considers the observational studies cited above and PROSPER which found no impact and the other intervention studies cited by Long *et al* which found 1% absolutes risk reduction from lipid lowering, then a different view of the significance of cholesterol in the context of the elderly emerges.

It therefore appears that there is no or a very weak statistically or clinically significant association between serum cholesterol levels and thus also LDL levels and CHD events in the elderly of either gender, although at very high levels there is only an inconsistent suggestion of the appearance of some risk.

Younger Men

There seems to be general agreement even among critics of the heart-cholesterol hypothesis that in this age group there is statistically significant association between the risk of CHD and serum cholesterol or LDL. The reason this age-gender group is different is unclear but one possibility is that psychological stress, its association with blood pressure and cholesterol levels, and in particular the cholesterol elevation associated with exaggerated blood pressure response to stress and aggravation may play a significant role [98]. This is the age group where men are subjected to high levels of stress associated with academic and career achievement, financial problems, domestic stress associated with the initial stages of raising children, and finally the severe stress associated with the breakup of a marriage or relationship. Stress is never considered quantitatively as a confounder in studies, but stress is recognized as a highly significant factor and trigger for acute coronary events and as well, coronary plaque progression [17]. Note that these same arguments were used and documented above in connection with the CARDIA study of LDL exposure and atherosclerosis in young individuals.

Back to the Paradox

Thus an attractive resolution of the above described paradox is that the association between serum cholesterol and thus LDL and the acute coronary events is weak or non-existent for women of all ages and the elderly, and cholesterol may only be a marker for stress in younger men where the association does appear to exist. However, younger men have a very low risk of acute CHD events compared to older individuals, and for those who experience sudden cardiac death, there is no correlation with cholesterol at all [15]. It is noteworthy that many studies do not stratify endpoint results by both age and gender, and furthermore, meta-analyses, which have profound influence on practice and guidelines, are also not generally stratified both by age and gender.

The paradox as outlined does not include a detailed discussion of the relative importance of non-calcified plaque, mixed calcified and non-calcified plaque and calcified plaque. Only recently has research started to differentiate these subtypes.

For the hypothesis that cholesterol causes acute heart disease related events, there appear to be quite a few black swans and it can be argued that there is no paradox at all. The greater absolute risk reduction in secondary statin therapy, which has had a strong but unjustified impact on primary prevention strategies, may be due to pleiotropic effects, and this view is reinforced by the very rapid impact of statin therapy seen in some studies subsequent to a major coronary event with statin naïve patients.

Zero Coronary Calcium

When large groups are screened, there will always be some where the radiologist cannot detect any coronary calcification and describes the arteries as "normal" or assigns a CACS of zero. Hecht has briefly reviewed prognostic studies where the CACS was zero [145]. From a pooling of three prospective studies with a median follow-up of about 4 years, the event rate per year of any adverse coronary event was 0.17% with a range of 0.11 to 0.9%. Hecht summarizes meta-analyses of studies involving over 49,000 individuals with a zero calcium score at baseline. A yearly event rate of 0.1% over 4.2 to 5.6 years follow-up was found.

In a review, Gottlieb et al. [146] discuss zero calcium scores in the context of diabetic and other high-risk patient populations. They cite one study showing that diabetic patients with zero coronary calcium had the same risk for events as non-diabetic patients after a mean follow-up of 5 years even though only 50% of the non-diabetic and 25% of the diabetic patients still had a zero calcium score. They cite two other studies consistent with these results.

In a recent study, Min *et al* [147] looked at the predictors of CAC in individuals with CAC = 0 progressing to a finite calcium score. A total of 25% of patients with CAC = 0 developed CAC during the 4-year follow-up. The mean age was 49 and the cohort was about equally divided between men and women. Progression from CAC = 0 was not linear but occurred at an increasing rate each year. Consistent with the studies reviewed above, cholesterol levels were not a significant factor in univariate analysis and thus omitted in multivariate analysis where only the presence of diabetes, smoking and age > 40 were significantly associated with the development of calcified plaque.

A zero calcium score, while an excellent indication of very low risk of acute cardiac events, is nevertheless no guarantee of the absence of non-calcified plaques or a major or minor stenosis [148]. In fact, coronary calcification is only marginally related to the extent of coronary stenosis and both obstructive and non-obstructive coronary artery disease can occur in the absence of calcification. Coronary stenosis is frequently not accompanied by calcification, highly calcified plaques are frequently non-obstructive and the calcium score is not suitable for ruling out obstructive CAD nor is relying on unenhanced CT justified when making the decision regarding discharge home for individuals presenting in the emergency department with suspected acute heart disease [146].

Non-Calcified and Mixed Plaque

For 20 years, electron beam computerized tomography (EBCT) without contrast media has been used to identify calcified coronary plaque. This has been of great value even though the scans do not pick up non-calcified plaque. The amount of coronary calcium correlates linearly with total coronary plaque burden and the higher the atherosclerotic burden, the higher the probability of acute events. The ability of the calcium score to predict CVD events in asymptomatic individuals has been confirmed in many clinical trials and studies indicate superiority over traditional risk stratification tools including carotid intima–media thickness (IMT) [146]. In fact, in one cohort study even patients who were in the greater than 75th percentile of carotid IMT but zero coronary calcium score had less than 1% per year risk for CVD events [149].

Recently improved CT technology termed computed coronary tomography angiography (CCTA), also called multislice computed tomographic angiography (MSCAT) or multidetector computed tomography (MDCT), has been developed and used in studies. This CT technology is used both with and without contrast enhancement. This makes it possible with a non-invasive technique to identify calcified, mixed and non-calcified plaque as well as stenosis. The study of plaque subtypes as compared to total CAC has only recently become an area of interest, and although the accumulated data is sparse compared to that associated with calcified coronary plaques quantified by conventional electron beam computed tomography, the situation is changing rapidly. CCTA or other improved coronary CT techniques provide a much more complete assessment of coronary atherosclerosis which then will make possible a re-examination of questions such as prevalence, progression, risk factors and factors impacting prognosis for each subtype.

A recent study has demonstrated that contrast-enhanced CCTA can also be used to measure CAC and found an excellent correlation with unenhanced CAC measurements. This suggests that two scans are unnecessary order to obtain a risk assessment which includes both non-calcified plaque and stenosis as well as a calcium score [150].

This is now an active area of research. Furthermore, this more sophisticated non-invasive technique has opened new avenues of research into the characteristics of vulnerable plaques. CCTA with contrast has been used mostly to study small groups of subjects with heart disease or symptoms strongly suggestive of this disorder. Studies have involved a variety of goals and information is accumulating, but it appears too early to attempt any general conclusions concerning risk factors or the impact of interventions for each plaque subtype or the distribution or seriousness of stenosis. Calcified plaque and the calcium score remain the only widely used and extensively studied surrogates for the presence, progression, response to medication and event risk evaluation of silent coronary atherosclerosis.

Preventing, Slowing or Reversing Coronary Plaque Progression

The traditional approach to studying progression and regression of atherosclerosis focused on the carotid arteries since ultrasound measurements were simple and non-invasive. This is still popular today although the clinical significance of small changes in carotid artery intima thickness or atheroma volume has never been demonstrated. The same is true for invasive studies using intravascular ultrasonography where a recent study found statin treatment reduced progression by measuring the percent change in atheroma volume [151]. One can question the clinical significance of a 1% decrease. The clinical significance of decreases in the CACS is also unknown, and in addition, the number of studies addressing reversing of halting CAC progression is limited.

A recent study involved dietary advice and combined intensive lipid management (statin plus niacin) along with supplementation with omega-3 fatty acids and increased vitamin D status. The targets were triglycerides ≤ 60 mg/dL, HDL ≥60 mg/dL, and 25-hydroxy vitamin D levels ≥50 ng/mL. Out of 45 male and female subjects with calcium scores ≥50 Agatston units, after about 18 months 20 subjects experienced a 15% drop in calcium score (maximum 64%), and 22 had their progression arrested or slowed to 12%, whereas a 22% to 52% increase in score per year was expected [152]. In another study involving hypertensive patients, a calcium channel blocker was found to significantly slow the progression of coronary calcification when the control was a diuretic [153]. Also, lowering the triglyceride/HDL ratio with the drug pioglitazone was associated with a beneficial impact on the progression of coronary atherosclerosis in diabetic patients [154]. This study suggests the importance of examining the impact of addressing the dyslipidemia of the metabolic syndrome with aggressive dietary intervention with the goal of reversing coronary atherosclerosis. In a mouse study, high HDL was found to promote rapid atherosclerosis regression and to alter the inflammatory properties of monocyte-derived plaque [155]. Potential modifiable risks factors associated with the severity or progression of coronary calcification also include physiological stress [156], depression [114] and sleep apnea [157]. Unfortunately, little effort has gone into aggressively addressing the problem of interventions that significantly slow or reverse directly measured coronary plaque progression and as well the impact on events, and yet this in fact is the real challenge facing those interested in CHD primary prevention.

Conclusion

Coronary atherosclerosis, which typically begins at a rather young age and progresses throughout life, appears independent of total cholesterol or LDL levels, which calls into doubt classical etiological models and should encourage the development and testing of new hypotheses [97]. Lowering LDL with statins has only a very small absolute effect on the risk of acute events in asymptomatic individuals, has proved slightly more useful in secondary prevention, but there remain numerous serious questions as to the importance of pleiotropic effects vs. lipid lowering, and the pleiotropic actions may be better achieved by other drugs or interventions. However, the risk of sudden cardiac death is independent of cholesterol levels, over 50% of all cardiac deaths are sudden and as discussed above and statins also do not appear to influence mortality [15]. Primary prevention lipid lowering drug trials remain controversial with criticism that has continued over several decades concerning issues such as age, gender, subject selection, cohort contamination by individuals with CHD, very high-risk subjects, very low absolute benefits, high numbers needed to treat to prevent one adverse event, no impact on overall mortality and indications of the prevalence of conflicts of interest and bias [96].

Diabetics represent a special case since there is little doubt this disease strongly enhances the risk of acute coronary events and in general, cardiovascular and peripheral vascular problems. Thus the obvious question. Is targeting LDL in diabetics indicated when it rarely appears as significant when one examines correlations with the prevalence or progression of silent coronary atherosclerosis or coronary event free survival, or when one takes into account the very small absolute benefits, similar to that found in non-diabetics, seen in true primary prevention statin intervention trials when the endpoint is fatal or non-fatal MI. It is interesting that in commentaries and reviews, ASCOT and ASPEN are frequently ignored in favour of HPS and CARDS, evidence of cherry picking for higher but still small absolute risk reductions. In a review concerning treatment of type 2 diabetics, the question addressed for lipids was "How low should we go?" Only CARDS and HPS were cited as justification for statin therapy, and only relative risk reductions were discussed. The authors did, however, comment on the limited data concerning taking cholesterol levels to very low values and suggest that this is an area for future trials [158]. But using relative risks, viewing HPS as a primary prevention trial without discussing the expanded endpoint, and omitting ASCOT and ASPEN inflated the suggested benefit.

In one recent comprehensive review on cardiovascular outcomes in type 2 diabetes which emphasized preventive therapies [159], the principal citation in the lipid section was the Cholesterol Treatment Trialists' Collaboration Study [160] which was viewed as robust evidence of the merits of statin intervention, pointing to the 18,000 subjects with diabetes out of a total of over 90,00 total participants. But in this meta-analysis of 14 studies, only one study involved true primary prevention (CARDS) and for a another trial (HPS), as discussed above there were problems separating primary from secondary prevention which were endpoint dependent. The analysis failed to include ASCOT and ASPEN. In fact, the use of large meta-analyses which involve mostly secondary prevention studies as justification for statin use in primary prevention is commonly encountered in review articles. Furthermore, while LDL targets are an integral part of guidelines and standard practice, there are no studies where the main objective was establishing the optimum LDL targets to go with the recommendations in the guidelines, especially for diabetics [158]. A recent review even suggested that type 2 diabetes should in fact not be considered a true risk equivalent for CHD [161].

LDL is universally regarded as the "bad" cholesterol. The issues discussed above suggest a different view. Why is it consistently absent as a factor in studies of the risk of prevalence and progression of silent atherosclerosis in both diabetics and non-diabetics? Furthermore, why does low LDL characterize half of hospital admissions for MI? In addition, non-statin drugs that lower LDL do not reduce event risk? Why are the numbers needed to treat so high in true primary prevention? If the NNT found in intervention studies is 50 or 100, or even 25, there are 49, 99 or 24 who were treated, typically over 4 years, but did not benefit from lowering of circulating LDL. Then there are the statin adverse effects. It is widely recognized, post-introduction side effect monitoring is notoriously inefficient. In fact, the actual prevalence of side effects of statins is unknown and an area of active investigation.

The focus on relative rather than absolute risk reduction has resulted in widespread inflated perceptions of benefit, confused the risk/benefit analysis and produced a false sense of security among the millions of statin users. The extensive use of relative risk in this field has been the subject of criticism for several decades. A 20-30% relative risk reduction is impressive and strongly influences therapeutic decisions, but it can be associated with a 1%-2% or even smaller absolute event risk reduction which is not impressive [162, 163].

There seems to be no consensus regarding the magnitude of an absolute risk reduction that is clinically significant. This is understandable since many factors come into play. It can be argued that a low-cost, low-risk preventive measure for a potentially disabling or fatal disease can have a high threshold for NNT. However, if a treatment carries high risk and high cost, this can in the view of some clinicians reduce the limit of the NNT to quite a low number above which treatment is not justified [162]. It can be argued that patients need to be advised on the basis of absolute risk reductions, but not only do the above factors enter in, but the particular situation presented by the individual patient needs to be considered to ascertain if study-derived NNTs are applicable or if the probability of benefit may be much higher or lower [163]. Furthermore, underreporting of adverse effects makes a meaningful risk/benefit analysis impossible.

The notion is gaining support that widespread screening for the presence and extent of coronary calcium is indicated, especially for those of intermediate risk by the Framingham Risk Score. The results are intended to guide the degree of treatment aggressiveness. But there is almost no data regarding how to significantly arrest or reverse the progression of atherosclerosis nor the associated clinical benefit. The few glimmers of hope, amplified into suggestions of significant success, have been based on very small changes in targeted carotid or coronary artery atheromas or in carotid intima media thickness. The significance of these very small changes appear to be of questionable clinical significance and there is a poor correlation between atherosclerosis in these two vascular beds. Neither statins, most antihypertensive drugs or sevelamer in the case of those with chronic kidney disease have shown any impact on progression of CAC [164].

There do not appear to be studies in the context of arresting or reversing coronary atherosclerosis measured by coronary calcium which provide guidance regarding interventions such as cessation of smoking, exercise, a Mediterranean diet, moderate alcohol consumption, optimal vitamin D status, consumption of ample long-chain omega-3 fatty acid and reducing psychological stress, actions suggested by observational studies which are associated with reduced risk of acute events, especially when combined into an integrated program. One study discussed above did find substantial regression of CAC associated with triglyceride targets combined with omega-3 fatty acid and vitamin D supplementation, but much more research is obviously needed.

The difficulties individuals experience in loosing weight, adopting dietary strategies that might assist in weight loss and improve nutrition, avoiding the development or reversing the metabolic syndrome, diabetes and the associated characteristic dyslipidemia, and stopping smoking appear to be a serious impediment to progress in prevention. Even a strengthened evidence base for the merits of such actions based on intervention studies with both event and CAC endpoints may not help motivate patients. Professional advice and encouragement appear to have limited impact.

The literature cited and discussed above suggests that a new paradigm is urgently needed, especially in the context of primary prevention of CHD [17, 86]. This issues has been recently discussed and documented by Ravnskov and others [4, 18, 97, 165, 166], and a new hypothesis has been advanced by Ravnskov and McCully which focuses on action in the arterial media initiated mostly by agents entering via or blocking the vasa vasorum with only monocytes crossing the endothelial barrier to enter the media. The hypothesis addresses many of the ongoing issues [97]. Any new paradigm will also have to accommodate the information now accumulating regarding plaque subtypes and vulnerable vs. non-vulnerable plaques. It is noteworthy since the paper by Ravnskov and McCully was published in 2009, there is virtually no activity in the area of new hypotheses. It is suggested that this lack of progress is due to the still unquestioned primacy of the cholesterol-heart hypothesis, the associated cholesterol-atherosclerosis hypothesis, and contentment with the current model of atherosclerosis. Cholesterol appears to only be a distraction and, given the large body of evidence suggesting that it is irrelevant in the context of atherosclerosis and a weak or non-existent factor when acute coronary event risks are considered. It is unlikely that additional evidence will be brought forward that neutralizes this large body of significant evidence that calls into question the cholesterol-heart hypothesis.

Science becomes dysfunctional when dogma and vested interests trump critical analysis and constant questioning of the conventional wisdom. Yet critics believe that there is a culture today in medical science, which aggressively and successfully resists new ideas and challenges to widespread beliefs and the conventional wisdom, and it can be argued that this is obviously not in the best interests of patients and inhibits meaningful scientific progress. It is time for a change.

References

[1] Lande K, Sperry W: Human Atherosclerosis in Relation to the Cholesterol Content of the Blood Serum. *Archives of Pathology* 1936; 22:301-312.

[2] Pedersen HS, Mulvad G, Newman WP, III, Boudreau DA: Atherosclerosis in coronary arteries and aorta among Greenlanders: an autopsy study. *Atherosclerosis* 2003; 170(1):93-103.

[3] Mathur K, Patney N, Kumar V, Sharma R: Serum Cholesterol and Atherosclerosis in Man. *Circulation* 1961; 23(6):847-852.

[4] Rosch PJ: Cholesterol does not cause coronary heart disease in contrast to stress. *Scand. Cardiovasc. J.* 2008; 42(4):244-249.

[5] Smith R, Pinckney E: Diet, blood cholesterol and coronary heart disease: *A critical review of the literature*. Sherman Oaks, CA, Vector enterprises, 1991.

[6] Lecerf JM, de LM: Dietary cholesterol: from physiology to cardiovascular risk. *Br. J. Nutr.* 2011; 106(1):6-14.

[7] Kannel WB, Castelli WP, Gordon T: Cholesterol in the prediction of atherosclerotic disease. New perspectives based on the Framingham study. *Ann. Intern. Med.* 1979; 90(1):85-91.

[8] Anderson KM, Castelli WP, Levy D: Cholesterol and mortality. 30 years of follow-up from the Framingham study. *JAMA* 1987; 257(16):2176-2180.

[9] Castelli WP: Concerning the possibility of a nut.. *Arch. Intern. Med.* 1992; 152(7):1371-1372.

[10] Stamler J, Wentworth D, Neaton JD: Is relationship between serum cholesterol and risk of premature death from coronary heart disease continuous and graded? Findings in 356,222 primary screenees of the Multiple Risk Factor Intervention Trial (MRFIT). *JAMA* 1986; 256(20):2823-2828.

[11] Liao JK, Laufs U: Pleiotropic effects of statins. *Annu. Rev. Pharmacol. Toxicol.* 2005; 45:89-118.

[12] Sadowitz B, Maier KG, Gahtan V: Basic science review: Statin therapy--Part I: The pleiotropic effects of statins in cardiovascular disease. *Vasc. Endovascular. Surg.* 2010; 44(4):241-251.

[13] Mihos CG, Salas MJ, Santana O: The pleiotropic effects of the hydroxy-methyl-glutaryl-CoA reductase inhibitors in cardiovascular disease: a comprehensive review. *Cardiol. Rev.* 2010; 18(6):298-304.

[14] de Lorgeril M: Disappointing recent cholesterol-lowering drug trials: is it not time for a full reappraisal of the cholesterol theory? *http://michel delorgeril info/dwnl/wrnd/ DisappointingCholDrugTrials_wrnd2009 pdf) World Rev. Nutr. Diet* 2009; 100:80-89.

[15] de Lorgeril M, Salen P: Cholesterol lowering, sudden cardiac death and mortality. *Scand. Cardiovasc. J.* 2008; 42(4):264-267.

[16] Yusuf S, Hawken S, Ounpuu S, Dans T, Avezum A, Lanas F, McQueen M, Budaj A, Pais P, Varigos J, Lisheng L: Effect of potentially modifiable risk factors associated with myocardial infarction in 52 countries (the INTERHEART study): case-control study. *Lancet* 2004; 364(9438):937-952.

[17] Ware WR: Psychological stress, insulin resistance, inflammation and the assessment of heart disease risk. Time for a paradigm shift? *Med. Hypotheses* 2008; 71(1):45-52.

[18] Kendrick M: *The Great Cholesterol Con*. London, John Blake Publishing,Ltd, 2007.

[19] Ravnskov U: *The Cholesterol Myths*. Washington, NewTrends Publishing, Inc, 2000.

[20] Ravnskov U: *Fat and Cholesterol are Good For You*. Sweden, GB Publishing, 2009.

[21] Taubes G: Good Calories, Bad Calories. *Challenging the conventional wisdom on diet, weight control and disease*. New York, Alfred A. Knopf, 2007.

[22] Executive Summary of The Third Report of The National Cholesterol Education Program (NCEP) Expert Panel on Detection, Evaluation, And Treatment of High Blood Cholesterol In Adults (Adult Treatment Panel III): *JAMA* 2001; 285(19):2486-2497.

[23] Sinatra S, Roberts JC: *Reverse Heart Diease Now*. New Jersey, John Wiley and Sons, 2007.

[24] Sinatra ST: Metabolic cardiology: the missing link in cardiovascular disease. *Altern. Ther. Health Med.* 2009; 15(2):48-50.

[25] Polonsky TS, McClelland RL, Jorgensen NW, Bild DE, Burke GL, Guerci AD, Greenland P: Coronary Artery Calcium Score and Risk Classification for Coronary Heart Disease Prediction. *JAMA* 2010; 303(16):1610-1616.

[26] Scott BR, Sanders CL, Mitchel REJ, Boreham DR. CT scans may reduce rather than increase the risk of cancer.(Report). *Journal of American Physicians and Surgeons* 13[1], 8. 22-3-2008. Ref Type: Magazine Article.

[27] Gori T, Munzel T: Biological effects of low-dose radiation: of harm and hormesis. *Eur. Heart J.* 2011.

[28] Jaworowski Z: Radiation hormesis--a remedy for fear. *Hum. Exp. Toxicol.* 2010; 29(4):263-270.

[29] Jolly D, Meyer J: A brief review of radiation hormesis. *Australas. Phys. Eng. Sci. Med.* 2009; 32(4):180-187.

[30] Elkeles RS, Godsland IF, Feher MD, Rubens MB, Roughton M, Nugara F, Humphries SE, Richmond W, Flather MD: Coronary calcium measurement improves prediction of cardiovascular events in asymptomatic patients with type 2 diabetes: the PREDICT study. *Eur. Heart J.* 2008.

[31] Bots ML, Baldassarre D, Simon A, de GE, O'Leary DH, Riley W, Kastelein JJ, Grobbee DE: Carotid intima-media thickness and coronary atherosclerosis: weak or strong relations? *Eur. Heart J.* 2007; 28(4):398-406.

[32] Grundy SM: Promise of low-density lipoprotein-lowering therapy for primary and secondary prevention. *Circulation* 2008; 117(4):569-573.

[33] Ware WR: The mainstream hypothesis that LDL cholesterol drives atherosclerosis may have been falsified by non-invasive imaging of coronary artery plaque burden and progression. *Med. Hypotheses* 2009; 73(4):596-600.

[34] Church TS, Levine BD, McGuire DK, Lamonte MJ, Fitzgerald SJ, Cheng YJ, Kimball TE, Blair SN, Gibbons LW, Nichaman MZ: Coronary artery calcium score, risk factors, and incident coronary heart disease events. *Atherosclerosis* 2007; 190(1):224-231.

[35] Greenland P, Bonow RO: How low-risk is a coronary calcium score of zero? The importance of conditional probability. *Circulation* 2008; 117(13):1627-1629.

[36] Hecht HS, Superko HR, Smith LK, McColgan BP: Relation of coronary artery calcium identified by electron beam tomography to serum lipoprotein levels and implications for treatment. *The American Journal of Cardiology* 2001; 87(4):406-412.

[37] Hecht HS, Superko HR: Electron beam tomography and national cholesterol education program guidelines in asymptomatic women. *Journal of the American College of Cardiology* 2001; 37(6):1506-1511.

[38] Johnson KM, Dowe DA, Brink JA: Traditional clinical risk assessment tools do not accurately predict coronary atherosclerotic plaque burden: a CT angiography study. *AJR Am. J. Roentgenol.* 2009; 192(1):235-243.

[39] Kop WJ, Berman DS, Gransar H, Wong ND, Miranda-Peats R, White MD, Shin M, Bruce M, Krantz DS, Rozanski A: Social network and coronary artery calcification in asymptomatic individuals. *Psychosom. Med.* 2005; 67(3):343-352.

[40] Arad Y, Goodman KJ, Roth M, Newstein D, Guerci AD: Coronary calcification, coronary disease risk factors, C-reactive protein, and atherosclerotic cardiovascular disease events: the St. Francis Heart Study. *J. Am. Coll. Cardiol.* 2005; 46(1):158-165.

[41] Jensen JM, Gerdes LU, Jensen HK, Christiansen TM, Brorholt-Petersen JU, Faergeman O: Association of coronary heart disease with age-adjusted aortocoronary calcification in patients with familial hypercholesterolaemia. *J. Intern. Med.* 2000; 247(4):479-484.

[42] Kronmal RA, McClelland RL, Detrano R, Shea S, Lima JA, Cushman M, Bild DE, Burke GL: Risk factors for the progression of coronary artery calcification in asymptomatic subjects: results from the Multi-Ethnic Study of Atherosclerosis (MESA). *Circulation* 2007; 115(21):2722-2730.

[43] Sung J, Lim SJ, Choe Y, Choi YH, Lee MK, Lee SH, Hong KP, Park JE: Comparison of the coronary calcium score with the estimated coronary risk. *Coron. Artery Dis.* 2008; 19(7):475-479.

[44] Ramadan MM, Mahfouz EM, Gomaa GF, El-Diasty TA, Alldawi L, Ikrar T, Limin D, Kodama M, Aizawa Y: Evaluation of coronary calcium score by multidetector computed tomography in relation to endothelial function and inflammatory markers in asymptomatic individuals. *Circ. J.* 2008; 72(5):778-785.

[45] Takamiya T, Zaky WR, Edmundowics D, Kadowaki T, Ueshima H, Kuller LH, Sekikawa A: World Health Organization-defined metabolic syndrome is a better predictor of coronary calcium than the adult treatment panel III criteria in American men aged 40-49 years. *Diabetes Care* 2004; 27(12):2977-2979.

[46] Lee KK, Fortmann SP, Fair JM, Iribarren C, Rubin GD, Varady A, Go AS, Quertermous T, Hlatky MA: Insulin resistance independently predicts the progression of coronary artery calcification. *American Heart Journal* 2009; 157(5):939-945.

[47] Budoff MJ, Hokanson JE, Nasir K, Shaw LJ, Kinney GL, Chow D, Demoss D, Nuguri V, Nabavi V, Ratakonda R, Berman DS, Raggi P: Progression of coronary artery calcium predicts all-cause mortality. *JACC Cardiovasc. Imaging* 2010; 3(12):1229-1236.

[48] Park HE, Kim MK, Choi SY, Lee W, Shin CS, Cho SH, Oh BH: The prevalence and distribution of coronary artery calcium in asymptomatic Korean population. *Int. J. Cardiovasc. Imaging* 2011.

[49] Lee HT, Shin J, Lim YH, Kim BK, Kim YT, Lee JU, Hong S, Song SY, Cho SH: The relationship between coronary artery calcification and bone mineral density in patients according to their metabolic syndrome status. *Korean Circ. J.* 2011; 41(2):76-82.

[50] Jeon GH, Kim SH, Yun SC, Chae HD, Kim CH, Kang BM: Association between serum estradiol level and coronary artery calcification in postmenopausal women. *Menopause* 2010; 17(5):902-907.

[51] Rondanelli M, Giacosa A, Opizzi A, Pelucchi C, La VC, Montorfano G, Negroni M, Berra B, Politi P, Rizzo AM: Long chain omega 3 polyunsaturated fatty acids supplementation in the treatment of elderly depression: effects on depressive symptoms, on phospholipids fatty acids profile and on health-related quality of life. *J. Nutr. Health Aging* 2011; 15(1):37-44.

[52] Coylewright M, Rice K, Budoff MJ, Blumenthal RS, Greenland P, Kronmal R, Barr RG, Burke GL, Tracy R, Post WS: Differentiation of severe coronary artery calcification in the Multi-Ethnic Study of Atherosclerosis. *Atherosclerosis* 2011.

[53] Elkeles RS, Godsland IF, Rubens MB, Feher MD, Nugara F, Flather MD: The progress of coronary heart disease in Type 2 diabetes as measured by coronary calcium score from electron beam computed tomography (EBCT): the PREDICT study. *Atherosclerosis* 2008; 197(2):777-783.

[54] Wong ND, Kawakubo M, Labree L, Azen SP, Xiang M, Detrano R: Relation of coronary calcium progression and control of lipids according to National Cholesterol Education Program guidelines. *Am. J. Cardiol.* 2004; 94(4):431-436.

[55] Taylor AJ, Bindeman J, Le TP, Bauer K, Byrd C, Feuerstein IM, Wu H, O'Malley PG: Progression of calcified coronary atherosclerosis: relationship to coronary risk factors and carotid intima-media thickness. *Atherosclerosis* 2008; 197(1):339-345.

[56] Sutton-Tyrrell K, Kuller LH, Edmundowicz D, Feldman A, Holubkov R, Givens L, Matthews KA: Usefulness of electron beam tomography to detect progression of coronary and aortic calcium in middle-aged women. *Am. J. Cardiol.* 2001; 87(5):560-564.

[57] Gopal A, Nasir K, Liu ST, Flores FR, Chen L, Budoff MJ: Coronary calcium progression rates with a zero initial score by electron beam tomography. *Int. J. Cardiol.* 2007; 117(2):227-231.

[58] Yoon HC, Emerick AM, Hill JA, Gjertson DW, Goldin JG: Calcium begets calcium: progression of coronary artery calcification in asymptomatic subjects. *Radiology* 2002; 224(1):236-241.

[59] Hsia J, Klouj A, Prasad A, Burt J, ms-Campbell LL, Howard BV: Progression of coronary calcification in healthy postmenopausal women. *BMC Cardiovasc. Disord.* 2004; 4:21.

[60] Raggi P, Cooil B, Ratti C, Callister TQ, Budoff M: Progression of coronary artery calcium and occurrence of myocardial infarction in patients with and without diabetes mellitus. *Hypertension* 2005; 46(1):238-243.

[61] Chironi G, Simon A, Denarie N, Vedie B, Sene V, Megnien JL, Levenson J: Determinants of progression of coronary artery calcifications in asymptomatic men at high cardiovascular risk. *Angiology* 2002; 53(6):677-683.

[62] Paramsothy P, Knopp RH, Bertoni AG, Blumenthal RS, Wasserman BA, Tsai MY, Rue T, Wong ND, Heckbert SR: Association of combinations of lipid parameters with carotid intima-media thickness and coronary artery calcium in the MESA (Multi-Ethnic Study of Atherosclerosis). *J Am Coll Cardiol* 2010; 56(13):1034-1041.

[63] Pletcher MJ, Bibbins-Domingo K, Liu K, Sidney S, Lin F, Vittinghoff E, Hulley SB: Nonoptimal lipids commonly present in young adults and coronary calcium later in life: the CARDIA (Coronary Artery Risk Development in Young Adults) study. *Ann. Intern. Med.* 2010; 153(3):137-146.

[64] Francis KT: Psychologic correlates of serum indicators of stress in man: a longitudinal study. *Psychosom. Med.* 1979; 41(8):617-628.

[65] Bijlani RL, Sud S, Gandhi BM, Tandon BN: Relationship of examination stress to serum lipid profile. *Indian J. Physiol. Pharmacol.* 1986; 30(1):22-30.

[66] Scheuch K, Pietruschka WD, Eckhardt G, Reinelt D, Richter V, Reuter W: [HDL and LDL cholesterol changes in psychological stress in relation to stress experience]. *Z. Gesamte. Inn. Med.* 1984; 39(12):273-277.

[67] Matthews KA, Zhu S, Tucker DC, Whooley MA: Blood Pressure Reactivity to Psychological Stress and Coronary Calcification in the Coronary Artery Risk Development in Young Adults Study. *Hypertension* 2006; 47(3):391-395.

[68] Schmid M, Achenbach S, Ropers D, Komatsu S, Ropers U, Daniel WG, Pflederer T: Assessment of Changes in Non-Calcified Atherosclerotic Plaque Volume in the Left

Main and Left Anterior Descending Coronary Arteries over Time by 64-Slice Computed Tomography. *The American Journal of Cardiology* 2008; 101(5):579-584.

[69] Ravnskov U: The questionable role of saturated and polyunsaturated fatty acids in cardiovascular disease. *J. Clin. Epidemiol.* 1998; 51(6):443-460.

[70] Jakobsen MU, Dethlefsen C, Joensen AM, Stegger J, Tjonneland A, Schmidt EB, Overvad K: Intake of carbohydrates compared with intake of saturated fatty acids and risk of myocardial infarction: importance of the glycemic index. *Am. J. Clin. Nutr.* 2010; 91(6):1764-1768.

[71] Siri-Tarino PW, Sun Q, Hu FB, Krauss RM: Meta-analysis of prospective cohort studies evaluating the association of saturated fat with cardiovascular disease. *Am. J. Clin. Nutr.* 2010; 91(3):535-546.

[72] Yamagishi K, Iso H, Yatsuya H, Tanabe N, Date C, Kikuchi S, Yamamoto A, Inaba Y, Tamakoshi A, for the JACC Study Group: Dietary intake of saturated fatty acids and mortality from cardiovascular disease in Japanese: the Japan Collaborative Cohort Study for Evaluation of Cancer Risk (JACC) Study. *Am. J. Clin. Nutr.* 2010; 92(4):759-765.

[73] Hu FB: Are refined carbohydrates worse than saturated fat? *Am. J. Clin. Nutr.* 2010; 91(6):1541-1542.

[74] Accurso A, Bernstein RK, Dahlqvist A, Draznin B, Feinman RD, Fine EJ, Gleed A, Jacobs DB, Larson G, Lustig RH, Manninen AH, McFarlane SI, Morrison K, Nielsen JV, Ravnskov U, Roth KS, Silvestre R, Sowers JR, Sundberg R, Volek JS, Westman EC, Wood RJ, Wortman J, Vernon MC: Dietary carbohydrate restriction in type 2 diabetes mellitus and metabolic syndrome: time for a critical appraisal. *Nutr. Metab. (Lond)* 2008; 5:9.

[75] Moynihan R: Surrogates under scrutiny: fallible correlations, fatal consequences. *BMJ* 2011; 343:d5160.

[76] Koulaouzidis G, Henein M: Coronary Calcification and Hormones. *Angiology* 2011; Ahead of print, Mar 18, 2011.

[77] Naghavi M: Preventive Cardiology: the SHAPE of the future. A Synopsis from the Screening for Heart Attack Prevention and Education (SHAPE) Task Force report. *Herz.* 2007; 32(5):356-361.

[78] Nasir K, Vasamreddy C, Blumenthal RS, Rumberger JA: Comprehensive coronary risk determination in primary prevention: an imaging and clinical based definition combining computed tomographic coronary artery calcium score and national cholesterol education program risk score. *Int. J. Cardiol.* 2006; 110(2):129-136.

[79] Houslay ES, Cowell SJ, Prescott RJ, Reid J, Burton J, Northridge DB, Boon NA, Newby DE: Progressive coronary calcification despite intensive lipid-lowering treatment: a randomised controlled trial. *Heart* 2006; 92(9):1207-1212.

[80] Arad Y, Spadaro LA, Roth M, Newstein D, Guerci AD: Treatment of asymptomatic adults with elevated coronary calcium scores with atorvastatin, vitamin C, and vitamin E: the St. Francis Heart Study randomized clinical trial. *J. Am. Coll. Cardiol.* 2005; 46(1):166-172.

[81] Henein MY, Owen A: Statins moderate coronary stenoses but not coronary calcification: Results from meta-analyses. *Int. J. Cardiol.* 2010; Published ahead of print, September 4, 2010.

[82] Raggi P, Davidson M, Callister TQ, Welty FK, Bachmann GA, Hecht H, Rumberger JA: Aggressive versus moderate lipid-lowering therapy in hypercholesterolemic postmenopausal women: Beyond Endorsed Lipid Lowering with EBT Scanning (BELLES). *Circulation* 2005; 112(4):563-571.

[83] Schmermund A, Achenbach S, Budde T, Buziashvili Y, Forster A, Friedrich G, Henein M, Kerkhoff G, Knollmann F, Kukharchuk V, Lahiri A, Leischik R, Moshage W, Schartl M, Siffert W, Steinhagen-Thiessen E, Sinitsyn V, Vogt A, Wiedeking B, Erbel R: Effect of Intensive Versus Standard Lipid-Lowering Treatment With Atorvastatin on the Progression of Calcified Coronary Atherosclerosis Over 12 Months: A Multicenter, Randomized, Double-Blind Trial. *Circulation* 2006; 113(3):427-437.

[84] Jonathan E, Derrick B, Emma L, Sarah P, John D, Jane A, Rory C: C-reactive protein concentration and the vascular benefits of statin therapy: an analysis of 20,536 patients in the Heart Protection Study. *Lancet* 2011; 377(9764):469-476.

[85] Burgstahler C, Reimann A, Beck T, Kuettner A, Baumann D, Heuschmid M, Brodoefel H, Claussen CD, Kopp AF, Schroeder S: Influence of a lipid-lowering therapy on calcified and noncalcified coronary plaques monitored by multislice detector computed tomography: results of the New Age II Pilot Study. *Invest. Radiol.* 2007; 42(3):189-195.

[86] de Lorgeril M, Salen P: Cholesterol lowering and mortality: Time for a new paradigm? *Nutrition, Metabolism and Cardiovascular Diseases* 2006; 16(6):387-390.

[87] de Lorgeril M, Salen P, Corcos T, Defaye P, Juneau M, Pavy B, Saoudi N: Is moderate drinking as effective as cholesterol lowering in reducing mortality in high-risk coronary patients? *Eur. Heart J.* 2008; 29(1):4-6.

[88] Al-Mallah MH, Hatahet H, Cavalcante JL, Khanal S: Low admission LDL-cholesterol is associated with increased 3-year all-cause mortality in patients with non ST segment elevation myocardial infarction. *Cardiol. J.* 2009; 16(3):227-233.

[89] Ray KK, Seshasai SRK, Erqou S, Sever P, Jukema JW, Ford I, Sattar N: Statins and All-Cause Mortality in High-Risk Primary Prevention: A Meta-analysis of 11 Randomized Controlled Trials Involving 65 229 Participants. *Arch. Intern. Med.* 2010; 170(12):1024-1031.

[90] Ridker PM, Danielson E, Fonseca FA, Genest J, Gotto AM, Jr., Kastelein JJ, Koenig W, Libby P, Lorenzatti AJ, Macfadyen JG, Nordestgaard BG, Shepherd J, Willerson JT, Glynn RJ: Rosuvastatin to Prevent Vascular Events in Men and Women with Elevated C-Reactive Protein. *N. Engl. J. Med.* 2008; 359:2195-2207.

[91] Elias-Smale SE, Kardys I, Oudkerk M, Hofman A, Witteman JC: C-reactive protein is related to extent and progression of coronary and extra-coronary atherosclerosis; results from the Rotterdam study. *Atherosclerosis* 2007; 195(2):e195-e202.

[92] Hosseinsabet A, Mohebbi A, Almasi A: C-reactive protein and coronary calcium score association in coronary artery disease. *Cardiol. J.* 2008; 15(5):431-436.

[93] Blaha MJ, Budoff MJ, Defilippis AP, Blankstein R, Rivera JJ, Agatston A, O'Leary DH, Lima J, Blumenthal RS, Nasir K: Associations between C-reactive protein, coronary artery calcium, and cardiovascular events: implications for the JUPITER population from MESA, a population-based cohort study. *Lancet* 2011; 378(9792):684-692.

[94] de Lorgeril M, Salen P, Abramson J, Dodin S, Hamazaki T, Kostucki W, Okuyama H, Pavy B, Rabaeus M: Cholesterol Lowering, Cardiovascular Diseases, and the

Rosuvastatin-JUPITER Controversy: A Critical Reappraisal. *Arch. Intern. Med.* 2010; 170(12):1032-1036.

[95] Ware WR: The JUPITER lipid lowering trial and vitamin D. *Dermato-Endochrinology* 2010; 2(2):50-54.

[96] Wright J: Do statins have a role in primary prevention? An update. *Theraeutics Initative (Theraputics Letter)* 2010; 77(March-April 2010, http://ti.ubc.ca/letter77).

[97] Ravnskov U, McCully KS: Review and Hypothesis: Vulnerable plaque formation from obstruction of Vasa vasorum by homocysteinylated and oxidized lipoprotein aggregates complexed with microbial remnants and LDL autoantibodies. *Ann. Clin. Lab. Sci.* 2009; 39(1):3-16.

[98] Ware WR: High cholesterol and coronary heart disease in younger men: the potential role of stress induced exaggerated blood pressure response. *Med. Hypotheses* 2008; 70(3):543-547.

[99] Rosch PJ: Cholesterol does not cause coronary heart disease in contrast to stress. *Scand. Cardiovasc. J.* 2008; 42(4):244-249.

[100] Caro JJ, Ward AJ, O'Brien JA: Lifetime costs of complications resulting from type 2 diabetes in the U.S. *Diabetes Care* 2002; 25(3):476-481.

[101] American Diabetes Association: Standards of medical care in diabetes--2011. *Diabetes Care* 2011; 34 Suppl 1:S11-S61.

[102] Mazzone T, Meyer PM, Kondos GT, Davidson MH, Feinstein SB, D'Agostino RB, Sr., Perez A, Haffner SM: Relationship of traditional and nontraditional cardiovascular risk factors to coronary artery calcium in type 2 diabetes. *Diabetes* 2007; 56(3):849-855.

[103] Anand DV, Lim E, Hopkins D, Corder R, Shaw LJ, Sharp P, Lipkin D, Lahiri A: Risk stratification in uncomplicated type 2 diabetes: prospective evaluation of the combined use of coronary artery calcium imaging and selective myocardial perfusion scintigraphy. *Eur. Heart J.* 2006; 27(6):713-721.

[104] Elkeles RS, Feher MD, Flather MD, Godsland IF, Nugara F, Richmond W, Rubens MB, Wang D: The association of coronary calcium score and conventional cardiovascular risk factors in Type 2 diabetic subjects asymptomatic for coronary heart disease (The PREDICT Study). *Diabet. Med.* 2004; 21(10):1129-1134.

[105] Wolfe ML, Iqbal N, Gefter W, Mohler ER, III, Rader DJ, Reilly MP: Coronary artery calcification at electron beam computed tomography is increased in asymptomatic type 2 diabetics independent of traditional risk factors. *J. Cardiovasc. Risk* 2002; 9(6):369-376.

[106] Martin SS, Qasim AN, Mehta NN, Wolfe M, Terembula K, Schwartz S, Iqbal N, Schutta M, Bagheri R, Reilly MP: Apolipoprotein B but not LDL cholesterol is associated with coronary artery calcification in type 2 diabetic whites. *Diabetes* 2009; 58(8):1887-1892.

[107] Godsland IF, Elkeles RS, Feher MD, Nugara F, Rubens MB, Richmond W, Khan M, Donovan J, Anyaoku V, Flather MD: Coronary calcification, homocysteine, C-reactive protein and the metabolic syndrome in Type 2 diabetes: the Prospective Evaluation of Diabetic Ischaemic Heart Disease by Coronary Tomography (PREDICT) Study. *Diabet Med.* 2006; 23(11):1192-1200.

[108] Kobayashi S, Oka M, Maesato K, Ikee R, Mano T, Hidekazu M, Ohtake T: Coronary Artery Calcification, ADMA, and Insulin Resistance in CKD Patients. *Clinical Journal of the American Society of Nephrology* 2008; 3(5):1289-1295.

[109] Saremi A, Moritz TE, Anderson RJ, Abraira C, Duckworth WC, Reaven PD: Rates and determinants of coronary and abdominal aortic artery calcium progression in the Veterans Affairs Diabetes Trial (VADT). *Diabetes Care* 2010; 33(12):2642-2647.

[110] Kinney GL, Snell-Bergeon JK, Maahs DM, Eckel RH, Ehrlich J, Rewers M, Hokanson JE: Lipoprotein-associated phospholipase A activity predicts progression of subclinical coronary atherosclerosis. *Diabetes Technol. Ther.* 2011; 13(3):381-387.

[111] Anand DV, Lim E, Darko D, Bassett P, Hopkins D, Lipkin D, Corder R, Lahiri A: Determinants of progression of coronary artery calcification in type 2 diabetes role of glycemic control and inflammatory/vascular calcification markers. *J. Am. Coll. Cardiol.* 2007; 50(23):2218-2225.

[112] Elkeles RS, Godsland IF, Rubens MB, Feher MD, Nugara F, Flather MD: The progress of coronary heart disease in Type 2 diabetes as measured by coronary calcium score from electron beam computed tomography (EBCT): the PREDICT study. *Atherosclerosis* 2008; 197(2):777-783.

[113] Campayo A, Gomez-Biel C, Lobo A: Diabetes and Depression. *Current Psychiatry Reports* 2011; 13(1):26-30.

[114] Janssen I, Powell LH, Matthews KA, Cursio JF, Hollenberg SM, Sutton-Tyrrell K, Bromberger JT, Everson-Rose SA: Depressive symptoms are related to progression of coronary calcium in midlife women: The Study of Women's Health Across the Nation (SWAN) Heart Study. *Am. Heart J.* 2011; 161(6):1186-1191.

[115] Elkeles RS: Coronary artery calcium and cardiovascular risk in diabetes. *Atherosclerosis* 2010; 210(2):331-336.

[116] Sever PS, Poulter NR, Dahlof B, Wedel H, Collins R, Beevers G, Caulfield M, Kjeldsen SE, Kristinsson A, McInnes GT, Mehlsen J, Nieminen M, O'Brien E, Ostergren J: Reduction in cardiovascular events with atorvastatin in 2,532 patients with type 2 diabetes: Anglo-Scandinavian Cardiac Outcomes Trial--lipid-lowering arm (ASCOT-LLA). *Diabetes Care* 2005; 28(5):1151-1157.

[117] Knopp RH, d'Emden M, Smilde JG, Pocock SJ: Efficacy and safety of atorvastatin in the prevention of cardiovascular end points in subjects with type 2 diabetes: the Atorvastatin Study for Prevention of Coronary Heart Disease Endpoints in non-insulin-dependent diabetes mellitus (ASPEN). *Diabetes Care* 2006; 29(7):1478-1485.

[118] Colhoun HM, Betteridge DJ, Durrington PN, Hitman GA, Neil HA, Livingstone SJ, Thomason MJ, Mackness MI, Charlton-Menys V, Fuller JH: Primary prevention of cardiovascular disease with atorvastatin in type 2 diabetes in the Collaborative Atorvastatin Diabetes Study (CARDS): multicentre randomised placebo-controlled trial. *Lancet* 2004; 364(9435):685-696.

[119] Collins R, Armitage J, Parish S, Sleigh P, Peto R: MRC/BHF Heart Protection Study of cholesterol-lowering with simvastatin in 5963 people with diabetes: a randomised placebo-controlled trial. *Lancet* 2003; 361(9374):2005-2016.

[120] Cholesterol Treatment Trialists' (CTT) Collaborators: Efficacy of cholesterol-lowering therapy in 18□686 people with diabetes in 14 randomised trials of statins: a meta-analysis. *The Lancet* 2008; 371(9607):117-125.

[121] Taylor F, Ward K, Moore TH, Burke M, Davey SG, Casas JP, Ebrahim S: Statins for the primary prevention of cardiovascular disease. *Cochrane Database Syst. Rev.* 2011;(1):CD004816.

[122] Citrome L: Number needed to treat: what it is and what it isn't, and why every clinician should know how to calculate it. *J. Clin. Psychiatry* 2011; 72(3):412-413.

[123] Breau RH, Fergusson D, Dahm P: Evidence-based urology in practice: number needed to treat. *BJU Int.* 2009; 104(1):6-8.

[124] McAlister FA: The "number needed to treat" turns 20--and continues to be used and misused. *CMAJ* 2008; 179(6):549-553.

[125] Hippisley-Cox J, Coupland C: Individualising the risks of statins in men and women in England and Wales: population-based cohort study. *Heart* 2010; 96(12):939-947.

[126] Sattar N, Preiss D, Murray HM, Welsh P, Buckley BM, de Craen AJ, Seshasai SRK, McMurray JJ, Freeman DJ, Jukema JW, Macfarlane PW, Packard CJ, Stott DJ, Westendorp RG, Shepherd J, Davis BR, Pressel SL, Marchioli R, Marfisi RM, Maggioni AP, Tavazzi L, Tognoni G, Kjekshus J, Pedersen TR, Cook TJ, Gotto AM, Clearfield MB, Downs JR, Nakamura H, Ohashi Y, Mizuno K, Ray KK, Ford I: Statins and risk of incident diabetes: a collaborative meta-analysis of randomised statin trials. *The Lancet* 1927; 375(9716):735-742.

[127] Waters DD, Ho JE, DeMicco DA, Breazna A, Arsenault BJ, Wun CC, Kastelein JJ, Colhoun H, Barter P: Predictors of New-Onset Diabetes in Patients Treated With Atorvastatin: Results From 3 Large Randomized Clinical Trials. *Journal of the American College of Cardiology* 2011; 57(14):1535-1545.

[128] Keech A, Simes RJ, Barter P, Best J, Scott R, Taskinen MR, Forder P, Pillai A, Davis T, Glasziou P, Drury P, Kesaniemi YA, Sullivan D, Hunt D, Colman P, d'Emden M, Whiting M, Ehnholm C, Laakso M: Effects of long-term fenofibrate therapy on cardiovascular events in 9795 people with type 2 diabetes mellitus (the FIELD study): randomised controlled trial. *Lancet* 2005; 366(9500):1849-1861.

[129] Ansquer JC, Foucher C, Aubonnet P, Le MK: Fibrates and microvascular complications in diabetes--insight from the FIELD study. *Curr. Pharm. Des.* 2009; 15(5):537-552.

[130] Ginsberg HN, Elam MB, Lovato LC, Crouse JR, III, Leiter LA, Linz P, Friedewald WT, Buse JB, Gerstein HC, Probstfield J, Grimm RH, Ismail-Beigi F, Bigger JT, Goff DC, Jr., Cushman WC, Simons-Morton DG, Byington RP: Effects of combination lipid therapy in type 2 diabetes mellitus. *N. Engl. J. Med.* 2010; 362(17):1563-1574.

[131] Greenland P, Bonow RO, Brundage BH, Budoff MJ, Eisenberg MJ, Grundy SM, Lauer MS, Post WS, Raggi P, Redberg RF, Rodgers GP, Shaw LJ, Taylor AJ, Weintraub WS: ACCF/AHA 2007 clinical expert consensus document on coronary artery calcium scoring by computed tomography in global cardiovascular risk assessment and in evaluation of patients with chest pain: a report of the American College of Cardiology Foundation Clinical Expert Consensus Task Force (ACCF/AHA Writing Committee to Update the 2000 Expert Consensus Document on Electron Beam Computed Tomography) developed in collaboration with the Society of Atherosclerosis Imaging and Prevention and the Society of Cardiovascular Computed Tomography. *J. Am. Coll. Cardiol.* 2007; 49(3):378-402.

[132] Jacobs D, Blackburn H, Higgins M, Reed D, Iso H, McMillan G, Neaton J, Nelson J, Potter J, Rifkind B, .: Report of the Conference on Low Blood Cholesterol: Mortality Associations. *Circulation* 1992; 86(3):1046-1060.

[133] Walsh JM, Pignone M: Drug treatment of hyperlipidemia in women. *JAMA* 2004; 291(18):2243-2252.

[134] Petretta M, Costanzo P, Perrone-Filardi P, Chiariello M: Impact of gender in primary prevention of coronary heart disease with statin therapy: a meta-analysis. *Int. J. Cardiol.* 2010; 138(1):25-31.

[135] Eisenberg T, Wells M: Statins and Adverse Cardiovascular Events in Moderate-risk Females: A Statistical and Legal Analysis with Implication for FDA Preemption Claims. *J. Emperical Legal Studies* 2008; 5(3):507-550.

[136] Ridker PM, Danielson E, Fonseca FA, Genest J, Gotto AM, Jr., Kastelein JJ, Koenig W, Libby P, Lorenzatti AJ, Macfadyen JG, Nordestgaard BG, Shepherd J, Willerson JT, Glynn RJ: Rosuvastatin to prevent vascular events in men and women with elevated C-reactive protein. *N. Engl. J. Med.* 2008; 359(21):2195-2207.

[137] de Lorgeril M, Salen P, Abramson J, Dodin S, Hamazaki T, Kostucki W, Okuyama H, Pavy B, Rabaeus M: Cholesterol Lowering, Cardiovascular Diseases, and the Rosuvastatin-JUPITER Controversy: A Critical Reappraisal. *Arch. Intern. Med.* 2010; 170(12):1032-1036.

[138] Larson MG: Assessment of cardiovascular risk factors in the elderly: the Framingham Heart Study. *Stat. Med.* 1995; 14(16):1745-1756.

[139] Nissinen A, Pekkanen J, Porath A, Punsar S, Karvonen MJ: Risk factors for cardiovascular disease among 55 to 74 year-old Finnish men: a 10-year follow-up. *Ann. Med.* 1989; 21(3):239-240.

[140] Siegel D, Kuller L, Lazarus NB, Black D, Feigal D, Hughes G, Schoenberger JA, Hulley SB: Predictors of cardiovascular events and mortality in the Systolic Hypertension in the Elderly Program pilot project. *Am. J. Epidemiol.* 1987; 126(3):385-399.

[141] Krumholz HM, Seeman TE, Merrill SS, Mendes de Leon CF, Vaccarino V, Silverman DI, Tsukahara R, Ostfeld AM, Berkman LF: Lack of association between cholesterol and coronary heart disease mortality and morbidity and all-cause mortality in persons older than 70 years. *JAMA* 1994; 272(17):1335-1340.

[142] Simons LA, Simons J, Friedlander Y, McCallum J: Cholesterol and other lipids predict coronary heart disease and ischaemic stroke in the elderly, but only in those below 70 years. *Atherosclerosis* 2001; 159(1):201-208.

[143] Shepherd J, Blauw GJ, Murphy MB, Bollen EL, Buckley BM, Cobbe SM, Ford I, Gaw A, Hyland M, Jukema JW, Kamper AM, Macfarlane PW, Meinders AE, Norrie J, Packard CJ, Perry IJ, Stott DJ, Sweeney BJ, Twomey C, Westendorp RG: Pravastatin in elderly individuals at risk of vascular disease (PROSPER): a randomised controlled trial. *Lancet* 2002; 360(9346):1623-1630.

[144] Long SB, Blaha MJ, Blumenthal RS, Michos ED: Clinical utility of rosuvastatin and other statins for cardiovascular risk reduction among the elderly. *Clin. Interv. Aging* 2011; 6:27-35.

[145] Hecht HS: A zero coronary artery calcium score: priceless. *J. Am. Coll. Cardiol.* 2010; 55(11):1118-1120.

[146] Gottlieb I, Sara L, Brinker J, Lima J, Rochitte C: CT Coronary Calcification: What Does a Score of □ Mean? *Current Cardiology Reports* 2011; 13(1):49-56.

[147] Min JK, Lin FY, Gidseg DS, Weinsaft JW, Berman DS, Shaw LJ, Rozanski A, Callister TQ: Determinants of Coronary Calcium Conversion Among Patients With a Normal Coronary Calcium Scan: What Is the ΓÇ£Warranty PeriodΓÇØ for Remaining Normal? *Journal of the American College of Cardiology* 2010; 55(11):1110-1117.

[148] Cheng VY, Lepor NE, Madyoon H, Eshaghian S, Naraghi AL, Shah PK: Presence and Severity of Noncalcified Coronary Plaque on 64-Slice Computed Tomographic Coronary Angiography in Patients With Zero and Low Coronary Artery Calcium. *The American Journal of Cardiology* 2007; 99(9):1183-1186.

[149] Folsom AR, Kronmal RA, Detrano RC, O'Leary DH, Bild DE, Bluemke DA, Budoff MJ, Liu K, Shea S, Szklo M, Tracy RP, Watson KE, Burke GL: Coronary artery calcification compared with carotid intima-media thickness in the prediction of cardiovascular disease incidence: the Multi-Ethnic Study of Atherosclerosis (MESA). *Arch. Intern. Med.* 2008; 168(12):1333-1339.

[150] Bischoff B, Kantert C, Meyer T, Hadamitzky M, Martinoff S, Schomig A, Hausleiter J: Cardiovascular risk assessment based on the quantification of coronary calcium in contrast-enhanced coronary computed tomography angiography. *Eur. J. Echocardiogr.* 2011.

[151] Nicholls SJ, Ballantyne CM, Barter PJ, Chapman MJ, Erbel RM, Libby P, Raichlen JS, Uno K, Borgman M, Wolski K, Nissen SE: Effect of two intensive statin regimens on progression of coronary disease. *N. Engl. J. Med.* 2011; 365(22):2078-2087.

[152] Davis W, Rockway S, Kwasny M: Effect of a Combined Therapeutic Approach of Intensive Lipid Management, Omega-3 Fatty Acid Supplementation, and Increased Serum 25 (OH) Vitamin D on Coronary Calcium Scores in Asymptomatic Adults. *Am. J. Ther.* 2009; 16(4):326-332.

[153] Motro M, Shemesh J: Calcium Channel Blocker Nifedipine Slows Down Progression of Coronary Calcification in Hypertensive Patients Compared With Diuretics. *Hypertension* 2001; 37(6):1410-1413.

[154] Nicholls SJ, Tuzcu EM, Wolski K, Bayturan O, Lavoie A, Uno K, Kupfer S, Perez A, Nesto R, Nissen SE: Lowering the triglyceride/high-density lipoprotein cholesterol ratio is associated with the beneficial impact of pioglitazone on progression of coronary atherosclerosis in diabetic patients: insights from the PERISCOPE (Pioglitazone Effect on Regression of Intravascular Sonographic Coronary Obstruction Prospective Evaluation) study. *J. Am. Coll. Cardiol.* 2011; 57(2):153-159.

[155] Feig JE, Rong JX, Shamir R, Sanson M, Vengrenyuk Y, Liu J, Rayner K, Moore K, Garabedian M, Fisher EA: HDL promotes rapid atherosclerosis regression in mice and alters inflammatory properties of plaque monocyte-derived cells. *Proc. Natl. Acad. Sci. U S A* 2011; 108(17):7166-7171.

[156] Seldenrijk A, Hamer M, Lahiri A, Penninx BW, Steptoe A: Psychological distress, cortisol stress response and subclinical coronary calcification. *Psychoneuroendocrinology* 2011; Published ahead of print May 28, 2011.

[157] Kepez A, Niksarlioglu EY, Hazirolan T, Hayran M, Kocabas U, Demir AU, Aytemir K, Tokgozoglu L, Nazli N: Evaluation of association between obstructive sleep apnea and coronary risk scores predicted by tomographic coronary calcium scoring in asymptomatic patients. *Anadolu Kardiyol. Derg.* 2011.

[158] Rutter MK, Nesto RW: Blood pressure, lipids and glucose in type 2 diabetes: how low should we go? Re-discovering personalized care. *Eur. Heart J.* 2011.

[159] Zoungas S, Patel A: Cardiovascular outcomes in type 2 diabetes: the impact of preventative therapies. *Ann. N Y Acad. Sci.* 2010; 1212:29-40.

[160] Baigent C, Keech A, Kearney PM, Blackwell L, Buck G, Pollicino C, Kirby A, Sourjina T, Peto R, Collins R, Simes R: Efficacy and safety of cholesterol-lowering

treatment: prospective meta-analysis of data from 90,056 participants in 14 randomised trials of statins. *Lancet* 2005; 366(9493):1267-1278.

[161] Riche DM, McClendon KS: Role of statins for the primary prevention of cardiovascular disease in patients with type 2 diabetes mellitus. *Am. J. Health Syst. Pharm.* 2007; 64(15):1603-1610.

[162] Gigerenzer G, Wegwarth O, Feufel M: Misleading communication of risk. *BMJ* 2010; 341:c4830.

[163] Citrome L: Relative vs. absolute measures of benefit and risk: what's the difference? *Acta Psychiatr. Scand.* 2010; 121(2):94-102.

[164] McCullough PA, Chinnaiyan KM: Annual Progression of Coronary Calcification in Trials of Preventive Therapies: A Systematic Review. *Arch. Intern. Med.* 2009; 169(22):2064-2070.

[165] Ravnskov U: Cholesterol was healthy in the end. *World Rev. Nutr. Diet.* 2009; 100:90-109.

[166] Ravnskov U: The fallacies of the lipid hypothesis. *Scand. Cardiovasc. J.* 2008; 42(4):236-239.

In: Horizons in World Cardiovascular Research. Vol. 6
Editor: Eleanor H. Bennington
ISBN: 978-1-63321-298-5

Chapter 6

Pulse Decomposition for Artery Pressure Waveforms: Using Three or Four Gaussian Functions?

Chengyu Liu[1,2,*]
[1]School of Control Science and Engineering and School of Information Science and Engineering, Shandong University, Jinan, China

Abstract

An early return of the reflection wave of the artery pressure waveform has been widely accepted as an important risk indicator of cardiovascular diseases. Waveform fitting method using Gaussian functions has been proven as a useful tool for decomposing the pressure waveform into sub-waves and hence assessing and quantifying the wave reflection. However, different researches employed different number of Gaussian functions and the appropriate number is still not determined. So the comparison for the parameters of Gaussian functions between using different Gaussian functions is essentially important for this Gaussian fitting method. The aim of this study is to compare the parameters differences between using three and four Gaussian functions. Fifty-six normal subjects and 51 heart failure subjects (New York Heart Association class II or III) were studied by noninvasive techniques applied to acquire the carotid artery pressure waveforms (CAPW) and radial artery pressure waveforms (RAPW). Then CAPW and RAPW signals were analyzed using Gaussian fitting and two-stage particle swarm optimizer to determine the parameters for each Gaussian function: peak time, peak amplitude and half-width. The results showed that for both normal and heart failure subjects, as well as for both CAPW and RAPW signals, the parameters from the first and second Gaussian functions have no significant statistical differences between using three and four Gaussians fitting (all $P>0.05$) whereas the parameters from the third Gaussian function have (all $P<0.01$). Further analysis showed that for both using three and four Gaussians fitting, as well as for both CAPW and RAPW signals, in comparison with normal subjects, heart failure subjects had significantly decreased peak amplitude of the

[*] E-mail: bestlcy@sdu.edu.cn.

first Gaussian function ($P<0.01$), significantly increased peak amplitude and significantly shorter peak times of the second Gaussian function (both $P<0.01$). This study is therefore an important step to further understand the underlying physiological mechanisms of the artery pressure waveform features using Gaussian functions.

1. Literature Review

The shape of artery pressure waveform is determined by the cardiac ejection function and the mechanical and geometric properties of the systemic arteries. It is mainly consisted of a forward-travelling pressure wave (incident wave) generated by left ventricular ejection and a backward-traveling pressure wave caused by reflection of the forward wave from sites of change in impedance within the peripheral arterial system (Laurent et al., 2007; Millasseau et al., 2006). Recent years, the backward-traveling pressure wave from the periphery to the heart, also called the reflected wave, has been widely accepted as an important risk indicator for cardiovascular diseases (Segers et al., 2012; Sugawara et al., 2010). Although the precise origin of the reflected wave is not directly identifiable, some studies have suggested that some significant decrease sites in diameter and a change in elasticity such as the juncture between thoracic and abdominal aorta, or between abdominal aorta and common iliac arteries, contribute to the pattern of wave reflection (Baruch et al., 2011; Kriz and Seba, 2008). Some researches also suggested that there are only the 'effective' reflection sites instead of precise origin in artery system (Segers et al., 2012). The pressure wave as measured at any location in the arterial tree will therefore consist of the superposition of these forward and backward components (Swillens and Segers, 2008; Baruch et al., 2011). Reflected wave affect the pressure and flow waveforms in aorta, and the impact depending on their return time (mainly determined by large arteries) and magnitude (determined by both periphery and large arteries) (Westerhof et al., 2006). In healthy subjects, the reflection wave normally returns to the central aorta in diastole and acts to maintain diastolic perfusion pressure in the coronary artery circulation. However, if the reflection wave comes back earlier to the heart (usually in the late systole), it will conduce the rise of the central systolic and pulse pressures and will depress the coronary perfusion pressure (Sugawara et al., 2010). For these reasons, the reflection wave has been well recognized as an important indicator of cardiovascular risk (Sugawara et al., 2010; Allen and Murray, 2002; Millasseau et al., 2006). So estimating and quantification of the amount of wave reflection should provide a better understanding of the pathophysiology of cardiovascular disease and a better assessment of cardiovascular risk in patients with hypertension, arteriosclerosis or peripheral vascular diseases (Sugawara et al., 2010; Westerhof et al., 2008; Westerhof et al., 2006; Mitchell et al., 2004).

It has been reported that early wave reflection is associated with ageing, with the reflection sites shifting proximally toward the heart (Segers et al., 2007; O'ourke and Nichols, 2004). On the contrary, a distal shift of reflection site was observed with advancing age (Mitchell et al., 2004). While other researchers reported that the major reflection sites only shifted distally from 65 years old and before that aging had no influence on the reflection site (Sugawara et al., 2010). These controversial conclusions are partly due to that different methods to identify the return time may yield substantially different parameter values (Segers et al., 2007). Because the identification methods are optional and non-uniform, it could induce a failure to compare the results from different researchers. Another explanation is that those methods are not sensitive enough to accurately represent the effect of wave reflection (Swillens and Segers, 2008). Therefore, developing the algorithms to accurately extract the reflection wave is clinically important.

Westerhof et al. demonstrated that the forward and backward components could be effectively acquired provided that aorta pressure and flow waveforms are known (Westerhof et al., 1972). This model analysis is considered as a gold standard method to assess wave reflection (Westerhof et al., 2006). However, assessing both aorta pressure and flow waveforms is usually inconvenient, so other methods to assess wave reflection have been proposed.

The most widespread method is the augmentation index (AI), expressing the ratio of the 'augmented pressure', attributed to the reflected wave, to the pulse pressure (O'ourke and Nichols, 2004; Kelly et al., 1989). AI relies on the measurement of the pressure waveform morphology only. Despite the many large studies where AI is measured, there is still no consensus on the prognostic value of AI in the general population. The drawback of AI is that it is a composite measure which is not only sensitive to the magnitude of wave reflection, but also by many other factors affecting the timing of the reflected waves, such as the height, the heart rate and the stiffness of the vessels (Segers et al., 2006).

The other common way to estimate the amount of wave reflection is by the derivative methods, which use the first (Millasseau et al., 2002) or second (Bortolotto et al., 2000) or third (Karamanoglu, 1997) derivatives of artery pressure waveform, or by the wave intensity analysis, which analyzes vascular hemodynamics in terms of traveling energy waves (Curtis et al., 2007; Zambanini et al., 2005). The advantages of the above mentioned methods are their simplicity and the possibility to be also used in real-time analysis. The disadvantage of them is that they are highly susceptible to noise and thus are limited to analyze the weak or noisy artery pressure waveforms, especially when the reflection wave in the diastole cannot be distinguished by sight.

To accurately obtain the characteristics of wave reflection, researchers have also modeled the arterial pressure waveform using pulse decomposition analysis (PDA), which decomposes a pulse waveform into several independent sub-waves. PDA methods are based on the physiological mechanism since the pulse waveform in a whole cardiac cycle is usually consisted of several sub-waves (Denardo et al., 2010; Su et al., 2009). So it is just in accordance with the emphasis by Millasseau for the fundamental question of what determines the contour of the pulse waveform and becomes a promising method for quantification of wave reflection (Millasseau et al., 2006).

Westerhof et al. separated a pulse waveform into two parts by a triangular wave of duration equal to the ejection time (Westerhof et al., 2006). Goswami et al. presented a two-pulse synthesis model to reconstruct the pulse waveform (Goswami et al., 2010). However, when the pulse waveforms become complicated, especially three or more crests exist in waveforms, two sub-waves method will fail. So three sub-waves (Qian et al., 1994), four sub-waves (Rubins, 2008), even five sub-waves (Huotari et al., 2012, 2011; Baruch et al., 2011) were used for the pulse decomposition. Rubins fitted each of systolic and diastolic waveforms with the sum of two Gaussian functions respectively (Rubins, 2008). However, this method has two weaknesses: one is that the fitting accuracy is not high and the fitting error between the original pulse and the fitted curve is about 10%, which makes the accurate location of the reflection wave impossible; the other one is the inappropriate hypothesis that regarding the positions of the sub-waves as the same for the different pulses (ear and finger). Huotari et al.

analyzed the finger and toe photoplethysmographic (PPG) pulses using five logarithmic normal functions (Huotari et al., 2012, 2011). Actually, this work also had a poor fitting accuracy and only provided some examples with an average maximum fitting error of 4%. Xu et al. proposed a multi-Gaussian fitting method to fit the pulse waveform using an adaptive number (four or five) of sub-waves and made the fitting error less than 2% (Wang et al., 2013; Xu et al., 2011). However, this method needs an initial parameter setting step. The initial parameters are acquired using the traditional first or second derivatives methods. As mentioned above, derivatives methods are highly susceptible to noise. In addition, in Xu *et al*'s studies (Wang et al., 2013; Xu et al., 2011), although using the adaptive number (four or five) of sub-waves could make the fitting accuracy less than 2 %, they did not give a physiological explanation and comparison analysis for the differences of parameters between four and five different number of fitting functions, which is very important for the clinical use of Gaussian fitting method.

In our recent research, we used three Gaussian functions to act as the sub-waves to fit both the carotid and radial pulses and achieved a best fitting accuracy compared with the above PDA methods. The fitting errors are 1.2% and 1.3% for the carotid and radial pulses respectively (Liu et al., 2013). We did not use any derivative operation to initialize the parameters of Gaussian functions but set them as random values to remove the susceptible aspect to noise of derivative methods (Liu et al., 2013). The parameters of Gaussian functions were determined by the fully informed particle swarm algorithm (Mendes et al., 2004). Although the fine fitting accuracy is achieved, the optimization time is long and the calculating efficiency is low.

Therefore, we also developed a two-stage particle swarm optimizer to efficiently determine the optimal parameters of Gaussian functions. To the best of our knowledge, two-stage particle swarm optimizer is used for the first time to fit the arterial pressure waveform (Liu et al., 2014b).

In terms of the clinical significance of this Gaussian fitting method, we explored the differences of parameters from three Gaussian functions between normal subjects and heart failure patients and found that there were significant differences between two groups (Liu et al., 2014a).

Our obtained results indicated the clinical significance of the Gaussian fitting and particle swarm optimization methods, which should provide essential tools for further understanding the underlying physiological mechanisms of the artery pressure waveform. However, an important issue about comparing the differences of the parameters from different number of Gaussian functions is still not systematically studied. So the comparison for the parameters of Gaussian functions between using different Gaussian functions is essentially important for this Gaussian fitting method.

The aim of this study is to compare the parameters differences between using three and four Gaussian functions for the carotid artery pressure waveforms (CAPW) and radial artery pressure waveforms (RAPW) between normal and heart failure subjects.

2. Methods

2.1. Subjects

One hundred and seven subjects were enrolled and were divided into two groups, (i) the heart failure group (29 females and 22 males, median age 63 years; range, 40–75 years) and, (ii) the normal group (30 females and 26 males; median age, 58 years; range, 25–73 years). The subjects, either in the heart failure or the normal groups, should, (i) be aged between 18 and 75 years old, (ii) agree to sign the information consent form and, (iii) not have participated in any other 'clinical trials' within the previous three months. Individually, the heart failure group must be in accord with classes II-III of the New York Heart Association (NYHA) Functional Classification and have an LVEF<0.50 with an ultrasonic cardiogram (UCG) detection. The individual requirements for the normal group are that, (i) half the group should be older than 50 years for the age matching and, (ii) they should have normal results with a UCG, blood lipid and glucose checks and electrocardiogram (ECG). Subjects with severe organ damage or subjects with psychiatric disorders will be excluded.

The study obtained the full approval of the Clinical Ethics Committee of the Qilu Hospitals of Shandong University. All of the potential risks and procedures of the study were explained to the subjects, and they gave their written informed consent to participate in the study.

2.2. Experimental Procedure

Figure 1. gives a schematic diagram illustrating the measurement system and experimental procedure. All the measurements were undertaken in a quiet, temperature-controlled measurement room in Shandong University Qilu Hospital, which provided a stable temperature at the level of 25 ± 3°C. Before the formal recording, each subject lay supine on a measurement bed for a 10 min rest period to allow cardiovascular stabilization.

Three electrocardio-electrode clamps were attached to the right wrist, the right ankle and the left ankle respectively, to acquire the standard limb Ⅱ-lead ECG signal. Two piezoresistive sensors were attached to the neck and the right wrist to acquire the CAPW and RAPW signals respectively. A cuff of mercurial sphygmomanometer was wrapped on the subject's right brachia for the auscultatory blood pressures measurement manually, i.e., Systolic Blood Pressure (SBP) and Diastolic Blood Pressure (DBP). All the measurements were performed by an experienced operator to ensure the electrocardio-electrode clamps, piezoresistive sensors and the cuff were attached well. For each study on a particular subject, ECG, CAPW and RAPW signals were synchronously recorded for 5 min, named 1st min, 2nd min, 3rd min, 4th min and 5th min signals in turn. During the recording session, the subjects were told to keep the regular and gentle breathing. Auscultatory SBP and DBP were recorded manually at the beginning and end of the signal recording from the right upper arm. The Mean Arterial Pressure (MAP) and Pulse Pressure (PP) were calculated using the classic formula: MAP = DBP + (SBP−DBP)/3 and PP = SBP-DBP. For each subject, SBP, DBP, MAP and PP all used the mean value of two measures. The overall mean and standard deviation (SD) values of SBP, DBP, MAP and PP were given in Table 1.

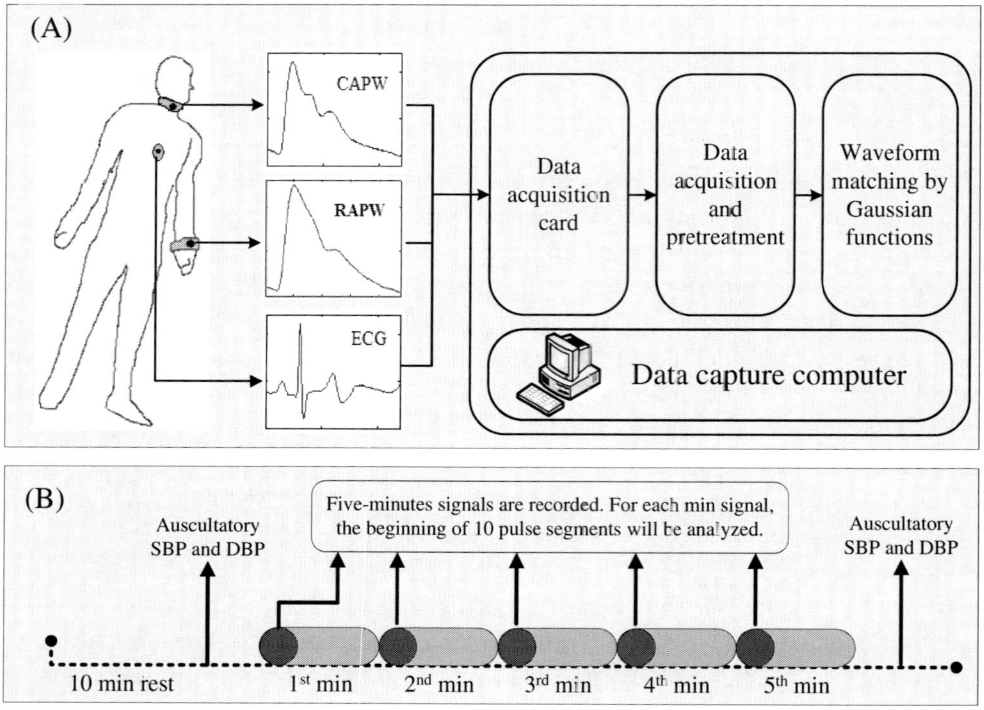

Figure 1. Schematic diagram of the measurement system (A), and the experimental procedure (B).

Table 1. Selected physiological characteristic of all subjects. The *P*-values measure the separation between normal and heart failure subjects

Variables	Normal subjects	Heart failure subjects	*P*-Values
No.	56	51	–
Men (%)	26 (46)	22 (43)	0.87
Age, year	58 ± 10	63 ± 9	0.06
Height, cm	169 ± 9	166 ± 8	0.40
Body mass, kg	71 ± 9	68 ± 9	0.46
Body Mass Index (BMI), kg/m^2	22.9 ± 3.1	23.8 ± 3.3	0.11
Heart Rate (HR), beats/min	70 ± 10	67 ± 8	0.44
NYHA, class II/III (%)	ND	30 (59)/21 (41)	–
Left Ventricular Ejection Fraction (LVEF), %	59 ± 12	38 ± 14	< 0.01
Systolic Blood Pressure (SBP), mmHg	122 ± 15	127 ± 13	0.37
Diastolic Blood Pressure (DBP), mmHg	74 ± 12	72 ± 9	0.65
Mean Arterial Pressure (MAP), mmHg	97 ± 11	96 ± 12	0.90
Pulse Pressure (PP) , mmHg	49 ± 13	56 ± 11	0.06

Note: Data are expressed as number or mean ± standard deviation (SD). NYHA, New York Heart Association; ND, no data.

2.3. Data Acquisition and Pretreatment

In each measurement, the ECG, CAPW and RAPW signals were converted simultaneously into digital signals using a 16-bit A/D data acquisition card (National Instruments, USA) and were recorded at a sample rate of 1000 Hz (Figure 2). Subsequently, the off-line analysis was performed by a custom designed computer program using the MATLAB software (Version R2009a, MathWorks Inc., USA). First, the slow varying components (0~0.05 Hz) were removed from the ECG, CAPW and RAPW signals respectively. Second, the R-wave peaks of the ECG were detected using the Wavelet Transform Modulus Maxima (WTMM) method (Martinez et al., 2004). Ectopic ECG beats were excluded (Liu et al., 2012). With the location of R-wave peaks, all feet (i.e., starting points) of the CAPW and RAPW signals were found (Solà et al., 2009). Then, the CAPW and RAPW signals were segmented using the starting points of two consecutive pulses respectively. Each pulse segment corresponded to one cardiac cycle (Figure 2). The pulse episodes with 10 successive pulses at the beginning of each min signal without ectopic beats were selected for the subsequent analysis. For each pulse, it will be treated with the length and amplitude normalization with the same length 1000 and the same amplitude range between 0 and 1 V.

2.4. Waveform Fitting Method

Each normalized pulse $S(n)$ will be fitted by three or four Gaussian functions. The Gaussian functions were denoted as $f_1(n)$, $f_2(n)$ and $f_3(n)$ when using three Gaussian functions and as $f_1(n)$, $f_2(n)$, $f_3(n)$ and $f_4(n)$ when using four Gaussian functions.

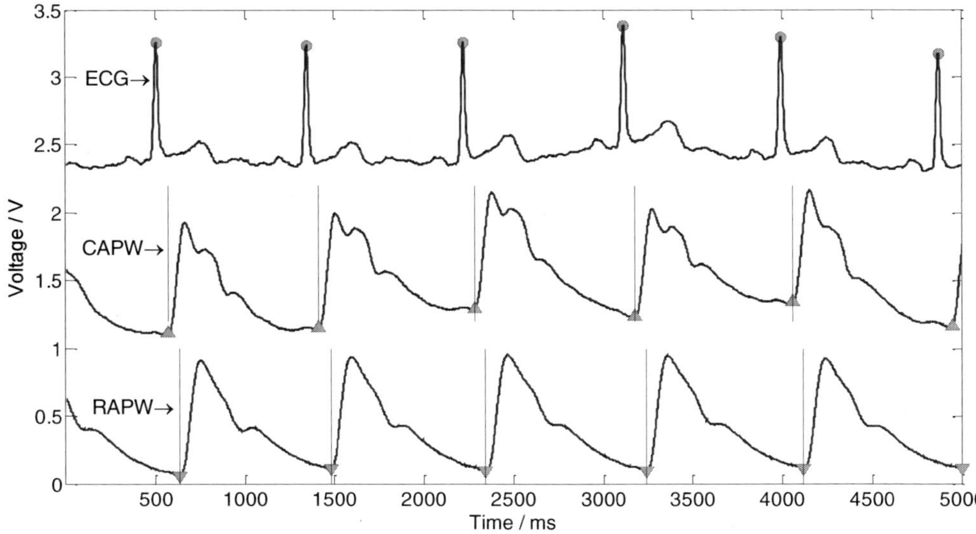

Figure 2. The simultaneously measured ECG, CAPW and RAPW signals. The detected R-wave peaks were denoted as "●", and the starting points of CAPW and RAPW signals were denoted as "▲" and "▼" respectively. The CAPW and RAPW signals were segmented to diffreret pulse segments from the current starting point to the next one.

The first Gaussian function $f_1(n)$ denoted the forward wave and the others might denoted the reflection waves.

Each Gaussian function $f_k(n)$ had 1000 points (n=1,2,…, 1000) and was determined by three parameters: peak time C_k, peak amplitude H_k and half-width W_k.

It was defined as follows:

$$f_k(n) = H_k \times \exp\left(-\frac{2(n-C_k)^2}{W_k^{\,2}}\right), \tag{1}$$

where n=1, 2, ···, 1000, k=1, 2, 3 or 1, 2, ···, 4.

After the parameters C_k, H_k and W_k were determined, the superimposed curve $f(n, x)$ of Gaussian functions was regarded as the fitted curve for the original pulse $S(n)$.

$$f(n,x) = \sum_{k=1}^{3 \text{ or } 4} f_k(n) \tag{2}$$

where $x=[C_k, H_k, W_k]$ (k=1, 2, 3 or 1, 2, ···, 4.) was the parameter vector.

The above mentioned waveform fitting problem with a superposition of three or four Gaussians is essentially an optimization problem. The objective function could be expressed as follows:

$$\text{Min} \quad F(x) = \sum_{n=1}^{1000} [f(n,x) - S(n)]^2, \tag{3}$$

where x is the parameter vector to be optimized. In the present study, we used the two-stage particle swarm optimizer to solve the optimization problem in Eq. (3) (Liu et al., 2014b). The fitting accuracy was controlled by the values of mean absolute error (MAE), which was expressed as follows:

$$\text{MAE} = \frac{\sum_{n=1}^{N} |f(n,x) - S(n)|}{N} \times 100\%. \tag{4}$$

where $f(n, x)$ is the fitting result using three or four Gaussian functions, $S(n)$ is the original pulse and N is the total number of sample points and is 1000 in this study. The parameter optimization will be ceased once MAE is less than 1.5%, which is accurate enough for the waveform matching (Liu et al., 2014a; Liu et al., 2013).

2.5. Statistical Analysis

Data were reported as mean ± standard deviation (SD) as specified. Unpaired Student's t-tests (2-tailed) or one-way ANOVA were used to calculate the statistical significance. Statistical significance was set a priori at P<0.05.

All statistical analyses were performed using the Statistical Package for Social Sciences (V19, SPSS Inc., Chicago, IL, USA).

3. Results

3.1. Physiological Characteristics of Subjects

Heart failure subjects are usually older. So the individual requirement for normal subjects, i.e., half should be older than 50 years, could ensure the age matching (P=0.06). LVEF was significantly reduced in heart failure subjects compared with that of normal subjects duo to the pathological reason (P<0.01), but, in other respects, two groups were well matched (Table 1). SBP (P=0.37), DBP (P=0.65) and MAP (P=0.90) did not differ between normal and heart failure subjects.

Heart failure was associated with an increase in PP (P=0.06), which was near of the borderline statistical significance (Table 1).

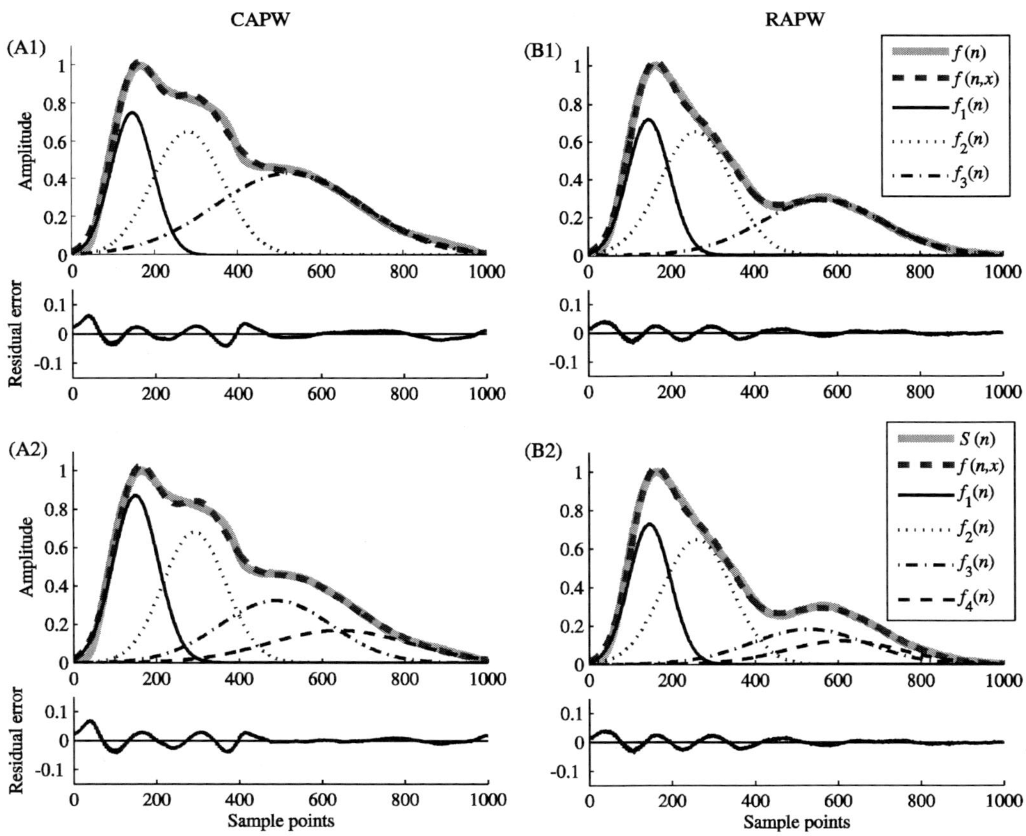

Figure 3. Examples of waveform fitting results from a normalized CAPW pulse (A1 for three gaussians fitting and A2 for four gaussians fitting) and a normalized RAPW pulse (B1 for three gaussians fitting and B2 for four gaussians fitting). In each sub-figure, the upper panel shows the original normalized pulse $S(n)$, the fitting curve $f(n,x)$ and the corresponding Gaussian functions. The bottom panel shows the corresponding residual error. All fitting error of MAE values are less than 1.5%.

3.2. Fitting Examples

Figure 3 shows the examples of waveform fitting results from a normalized CAPW pulse and a normalized RAPW pulse when using three and four Gaussian functions. The algorithm will be ceased if the fitting error of MAE value is less than 1.5%.

In each sub-figure, the upper panel shows the original normalized pulse $S(n)$ (bold solid line, green), the fitting curve $f(n,x)$ (bold dotted line, blue) and the corresponding three or four Gaussian functions: $f_1(n)$ (thin solid line), $f_2(n)$ (thin dotted line), $f_3(n)$ (thin broken line) and $f_4(n)$ (thin dashed line). The bottom panel shows the corresponding residual error. It is clear that the fitting results with MAE values less than 1.5% have fine visual fitting accuracy.

3.3. Effect of Different Recording Time on Parameters Results

In this section we will test the statistical stability for the parameters at different recordings time (1st min, 2nd min, 3rd min, 4th min and 5th min). For each parameter, the average value was firstly calculated from the 10 pulses in each minute. Then the overall mean and SD values were obtained across all subjects of the normal or heart failure group. One-way ANOVA was used to compare the statistical differences among five different recording times. Table 2 shows the example of the parameter results from normal subjects for CAPW and RAPW signals respectively when using three Gaussians fitting.

Table 2. The statistical results of nine parameters from normal subjects when using three Gaussians. The *P*-values measure the separation among the different recordings times

Variables		Different recording times					*P*-Values
		1st min	2nd min	3rd min	4th min	5th min	
CAPW	C_1, ms	127 ± 11	131 ± 12	126 ± 12	129 ± 13	130 ± 9	NS
	C_2, ms	272 ± 10	273 ± 9	269 ± 11	272 ± 11	267 ± 10	NS
	C_3, ms	518 ± 27	526 ± 29	529 ± 25	519 ± 31	522 ± 24	NS
	H_1	0.80 ± 0.11	0.78 ± 0.09	0.83 ± 0.13	0.81 ± 0.12	0.79 ± 0.13	NS
	H_2	0.78 ± 0.10	0.74 ± 0.12	0.81 ± 0.08	0.76 ± 0.11	0.82 ± 0.09	NS
	H_3	0.45 ± 0.09	0.41 ± 0.11	0.42 ± 0.10	0.40 ± 0.08	0.42 ± 0.09	NS
	W_1, ms	89 ± 11	92 ± 13	94 ± 11	91 ± 13	89 ± 12	NS
	W_2, ms	151 ± 14	157 ± 11	149 ± 14	153 ± 12	156 ± 13	NS
	W_3, ms	321 ± 37	318 ± 32	337 ± 29	332 ± 42	326 ± 27	NS
RAPW	C_1, ms	121 ± 12	117 ± 11	120 ± 10	121 ± 12	118 ± 11	NS
	C_2, ms	259 ± 11	261 ± 10	253 ± 9	255 ± 13	260 ± 11	NS
	C_3, ms	600 ± 25	597 ± 24	588 ± 26	592 ± 25	602 ± 31	NS
	H_1	0.75 ± 0.12	0.71 ± 0.10	0.73 ± 0.08	0.69 ± 0.12	0.71 ± 0.11	NS
	H_2	0.68 ± 0.11	0.73 ± 0.12	0.74 ± 0.10	0.68 ± 0.11	0.67 ± 0.12	NS
	H_3	0.33 ± 0.10	0.32 ± 0.10	0.32 ± 0.09	0.30 ± 0.11	0.34 ± 0.12	NS
	W_1, ms	93 ± 12	91 ± 10	90 ± 14	89 ± 11	90 ± 11	NS
	W_2, ms	150 ± 12	145 ± 13	153 ± 12	151 ± 11	147 ± 12	NS
	W_3, ms	331 ± 45	324 ± 34	339 ± 28	343 ± 38	339 ± 41	NS

Note: Data are expressed as number or mean ±standard deviation (SD). NS means there is no significant differences between different recording times (all $P>0.05$).

For all nine parameters, there are no significant differences among the different recording times (all $P>0.05$), which show the fine statistical stability of Gaussian parameters. When using four Gaussians fitting for normal subjects, all twelve parameters also have no significant differences among the different recording times (all $P>0.05$). The similar results could be obtained for heart failure subjects. So in the next sections, the mean values of the Gaussian parameters during 5 min were used for the analysis and comparison.

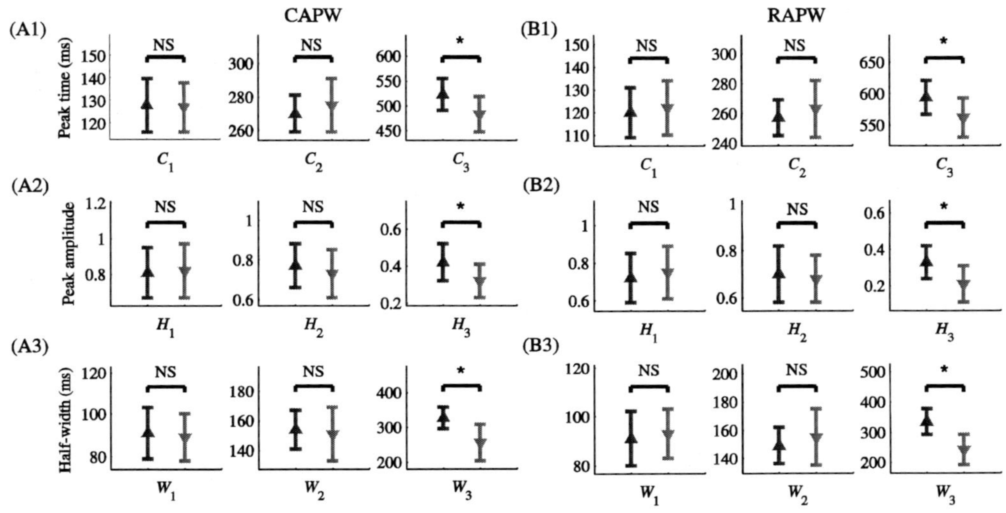

Figure 4. Error bars of nine parameters (C_1, C_2, C_3, H_1, H_2, H_3, W_1, W_2 and W_3) for normal subjects when using three and four Gaussian functions for both CAPW and RAPW signals. Blue '▲' shows the mean and stadard deviation (SD) when using three Gaussians fitting. Red '▼' shows the mean and SD when using four Gaussians fitting. NS means there is no significant differences ($P>0.05$) whereas '*' means there is ($P<0.01$).

3.4. Parameters Comparison between Using Three and Four Gaussian Functions

In this section we will compare the statistical differences for nine parameters (C_1, C_2, C_3, H_1, H_2, H_3, W_1, W_2 and W_3) between using three and four Gaussian functions. Figure 4 shows the error bars of the statistical results for normal subjects. For both CAPW and RAPW signals, the six parameters from the first Gaussian function $f_1(n)$ and second Gaussian function $f_2(n)$, i.e., C_1, C_2, H_1, H_2, W_1 and W_2, have no significant statistical differences between using three and four Gaussians fitting (all $P>0.05$). The thrree parameters from the third Gaussian function $f_3(n)$, i.e., C_3, H_3 and W_3, have significant statistical differences between using three and four Gaussians fitting (all $P<0.01$). Figure 5 shows the error bars of the statistical results of heart failure subjects, which are much similar with the results of normal subjects: six parameters from the first and second Gaussian functions have no significant statistical differences between using three and four Gaussians fitting (all $P>0.05$) whereas three parameters from the third Gaussian function have (all $P<0.01$). It is worth to note that for both normal and heart failure subjects, when using three Gaussians fitting, all three parameters from the third Gaussian function $f_3(n)$ are larger than those from using four

Gaussians fitting, which indicates that using four Gaussians fitting makes the third Gaussian function move forward and exhibit low amplitude and narrow half-width.

Because the parameter from third Gaussian function are different between using different numbers of Gaussian functions, so in the next section, only the six parameters from the first and second Gaussian functions are used for the comparison analysis between the normal and heart failure subjects.

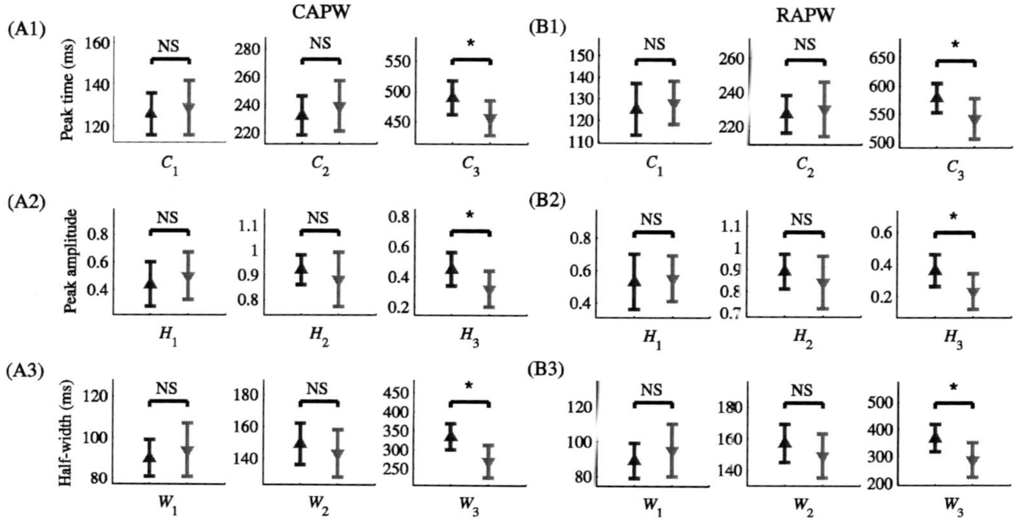

Figure 5. Error bars of nine parameters (C_1, C_2, C_3, H_1, H_2, H_3, W_1, W_2 and W_3) for heart failure subjects when using three and four Gaussian functions for both CAPW and RAPW signals. Blue '▲' shows the mean and stadard deviation (SD) when using three Gaussians fitting. Red '▼' shows the mean and SD when using four Gaussians fitting. NS means there is no significant differences (P>0.05) whereas '*' means there is (P<0.01).

3.5. Parameters Comparison between Normal and Heart Failure Subjects

Table 3 shows the statistical results of the selected six parameters (C_1, C_2, H_1, H_2, W_1 and W_2) between normal and heart failure subjects for both CAPW and RAPW signals when using three and four Gaussians fitting respectively. As shown in Table 3, no matter using three Gaussians fitting, or using four Gaussians fitting, heart failure was both associated with a marked advance in the peak time C_2 (P<0.01), while the peak time C_1 has no significant difference between two groups in either CAPW (P=0.9 for both three and four Gaussians fitting) or RAPW signals (P=0.7 for three Gaussians fitting and P=0.6 for four Gaussians fitting).

Heart failure was associated with a marked reduction in the peak amplitude H_1 and was associated with a marked rise in the peak amplitude H_2. All these two variables H_1 and H_2 had significant differences between two groups in either CAPW or RAPW signal (all P<0.01). Although the peak time of C_2 was reduced in heart failure, the width value W_2 was similar between normal and heart failure subjects in either CAPW or RAPW signal. The width value W_1 was also similar between two groups.

3.6. Parameters Stability Comparison between Setting Fitting Accuracy MAE≤1.5% and MAE≤5%

The parameters stability from Gaussian functions is essentially important for the Gaussian fitting method.

Table 3. Parameters comparison between two groups for both CAPW and RAPW signals when using three and four Gaussians fitting respectively. The *P*-values measure the separation between normal and heart failure subjects

Variables		CAPW				RAPW		
		Normal	Heart Failure	*P*-Values		Normal	Heart Failure	*P*-Values
Using three Gaussians fitting								
Peak time	C_1, ms	128 ± 12	126 ± 10	0.9		120 ± 11	125 ± 12	0.7
	C_2, ms	270 ± 11	232 ± 14*	< 0.01		257 ± 12	227 ± 11*	< 0.01
Peak amplitude	H_1	0.81 ± 0.14	0.44 ± 0.16*	< 0.01		0.72 ± 0.13	0.53 ± 0.17*	< 0.01
	H_2	0.77 ± 0.11	0.92 ± 0.06*	< 0.01		0.70 ± 0.12	0.89 ± 0.08*	< 0.01
Half-width	W_1, ms	91 ± 12	90 ± 9	0.9		91 ± 11	89 ± 10	0.9
	W_2, ms	154 ± 13	149 ± 13	0.8		149 ± 13	157 ± 12	0.1
Using four Gaussians fitting								
Peak time	C_1, ms	127 ± 11	129 ± 13	0.9		122 ± 12	128 ± 10	0.6
	C_2, ms	275 ± 16	239 ± 18*	< 0.01		263 ± 19	230 ± 16*	< 0.01
Peak amplitude	H_1	0.82 ± 0.15	0.50 ± 0.17*	< 0.01		0.75 ± 0.14	0.55 ± 0.14*	< 0.01
	H_2	0.73 ± 0.12	0.88 ± 0.11*	< 0.01		0.68 ± 0.10	0.84 ± 0.12*	< 0.01
Half-width	W_1, ms	89 ± 11	94 ± 13	0.3		93 ± 10	95 ± 15	0.5
	W_2, ms	151 ± 18	143 ± 15	0.2		155 ± 20	149 ± 14	0.4

Note: Data are expressed as number or mean ±standard deviation (SD).

In the present study, we set the optimization criterion for fitting accuracy as MAE≤1.5%. To certify this strict criterion is necessary for the stable fitting results, we compared results of three parameters from the first Gaussian function $f_1(n)$ for random selected five normal subjects when setting MAE≤1.5% and MAE≤5% respectively.

These three parameters are: the peak time C_1, the peak amplitude H_1 and the half-width W_1. For each subject, fifty pulses of CAPW signals (ten pulses in each min and five min signals in total) were used for this test. Figure 6 gives the boxplots of these three parameters when using three Gaussians fitting. It is clear that each parameter has a poor statistical stability when setting the optimization criterion as MAE≤5%. The better statistical stability can be found when setting MAE≤1.5%, which shows the necessity of the strict criterion (MAE≤1.5%) of fitting accuracy. Figure 7 shows the boxplots of these three parameters when using four Gaussians fitting. The similar results with Figure 6 could also be obtained.

4. Discussion

Major findings of this study are as follows. First, we have employed the Gaussian functions and the two-stage particle swarm optimizer (Liu et al., 2014b) to fit both the carotid and radial artery pressure waveforms (CAPW and RAPW) between normal and heart failure subjects. Fine fitting accuracy (MAE<1.5%) has been acquired when using both three and four Gaussian functions.

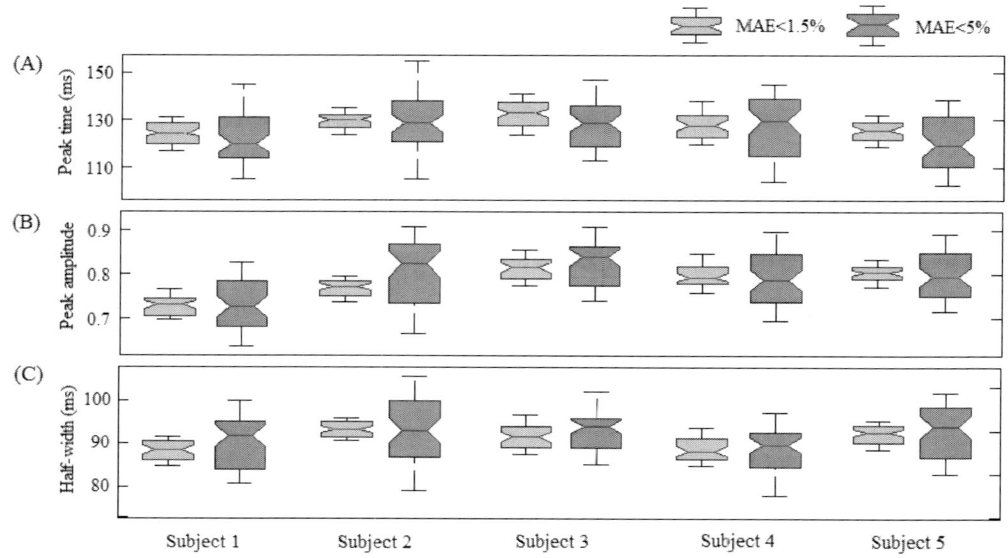

Figure 6. The boxplots of three parameters C_1 (A), H_1 (B) and W_1 (C) when using three Gaussians fitting by setting the optimizaiton criterion as MAE≤1.5% and MAE≤5% respectively.

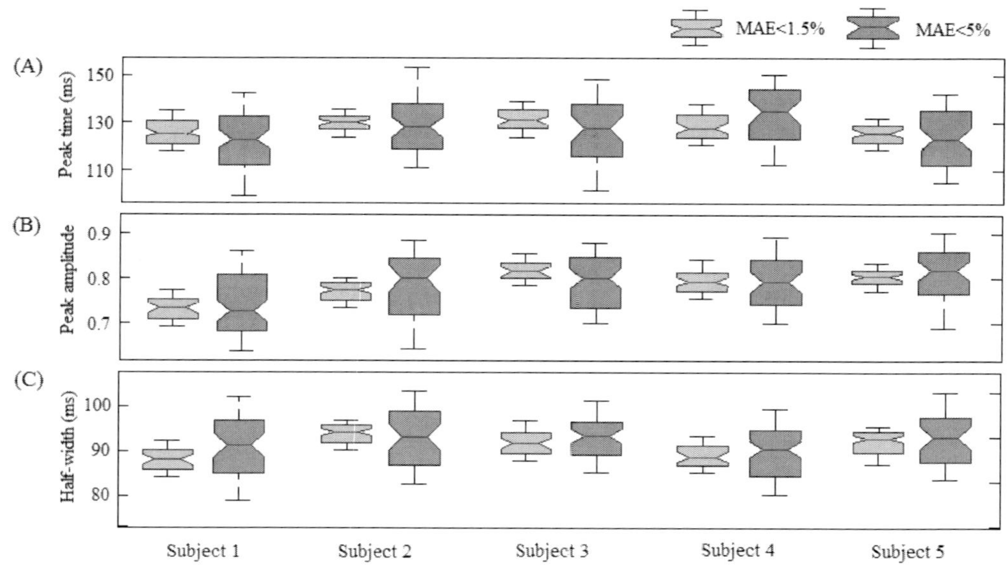

Figure 7. The boxplots of three parameters C_1 (A), H_1 (B) and W_1 (C) when using four Gaussians fitting by setting the optimizaiton criterion as MAE≤1.5% and MAE≤5% respectively.

The fitting results performs better than previous studies (Wang et al., 2013; Huotari et al., 2011; Goswami et al., 2010; Rubins, 2008; Westerhof et al., 2006; Qian et al., 1994), which forms a solid foundation for exploring the generation and reflection characteristics of arterial pressure waveforms from the connotative Gaussian functions.

Second but most important, we have compared the distribution characteristics of parameters between using three and four Gaussian functions for normal and heart failure subjects respectively.

For both CAPW and RAPW signals, the parameters from the first and second Gaussian function have no significant statistical differences between using three and four Gaussians fitting whereas the parameters from the third Gaussian function have (all $P<0.001$ for three parameters). This indicates that the join of the fourth Gaussian function could make the obvious change for the third Gaussian function, not only in time but also in amplitude and shape. However, the fourth Gaussian function has a little influence on the first and second Gaussian functions. However, the fourth Gaussian function has a little influence on the first and second Gaussian functions. Third, we compared the differences of six parameters from the first and second Gaussian functions between normal and heart failure subjects when using three and four Gaussian fitting respectively. For both using three and four Gaussian fitting, as well as for both CAPW and RAPW signals, in comparison with normal subjects, heart failure subjects had significantly decreased peak amplitude of the first Gaussian function ($P<0.001$), significantly increased peak amplitude and significantly shorter peak times of the second Gaussian function (both $P<0.001$).

Finally, we compared the parameters stability between setting the optimizaiton criterion as MAE≤1.5% and setting it as MAE≤5% and found just the strict optimizaiton criterion MAE≤1.5% could make the parameters stable with small standard deviation, which shows the fine fitting accuracy is essentially important for pulse decomposition methods. This study is therefore an important step to further understand the underlying physiological mechanisms of the artery pressure waveform features using Gaussian functions.

Previous studies about wave reflection have employed wave separation analysis (Westerhof et al., 2006; Westerhof et al., 1972), AI index assessment (O'ourke and Nichols, 2004; Kelly et al., 1989), frequency-based method (Kromer and Riegger, 1992), the first derivative (Millasseau et al., 2002), second derivative (Bortolotto et al., 2000), third derivative (Karamanoglu, 1997) and wave intensity analysis (Curtis et al., 2007; Zambanini et al., 2005), and so on. The achieved conclusions, such as the characteristics of wave reflection associated with ageing, have still had conflicting results (Laurent et al., 2007; Millasseau et al., 2006; Sugawara et al., 2010). It has been reported that early wave reflection is shifting proximally toward the heart (O'ourke and Nichols, 2004). On the contrary, a distal shift of reflection site was observed (Mitchell et al., 2004). While other researchers reported that the major reflection sites only shifted distally from 65 years old and before that aging had no influence on the reflection site (Sugawara et al., 2010). These controversial conclusions are partly due to that different methods to identify the return time may yield substantially different parameter values (Segers et al., 2007). Another explanation is that those methods are not sensitive enough to accurately represent the effect of wave reflection (Swillens and Segers, 2008). As previously described (Parker et al., 1988; Parker and Jones, 1990; Sugawara et al., 1997; Zambanini et al., 2005), the normal pattern of artery pressure waveform consisted of a large initial forward-traveling wave (incident wave) due to the ventricular contraction and several backward-traveling waves (reflection wave) duo to the impedance mismatching from the peripheral vasculature. So pulse decomposition analysis methods, which decompose a pulse waveform into several independent sub-waves, have been successfully employed for assessment the wave reflection. Previous studies of the pulse decomposition analysis of the arterial pressure waveforms mainly included: Westerhof et al. separated a pulse waveform into two parts by a triangular wave of duration equal to the ejection time (Westerhof et al., 2006). Goswami et al. presented a two-pulse synthesis model to reconstruct the pulse waveform (Goswami et al., 2010). However, when the pulse waveforms become complicated, especially three or more crests exist in waveforms, two sub-waves method will fail. So three sub-waves (Qian et al., 1994), four sub-waves (Rubins, 2008), even five sub-waves (Huotari et al., 2012, 2011; Baruch et al., 2011) were used for the pulse decomposition. In terms of the fitting accuracy, Rubins reported that the residual error between the measured pulse and the fitted waveform did not exceed 10% (Rubins, 2008). Huotari's study provided only some examples with an average maximum residual error of 4% (Huotari et al., 2012, 2011). Xu et al. proposed a multi-Gaussian fitting method to fit the pulse waveform using an adaptive number (four or five) of sub-waves and made the fitting error less than 2% (Wang et al., 2013; Xu et al., 2011).

However, the initialization of parameters using derivatives methods makes all the above methods could not immune to noise. In addition, there is no reported research for the physiological explanation that why using three, four or five functions to fit the pulse. In Xu *et al*'s studies (Wang et al., 2013; Xu et al., 2011), although using the adaptive number (four or five) of sub-waves could make the fitting accuracy less than 2 %, the physiological explanation and comparison analysis for the differences of parameters between four and five different number of fitting functions become very difficulty. In this study, the fitting error MAE could be limited within 1.5% for using three or four Gaussian functions, which achieved the most accurate results.

The first Gaussian function mainly reflects the features of incident wave and the other Gaussian functions could denote the features of reflection wave. Incident wave is regarded as the force source to accelerate the blood flow and is denoted as the symbol of the contraction function of left ventricle. In the present study, the peak time C_1 and the half-width W_1 of first Gaussian function have no significant difference between normal and heart failure subjects in either CAPW or RAPW signal. However, the peak amplitude H_1 of first Gaussian function has, which shows the contraction functions of left ventricle of heart failure subjects decline distinctly. The peak time C_2 of second Gaussian function has advanced shifted markedly and the peak amplitude H_2 of second Gaussian function has risen obviously in heart failure subjects in either CAPW or RAPW signal. Along with the heart failure process, the central and peripheral arterial stiffness will be changed and the different impedance matching between central aorta and peripheral arteries could be occurred, which might lead to the advanced shifts and high amplitude of reflection wave (Mitchell et al., 2004; Sugawara et al., 2010). Both the advanced shift and increased amplitude of reflection wave are regarded as the divinable risk factors for the cardiovascular system (Sugawara et al., 2010; Curtis et al., 2007; Nichols et al., 2006; O'ourke and Nichols, 2004; Mitchell et al., 2004; Millasseau et al., 2002).

Possible limitations in the methodology should be emphasized. Although the matching error is very low, the obtained sub-waves, no matter using three or four Gaussian functions, have the unclear physiological meanings and the meanings are different when compared with the current wave intensity analysis method (Curtis et al., 2007; Zambanini et al., 2005;

Sugawara et al., 2009). Therefore, the inherent physiological meanings for all sub-waves should be in-depth studied.

Acknowledgment

This work was supported by the National Natural Science Foundation of China under Grant 61201049, the Excellent Young Scientist Awarded Foundation of Shandong Province in China under Grant BS2013DX029, the China Postdoctoral Science Foundation under Grant 2013M530323 and the Postdoctoral Innovation Foundation of Shandong Province in China under Grant 201303102. The authors also would like to thank all of the volunteers for providing the invaluable data.

References

Allen J. and Murray A., 2002, Age-related changes in peripheral pulse timing characteristics at the ears, fingers and toes. *Journal of Human Hypertension,* 16 711-7.

Baruch M. C., Warburton D. E., Bredin S. S., Cote A., Gerdt D. W. and Adkins C. M., 2011, Pulse decomposition analysis of the digital arterial pulse during hemorrhage simulation. *Nonlinear Biomedical Physics,* 5 1-15.

Bortolotto L. A., Blacher J., Kondo T., Takazawa K. and Safar M. E., 2000, Assessment of vascular aging and atherosclerosis in hypertensive subjects: second derivative of photoplethysmogram versus pulse wave velocity. *American Journal of Hypertension,* 13 165-71.

Curtis S. L., Zambanini A., Mayet J., McG Thom S. A., Foale R., Parker K. H. and Hughes A. D., 2007, Reduced systolic wave generation and increased peripheral wave reflection in chronic heart failure. *American Journal of Physiology - Heart and Circulatory Physiology,* 293 H557-62.

Denardo S. J., Nandyala R., Freeman G. L., Pierce G. L. and Nichols W. W. 2010 Pulse wave analysis of the aortic pressure waveform in severe left ventricular systolic dysfunction. *Circulation: Heart Failure,* 3 149-56.

Goswami D., Chaudhuri K. and Mukherjee J., 2010, A new two-pulse synthesis model for digital volume pulse signal analysis. *Cardiovascular Engineering,* 10 109-17.

Huotari M., Vehkaoja A., Määttä K. and Kostamovaara J., 2011, Photoplethysmography and its detailed pulse waveform analysis for arterial stiffness, *Journal of Structural Mechanics,* 44 345-62.

Huotari M., Vehkaoja A., Määttä K. and Kostamovaara J., 2012, Pulse waveforms are an indicator of the condition of vascular system In *Proceedings of World Congress on Medical Physics and Biomedical Engineering*: Beijing pp 526-9.

Karamanoglu M., 1997, A System for Analysis of Arterial Blood Pressure Waveforms in Humans. *Computers and Biomedical Research,* 30 244-55.

Kelly R., Hayward C., Avolio A. and O'Rourke M., 1989, Noninvasive determination of age-related changes in the human arterial pulse. *Circulation,* 80 1652-9.

Kriz J. and Seba P., 2008, Force plate monitoring of human hemodynamics. *Nonlinear Biomedical Physics,* 2 1-9.

Kromer E. P. and Riegger G. A. J., 1992, Aortic input impedance in mild to moderate chronic congestive heart failure: lack of interrelation with neurohormonal activation. *European Heart Journal,* 13 113-8.

Laurent S., Cockcroft J., Van Bortel L., Boutouyrie P., Giannattasio C., Hayoz D., Pannier B., Vlachopoulos C., Wilkinson I. and Struijker-Boudier H., 2007, Abridged version of the expert consensus document on arterial stiffness. *Artery Research,* 1 2-12.

Liu C. Y., Li L. P., Zhao L. N., Zheng D. C., Li P. and Liu C. C., 2012, A combination method of improved impulse rejection filter and template matching for identification of anomalous intervals in electrocardiographic RR sequences. *Journal of Medical and Biological Engineering,* 32 245-50.

Liu C. Y., Zheng D. C., Murray A. and Liu C. C., 2013, Modelling carotid and radial artery pulse pressure waveforms by curve fitting with Gaussian functions. *Biomedical Signal Processing and Control,* 8 449-54.

Liu C. Y., Zheng D. C., Zhao L. N. and Liu C. C., 2014a, Gaussian fitting for carotid and radial artery pressure waveforms: comparison between normal subjects and heart failure patients. *Bio-Medical Materials and Engineering,* 24 271-7.

Liu C. Y., Zhuang T., Zhao L. N., Chang F. L., Liu C. C., Wei S. S., Li Q. Q. and Zheng D. C., 2014b, Analysis of arterial pressure waveforms using Gaussians and two-stage particle swarm optimizer. *IEEE Transactions on Biomedical Engineering* In press*Submitted to Plos One.*

Martinez J. P., Almeida R., Olmos S., Rocha A. P. and Laguna P., 2004, A wavelet-based ECG delineator: evaluation on standard databases. *IEEE Transactions on Biomedical Engineering, IEEE Transactions on* 51 570-81.

Mendes R., Kennedy J. and Neves J., 2004, The fully informed particle swarm: simpler, maybe better. *IEEE Transactions on Evolutionary Computation, IEEE Transactions on* 8 204-10.

Millasseau S. C., Kelly R. P., Ritter J. M. and Chowienczyk P. J., 2002, Determination of age-related increases in large artery stiffness by digital pulse contour analysis. *Clinical Science,* 103 371-7.

Millasseau S. C., Ritter J. M., Takazawa K. and Chowienczyk P. J., 2006, Contour analysis of the photoplethysmographic pulse measured at the finger. *Journal of Hypertension,* 24 1449-56.

Mitchell G. F., Parise H., Benjamin E. J., Larson M. G., Keyes M. J., Vita J. A., Vasan R. S. and Levy D., 2004, Changes in arterial stiffness and wave reflection with advancing age in healthy men and women: the framingham heart study. *Hypertension,* 43 1239-45.

Nichols W. W., Estrada J. C., Braith R. W., Owens K. and Conti C. R., 2006, Enhanced external counterpulsation treatment improves arterial wall properties and wave reflection characteristics in patients with refractory angina. *Journal of the American College of Cardiology,* 48 1208-14.

O'ourke M. F. and Nichols W. W. 2004, Changes in wave reflection with advancing age in normal subjects. *Hypertension,* 44 E10-E1.

Parker K. H. and Jones C. J., 1990, Forward and backward running waves in the arteries: analysis using the method of characteristics. *Journal of Biomechanical Engineering,* 112 322-6.

Parker K. H., Jones C. J., Dawson J. R. and Gibson D. G. 1988, What stops the flow of blood from the heart? *Heart and Vessels,* 4 241-5.

Qian W. L., Xu L. Y., Chen F. Y. and Zheng R. L., 1994, Acquiring characteristics of pulse wave by Gauss function separation. *Chinese Journal of Biomedical Engineering,* 13 1-7.

Rubins U., 2008, Finger and ear photoplethysmogram waveform analysis by fitting with Gaussians. *Medical and Biological Engineering and Computing,* 46 1271-6.

Segers P., De Backer J., Devos D., Rabben S. I., Gillebert T. C., Van Bortel L. M., De Sutter J., De Paepe A. and Verdonck P. R. 2006, Aortic reflection coefficients and their association with global indexes of wave reflection in healthy controls and patients with Marfan's syndrome. *American Journal of Physiology - Heart and Circulatory Physiology,* 290 H2385-92.

Segers P., Mynard J., Taelman L., Vermeersch S. and Swillens A. 2012, Wave reflection: Myth or reality? *Artery Research,* 6 7-11.

Segers P., Rietzschel E., De Buyzere M., De Bacquer D., Van Bortel L., De Backer G., Gillebert T. and Verdonck P. 2007, Assessment of pressure wave reflection: getting the timing right! *Physiological Measurement,* 28 1045-56.

Solà J., Vetter R., Renevey P., Chételat O., Sartori C. and Rimoldi S. F., 2009, Parametric estimation of pulse arrival time: a robust approach to pulse wave velocity. *Physiological Measurement,* 30 603-15.

Su S. Y., Wei C. C., Hsieh C. L., Tsao J. Y., Li T. C., Lin T., Chang H. H. and Lo L. C., 2009, Influence of menstrual cycle on pulse pressure waveforms measured from the radial artery in biphasic healthy women. *Journal of Alternative and Complementary Medicine,* 15 645-52.

Sugawara J., Hayashi K. and Tanaka H., 2010, Distal shift of arterial pressure wave reflection sites with aging. *Hypertension,* 56 920-5.

Sugawara M., Niki K., Ohte N., Okada T. and Harada A., 2009, Clinical usefulness of wave intensity analysis. *Medical and Biological Engineering and Computing,* 47 197-206.

Sugawara M., Uchida K., Kondoh Y., Magosaki N., Niki K., Jones C., Sugimachi M. and Sunagawa K., 1997, Aortic blood momentum - the more the better for the ejecting heart in vivo? *Cardiovascular Research,* 33 433-46.

Swillens A. and Segers P., 2008, Assessment of arterial pressure wave reflection: Methodological considerations. *Artery Research,* 2 122-31.

Wang L., Xu L. S., Feng S. T., Meng M. Q.-H. and Wang K. Q., 2013, Multi-Gaussian fitting for pulse waveform using Weighted Least Squares and multi-criteria decision making method. *Computers in Biology and Medicine,* 43 1661-72.

Westerhof B. E., Guelen I., Westerhof N., Karemaker J. M. and Avolio A., 2006, Quantification of wave reflection in the human aorta from pressure alone: a proof of principle. *Hypertension,* 48 595-601.

Westerhof B. E., van den Wijngaard J. P., Murgo J. P. and Westerhof N., 2008, Location of a reflection site is elusive: consequences for the calculation of aortic pulse wave velocity. *Hypertension,* 52 478-83.

Westerhof N., Sipkema P., van den Bos C. G. and Elzinga G., 1972, Forward and backward waves in the arterial system. *Cardiovascular Research,* 6 648-56.

Xu L. S., Feng S. T., Zhong Y., Feng C., Meng M. Q.-H. and Yan H. C., 2011, Multi-Gaussian fitting for digital volume pulse using weighted least squares method In *Proceedings of IEEE International Conference on Information and Automation*: Shenzhen pp 544-9.

Zambanini A., Cunningham S. L., Parker K. H., Khir A. W., McG Thom S. A. and Hughes A. D., 2005, Wave-energy patterns in carotid, brachial, and radial arteries: a noninvasive approach using wave-intensity analysis. *American Journal of Physiology - Heart and Circulatory Physiology,* 289 H270-6.

In: Horizons in World Cardiovascular Research. Vol. 6
Editor: Eleanor H. Bennington
ISBN: 978-1-63321-298-5

Chapter 7

Multidetector Computed Tomography as a Potential Modality to Detect Subclinical Atherosclerosis

***Kohichiro Iwasaki*[1] *and Shozo Kusachi*[2]**
[1]Department of Cardiology, Okayama Kyokuto Hospital, Japan
[2]Department of Medical Technology, Okayama University Graduate School of Health Sciences, Japan

Abstract

Coronary artery disease is a leading cause of mortality and morbidity in the developing and developed countries. In approximately 50% of patients with newly diagnosed coronary artery disease, the first presentation is either acute myocardial infarction or sudden cardiac death. Global risk scores are developed to stratify the risk of coronary artery disease. However recent research has revealed that the global risk score significantly underestimates or misclassifies risk in key subsets of the population. Many data also demonstrate that the major determinant of risk for atherosclerotic cardiovascular disease in asymptomatic adults is the presence of the underlying disease itself, namely subclinical atherosclerosis.

Multidetector computed tomography (MDCT) has emerged as a promising modality to evaluate coronary artery disease. MDCT has an excellent capacity to detect hemodynamically relevant stenosis and its ability to detect and characterize coronary plaque noninvasively is increasingly recognized. Recent studies using MDCT demonstrate that the prevalence of subclinical atherosclerosis in asymptomatic patients with low to intermediate risk is high. Especially, asymptomatic diabetic patients and asymptomatic patients with abnormal carotid finding have high prevalence of subclinical atherosclerosis. Also recent studies demonstrate that the coronary plaques that are prone to subsequent acute coronary syndrome are often associated with positive remodeling and low attenuation plaque, suggesting that once a patient is identified to be at high risk of having an adverse cardiac event by clinical risk assessment, imaging with MDCT would help better identify those at greater risk of acute coronary events.

Thus it is time to change the paradigm for testing for coronary artery disease from detection of a symptomatic luminal obstruction to preclinical arterial wall atherosclerosis. There is increasing need to detect disease at earlier stages so that asymptomatic patients with atherosclerosis in need of aggressive medical management can be identified. We believe that MDCT has a potential to fulfill these needs.

Introduction

Coronary artery disease is a leading cause of mortality and morbidity in the developing and developed countries [1]. In approximately 50% of patients with newly diagnosed coronary artery disease, the first presentation is either acute myocardial infarction or sudden cardiac death, which means that early mortality is very high [2, 3].

Many studies demonstrate that most myocardial infarction and sudden cardiac death do not occur at the sites of significant coronary narrowing [4-7], and coronary revascularization therapy of coronary obstruction in patients with stable angina do not reduce the risk of myocardial infarction or cardiac death [8].

In addition the premise is well supported in the literature that the major determinant of risk for atherosclerotic cardiovascular disease in asymptomatic adults is the presence of the underlying disease itself, namely subclinical atherosclerosis [9]. Once subclinical atherosclerosis is detected, intensity of drug therapy, particularly statin therapy, could be adjusted for plaque burden.

Grundy summarized the promise of atherosclerotic imaging [10]. First, imaging individualizes risk assessment beyond use of age, which is a less reliable surrogate for atherosclerotic burden. Second, imaging provides an integrated assessment of the lifetime exposure to risk factors. Third, imaging identifies individuals who are susceptible to developing atherosclerosis beyond established risk factors. Fourth, in the absence of detectable atherosclerosis, short-term risk appears to be very low.

Multidetector computed tomography (MDCT) has emerged as a promising modality to evaluate coronary artery disease noninvasively. Its ability to assess obstructive coronary artery disease has been demonstrated to be excellent compared with conventional coronary angiography [11-14]. Recently its ability to detect coronary plaques and characterize plaque composition has been studied [15-21].

In this review, we describe the role of MDCT as a potential modality to detect subclinical atherosclerosis with referring to recent reports as well as our recent studies.

Multidetector Computed Tomography (MDCT)

The introduction of electron beam computed tomography in the early 1990s followed by the development of MDCT scanners substantially improved the ability to perform CT imaging of cardiac structures, especially the coronary arteries. Sixty-four MDCT (64-MDCT) systems are now considered the minimum prerequisite for high-quality cardiac and coronary artery imaging. Further developments include systems with more detector rows (up to 320 slices) [22] as well as systems with two tubes and detectors (dual source CT) [23], which further improve image quality beyond 64-MDCT.

MDCT offers two ways of assessing coronary atherosclerosis. When performed without contrast agent, coronary calcium can be detected and quantified. When performed with contrast agent, coronary plaques can be detected.

Coronary Calcium

The amount of calcium is quantified by the so-called Agatston score. Agatston score calculates the calcium burden by multiplying the area of the calcified lesion by a weighting factor dependent on the peak signal of the lesion [24]. Volume and mass scores are alternative methods to quantify coronary calcium but they are not widely used.

Coronary artery calcification signifies the presence of coronary atherosclerosis and a strong linear correlation exists between total coronary artery atherosclerotic plaque burden and the extent of coronary artery calcification [25-29]. The coronary artery calcification has been found to be the most powerful predictor of cardiac events, providing independent and incremental information over risk factor-based assessment of the asymptomatic patients [30, 31]. Patients without detectable calcium have a very low rate of coronary death or myocardial infarction (0.4%) over 3 to 5 years of observation [32-36].

ACCF/AHA 2007 Clinical Expert Consensus Document on Coronary Artery Calcium Scoring by Computed Tomography in Global Cardiovascular Risk Assessment and in Evaluation of Patients With Chest Pain reported relative risk ratios according to level of risk for coronary artery calcium score (CACS) [37]. The summary relative risk ratio of coronary death and myocardial infarction was 1.9, 4.3, 7.2, and 10.8 in patients with mild (CACS of 1 to 99), moderate (100 to 399), high (400 to 999), and very high risk (>1,000) patients when compared to patients with no coronary calcium.

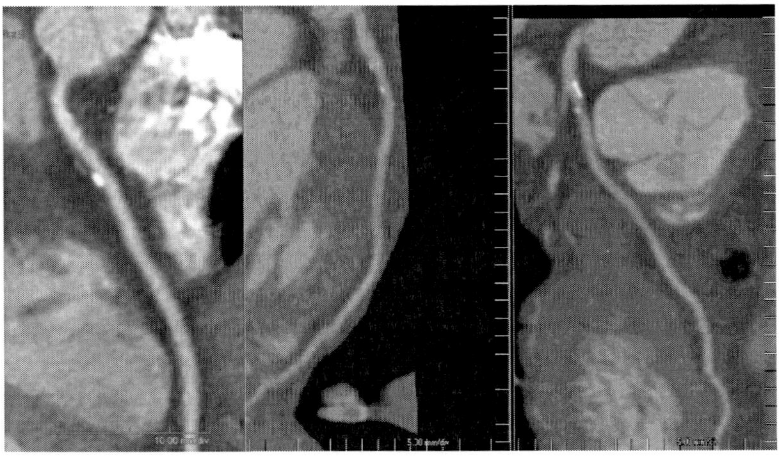

Figure 1. Representative case of coronary calcium 1. A coronary artery calcium score of this patient is 82. Abbreviations; LAD; left anterior descending coronary artery, LCX; left circumflex coronary artery, RCA; right coronary artery.

However, some caveats are needed. First, in spite of the relationship between coronary calcification and coronary plaque burden, there is only a weak correlation between the amount of coronary calcium and the angiographic severity of luminal stenosis. Second, calcification is neither the sign of stability nor instability of an individual plaque, and its presence or absence is not closely associated with the likelihood of an individual lesion to rupture and cause an event [38]. Patients who have calcified plaque are also more likely to have non-calcified or "soft" plaque that is prone to rupture and acute coronary syndrome.

It is the co-occurrence of calcified and non-calcified plaque that provides the means for estimating acute coronary events. Third, although the absence of coronary calcium makes the presence of significant luminal obstruction relatively unlikely, a zero calcium score cannot be used to rule out coronary artery stenosis in symptomatic individuals, especially when they present as young age and with acute symptoms [39, 40]. Fourth, in addition to plaque burden, plaque location should be considered as well, as vulnerable plaques are most often observed in proximal segments of the coronary artery tree. The presence of proximal lesion is therefore associated with an increased risk of vulnerable plaques.

Representative cases are shown in Figure 1 to 4.

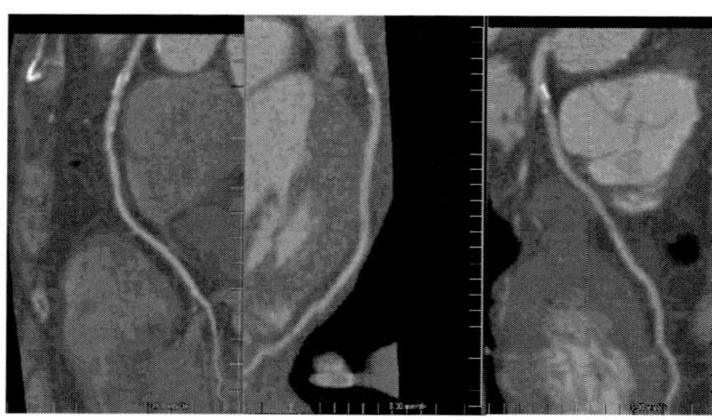
RCA LAD LCX

Figure 2. Representative case of coronary calcium 2. A coronary artery calcium score of this patient is 278. Abbreviations are the same as Figure 1.

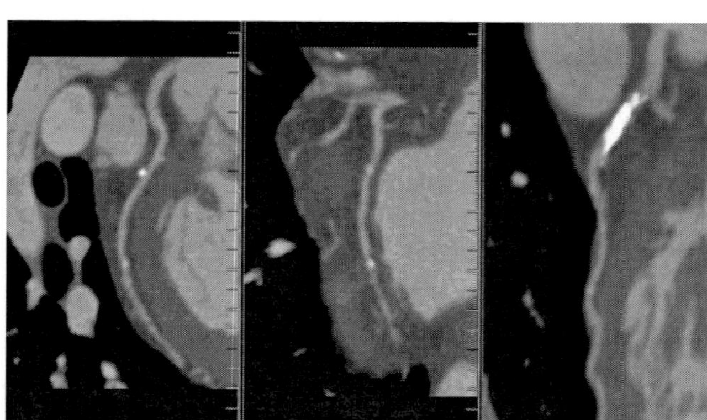
RCA LAD LCX

Figure 3. Representative case of coronary calcium 3. A coronary artery calcium score of this patient is 624. Abbreviations are the same as Figure 1.

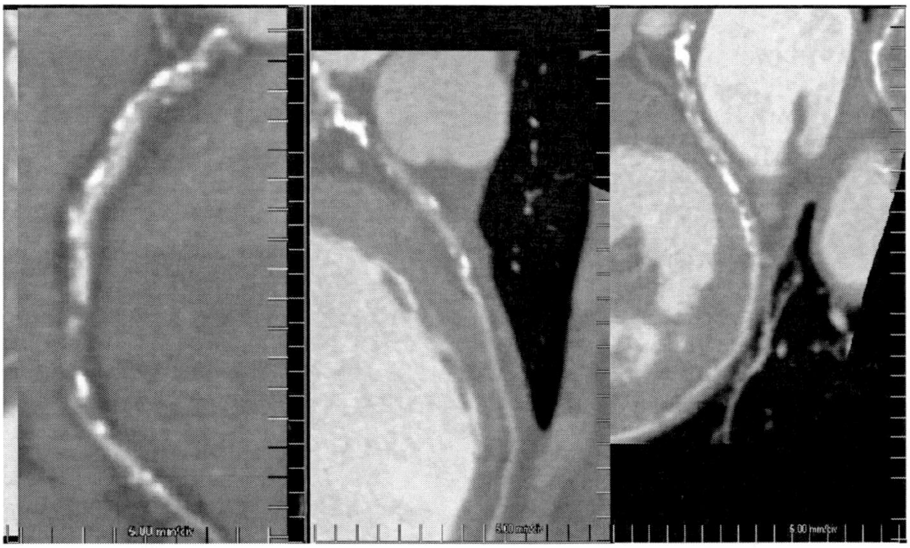

Figure 4. Representative case of coronary calcium 4. A coronary artery calcium score of this patient is 1,970. Abbreviations are the same as Figure 1.

Coronary Computed Tomography Angiography (CCTA)

Coronary computed tomography angiography (CCTA) demands excellent image quality without artifacts. Image quality is strongly dependent on heart rate and the patient's heart rate usually needs to be to less than 65bpm, which often needs beta-blocker administration.

With the last generation of 64-MDCT and adequate patient preparation, recent studies report the rates of sensitivity ranging from 91% to 99% and specificity between 93% and 98% for the detection of hemodynamically relevant stenoses in comparison with coronary angiography [11-14]. Thus the diagnostic accuracy of CCTA has already been definitively established. By well-performed prospective, multicenter studies, CCTA is an accurate diagnostic modality with superior diagnostic accuracy to detect and exclude anatomically obstructive coronary artery disease.

The high negative predictive value of 95% to 100% suggests that 64-MDCT would be a useful diagnostic technique to rule out the presence of coronary artery disease. The 64-MDCT has the advantage over myocardial perfusion imaging of being unlikely to underestimate or miss high-risk disease and the advantage over CT coronary calcium of visualizing and potentially characterizing non-calcified plaque [41, 42].

Recently, its ability to detect and characterize coronary plaques is increasingly recognized [15-21]. In studies that compared MDCT with intravascular ultrasound, sensitivities and specificities for the detection of coronary artery segments with plaque have been reported to be between 80 and 90% [15, 18, 19].

To some extent, MDCT allows assessment of plaque composition. As groups, lipid-rich, fibrous and calcified plaques display different Hounsfield units (HU), and could be differentiated reliably [15-21]. However, the variability of density measurement within plaque type is large and some studies did not find significant difference in CT attenuation between plaque types [43, 44]. Furthermore, density measurements within coronary plaques are heavily influenced by the contrast attenuation in the adjacent lumen, vessel size, and stenosis severity, and by image reconstruction parameters such as slice thickness and reconstruction kernel [45, 46]. Therefore, accurate classification of plaque composition by measuring the CT attenuation is currently not reliably possible.

Currently a differentiation can be made among non-calcified plaques having low attenuation, calcified plaques with high attenuation, and mixed plaques with both non-calcified and calcified elements [21]. Representative cases are shown in Figure 5 to 7.

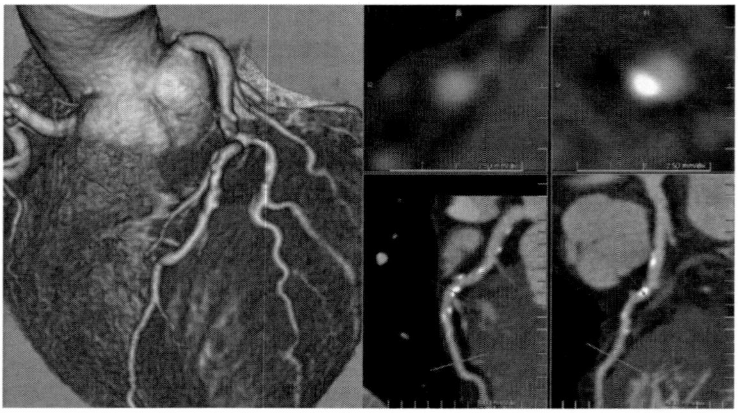

Figure 5. Representative case of coronary calcified plaque. A 65-year-old man with hypertension and hyperlipidemia underwent 64-MDCT. Volume rendering image (left panel) showed no significant stenosis with scattered calcification in the left anterior descending coronary artery. Curved multiplanar reconstruction image (right panel) revealed multiple calcified plaques.

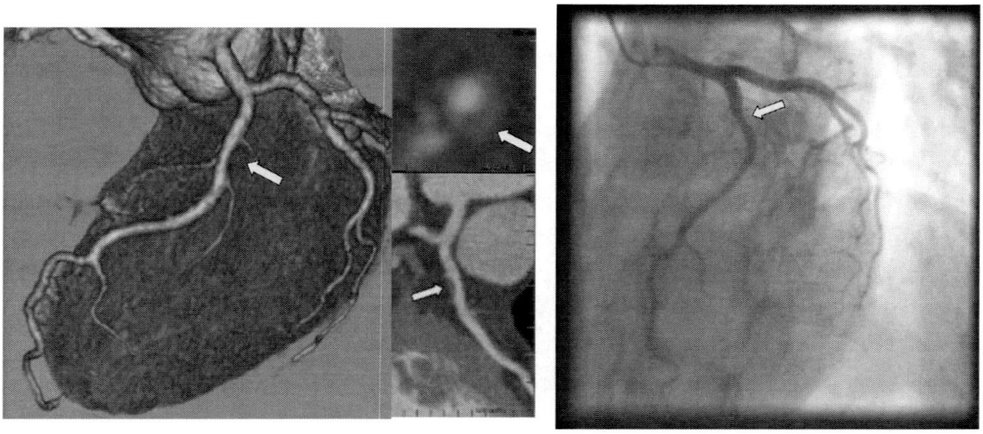

6A 6B

Figure 6. Representative case of coronary non-calcified plaque. A 50-year-old man with hyperlipidemia underwent 64-MDCT. Volume rendering image (Figure 6A, left panel) revealed moderate stenosis in the proximal portion of the left anterior descending coronary artery. Curved multiplanar reconstruction image (Figure 6A, right panel) showed non-calcified plaques with moderate stenosis in the same portion. A coronary angiography revealed moderate stenosis in the proximal portion of the left anterior descending coronary artery (Figure 6B).

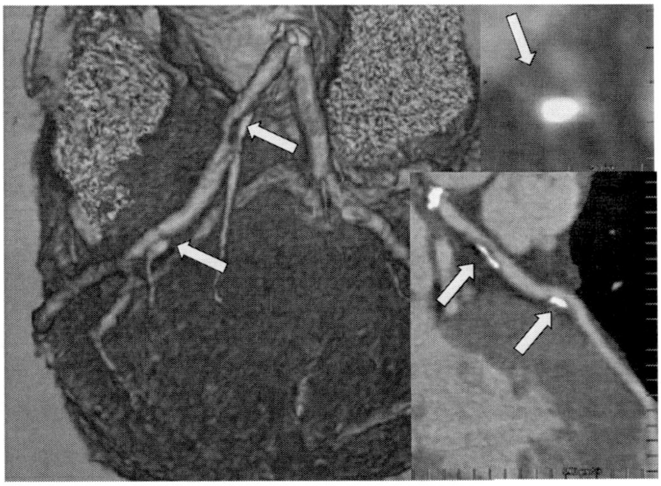

7A

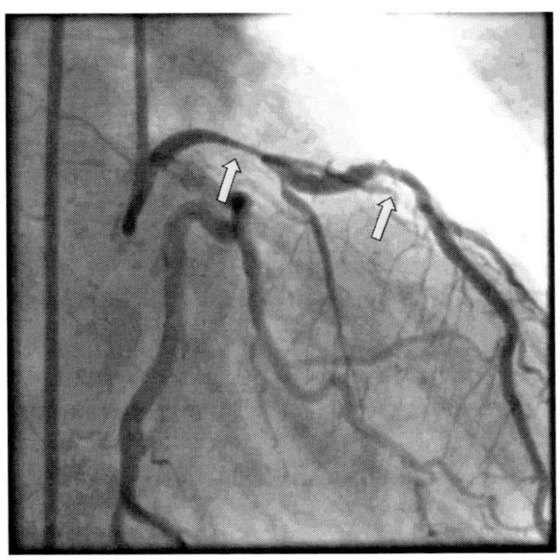

7B

Figure 7. Representative case of coronary mixed plaque. A 64-year-old man with hypertension underwent 64-MDCT. Volume rendering image (Figure 7A, left panel) revealed severe stenosis in the proximal portion and moderate stenosis in the mid portion of the left anterior descending coronary artery. Curved multiplanar reconstruction image (Figure 7A, right panel) showed calcified plaques with moderate to severe stenosis in the same portion. A coronary angiography (Figure 7B) revealed 75% stenosis in the proximal portion and 50% stenosis in the mid portion of the left anterior descending coronary artery. He underwent percutaneous coronary intervention.

Ionizing Radiation in Cardiac Imaging

MDCT has two major limitations. One is radiation exposure and the other is contrast-induced nephropathy.

A Society Advisory from the American Heart Association (AHA) Committee on Cardiac Imaging of the Council on Clinical Cardiology and Committee on Cardiovascular Imaging and Intervention of the Council on Cardiovascular Radiology and Intervention published a AHA Science Advisory entitled "Ionizing Radiation in Cardiac Imaging" [47].

According to this advisory, the estimated increase in the lifetime risk of dying of a malignancy associated with 10 mSv of ionizing radiation is ≈0.05%.

The relative risk of lung cancer ranges from 4.9 in individuals who smoked 1 to 15 cigarettes per day to 13.3 in individuals who smoked >25 cigarettes per day. By comparison, the relative risk of lung cancer associated with an effective dose of 1,000 mSv (approximately 50 to 100 CCTA) is 2.2. The relative risk of CCTA is small (1.02 to 1.06) compared with other well-documented risk factors for breast cancer, such as family history of breast cancer (2.1 to 3.6).

Because radiation-induced malignancies have a biological latency of approximately 10 to 40 years, they are less likely to manifest in older individuals. Conversely, if an imaging study uncovers a condition for which tailored management can improve patient outcomes, the imaging study may result in survival benefit without which the patient might not have lived long enough for a potential malignancy to develop.

This AHA Science Advisory states that "It is important to weigh the small hypothetical risk of inducing malignancies against the risk of not performing an imaging study, which may include misdiagnosis and failure to administer treatments that could improve medical outcomes."

Comparison with other Imaging Modalities

Table shows the advantage and disadvantage of several imaging modalities for the assessment of coronary artery disease.

Table. The advantage and disadvantage of imaging modalities for the assessment of coronary artery disease

Modality	Advantage	Disadvantage
MDCT	non-invasive	radiation exposure contrast media
CAG	defines therapeutic options	invasive no information on vessel wall
CMR	non-invasive no radiation exposure	low spatial resolution
IVUS	high spatial resolution	invasive
OCT	very high spatial resolution	invasive low penetration depth

Abbreviations: CAG; coronary angiography, CMR; cardiovascular magnetic resonance, IVUS; intravascular ultrasound, MDCT; multidetector computed tomography, OCT; optical coherence tomography.

Conventional Coronary Angiography

Conventional coronary angiography is still regarded as a gold standard for the evaluation of coronary artery disease. However a growing body of evidence suggests that coronary angiography is a luminography and has its own limitation [48]. The main causes of this limitation are coronary remodeling and diffuse involvement of coronary artery with atherosclerosis.

Arterial remodeling refers to a change in vessel size or cross-sectional area within the external elastic lamina. Positive remodeling denotes an increase in vessel size and negative remodeling denotes a reduction in vessel size. Most atherosclerotic segments exhibit some compensatory enlargement. Initially, the artery enlarges as plaque progresses and lumen size does no decrease. Early stages of lesion development may even be associated with overcompensation, which is increase in lumen size. However, at >40% lumen stenosis, the artery no longer enlarges at a rate sufficient to counterbalance the expansion of the atherosclerotic plaque, and lumen narrowing is no longer prevented [49-51].

Another limitation is that most patients with coronary artery disease have diffuse atherosclerosis involving the nearly entire coronary artery [52, 53].

Recent data demonstrate that there are many plaques detected by intravascular ultrasound but neglected by coronary angiography [52-54]. This means that coronary angiography misses many subclinical atherosclerosis. Thus coronary angiography is invasive, provides only a luminogram, and does not identify coronary plaques.

Cardiovascular Magnetic Resonance (CMR)

Although early study with magnetic resonance coronary angiography yielded favorable results [55], multiple subsequent studies could not reproduce the promising results of initial report [56-58]. Accuracy varies widely from study to study (sensitivity 38% to 83%, specificity 57% to 95%) even when the exams of patients with poor image quality are excluded [56-58].

Current limitations of spatial resolution and rapid coronary motion during the acquisition allow for only broad categorization of diameter stenosis. Coronary magnetic resonance imaging remains technically demanding, as respiratory and cardiac motion limits the useful data acquisition window. Imaging of the walls of coronary artery is particularly challenging because of their wall thickness, tortuous three-dimensional course of the coronary arteries, and close proximity of epicardial fat, coronary blood, and myocardium [59].

Intravascular Ultrasound (IVUS)

The IVUS image is the result of reflected ultrasound waves that are converted to electrical signals and sent to an external processing system for amplification [60]. Grayscale IVUS image is formed by the envelope of the radiofrequency signal. IVUS is commonly used to assess plaque burden, stenosis severity, lesion length, and stent deployment [61].

Some typical morphologic features of vulnerable plaque can be identified by IVUS. These are thin cap with large lipid core, fissured plaque, and positive remodeling [62-65].

Virtual histology IVUS (VH-IVUS) is based upon the radiofrequency analysis of the backscatter ultrasound signal and has been correlated with histology of various vascular types [65]. The reported accuracies are 91% for calcified regions, 90% for necrotic regions, 93% for fibrofatty regions, and 90% for fibrous regions [65].

Recently the potential value of VH-IVUS was evaluated in a multicenter prospective study, the Providing Regional Observations to Study Predictors of Events in the Coronary Tree (PROSPECT) study [66]. In patients who presented with an acute coronary syndrome and underwent percutaneous coronary intervention, major adverse cardiovascular events occurring during follow-up were equally attributable to recurrence at the site of culprit lesions and to nonculprit lesions. Although nonculprit lesions were frequently angiographically mild, most were thin-cap fibroatheromas or were characterized by a large plaque burden, a small luminal area, or some combination of these characteristics.

Optical Coherence Tomography (OCT)

Optical coherence tomography (OCT) is a technology that emits light with a wavelength of 1.3 μm to reflect off the vessel wall [67, 68]. The spatial resolution of OCT is 10-20 μm compared to 100 and 200 μm for IVUS and VH-IVUS, respectively.

Using OCT, plaque can be characterized as either lipid rich, fibrous, calcified, or thrombotic [68]. OCT is capable of accurately measuring fibrous cap thickness and identify those with thickness <65 μm, which from pathological studies is prone to rupture [69].

A major limitation of OCT is poor tissue penetration, which limits its ability to fully assess and quantify plaque burden or measure vessel dimensions [67, 68].

Limitations of Global Risk Scores

Global risk scores, such as the Framingham risk score (FRS), are developed to stratify the risk of cardiovascular disease [70, 71]. The assessment of traditional risk factors is the recommended initial step in risk assessment including a calculation of global scores. The National Cholesterol Educational Program (NCEP) Adult Treatment Panel (ATP)-III guidelines suggest the starting point in risk assessment in establishing the 10-year risk of myocardial infarction and cardiac death by use of the FRS. Risk is defined as follows; low, less than 10%; intermediate, between 10% and 20%, or high, greater than 20% [1, 72].

However recent research has revealed the limitation of the RFS and NCEP/ATP III guidelines.

Karim et al. [73] measured subclinical atherosclerosis in 498 healthy subjects and 69% of them had evidence of subclinical atherosclerosis in more than one of the three vascular beds (coronary, aortic, and carotid). Sixty-nine percent of the subjects categorized in the low risk FRS, 95% of the intermediate risk FRS, and 100% of the high risk FRS had subclinical atherosclerosis in more than one of the three vascular beds. Furthermore, of the 68 subjects with subclinical atherosclerosis in all three vascular beds, 35% had the low risk RFS, 41%

had the intermediate risk FRS, only 23% had the high risk FRS. Nasir et al. measured CACS in 1,611 asymptomatic individuals [74]. The CACS of 0, 1 to 99, 100 to 399, >400 was observed in 35%, 44%, 12%, and 9% of the patients, respectively. Overall, 59% and 78% of patients with CACS >400 and CACS >75th percentile were not identified as high risk and candidate for pharmacotherapy on the basis of NCEP categories. Furthermore, women as well as young individuals were less likely to be considered candidates for pharmacotherapy compared with men and older individuals in each CACS category. Ahmadi et al. studied mortality risk associated with CACS and FRS in 730 subjects classified as low risk versus high risk based on FRS [75]. Mortality rate was 18.5% in discordant low risk group (FRS <10% and CACS >100) compared with 7.7% in discordant high risk group (FRS >20% and CACS=0). Adjusted relative risk of mortality was 3.6 for discordant low risk group compared to discordant high risk group. Hadamitzky et al. studied the value of risk stratification with MDCT compared to FRS in a population of 1,256 patients during the follow-up of 18 months [76]. In patients without obstructive coronary artery disease on MDCT, the observed cardiac events were significantly lower than predicted by FRS. However significantly more events were observed in patients with obstructive coronary artery disease on MDCT compared to the predicted event rate.

Taken together, the limitations of the FRS and NCEP/ATPIII guidelines include a substantial underestimation of lifetime risk, especially women when only a 10-year risk model is used, misclassification of high-risk patients as low or intermediate risk, and misclassification of very low-risk subjects into higher strata of risk [77].

Furthermore, the following evidence has been recognized. A minority of patients with coronary artery disease has none of the traditional risk factors, but, more importantly, in a large proportion of patients with more than one risk factor, coronary artery disease does not develop [78, 79]. Only half of patients with acute myocardial infarction have hyperlipidemia. A substantial number (60% to 70%) of unheralded cardiovascular events occur in low and intermediate risk categories [80]. Therefore, a growing body of evidence supports the fact that global risk scores may be useful guides in predicting long term cardiovascular disease risk in healthy populations but often are suboptimal for individual risk estimation. It is apparent that risk prediction models relying on traditional risk factors, although adequate on the population level, have relatively low sensitivity and specificity for individual coronary artery disease. Assessment of conventional risk factor burden is necessary but may not accurately estimate risk of cardiovascular disease [81].

Importantly, implementing a high-risk strategy alone is unlikely to reduce the overall prevalence of coronary artery disease because the lower-risk population, which by sheer number is the larger group affected with heart disease, would compromise most events. Thus for societal purposes it is important to implement both high-risk prevention and population-based approaches [82].

Thus MDCT may contribute significantly to detect subclinical atherosclerosis.

MDCT and Subclinical Atherosclerosis

The sum of all atherosclerotic plaques in a subject defines the "plaque burden". The plaque burden increases with age and is positively associated with major risk factors for coronary artery disease. Plaque burden also correlates with the risk for acute coronary events. However, increased plaque burden is usually asymptomatic, and hence unrecognized and untreated, until a patient experiences the first event [83-85].

Although aggressive medical therapy is important, it will remain crucial to identify the individual patient with significant silent coronary artery disease. Tests for early detection of atherosclerotic vascular disease are therefore needed to better assess cardiovascular risk in asymptomatic individuals, the main focus of primary prevention.

Prevalence of Coronary Artery Disease in Asymptomatic Diabetic Patients by MDCT

Patients with type 2 diabetes have a 2- to 4-fold higher risk of a cardiovascular event than nondiabetic patients [86]. Previous studies have shown that the risk of myocardial infarction in a diabetic patient is comparable to the risk of recurrent infarction in a nondiabetic patient with a previous myocardial infarction [87]. In the recent report of the NCEP/ATP, type 2 diabetes was accorded a coronary artery disease risk-equivalent [88]. In type 2 diabetic patients myocardial ischemia is often asymptomatic and coronary artery disease is frequently in an advanced state when it becomes clinically manifest [89]. The available evidence suggest that occult coronary artery disease is a common finding among asymptomatic patients with diabetes, ranging from 20% in healthier subjects to >50% in patients with more complicated diabetes [90]. In the DIAD study [91], a prospective multicenter study in 1,124 truly asymptomatic patients with diabetes, of whom 522 were randomized to screening, Wackers et al. observed a 22% prevalence of silent coronary artery disease on adenosine myocardial perfusion imaging. Although most perfusion abnormalities were small, 6% of patients had moderate to large abnormalities.

Khaleeli et al. [92] performed electron beam tomography in 155 asymptomatic diabetic patients and found that 72% had coronary calcium and 48% had a CACS >102. Scholte et al. performed 64-MDCT in 70 asymptomatic diabetic patients [93]. A CACS of <10, 10-100, 101-400, and >400 was observed in 44%, 20%, 17%, and 19% of patients, respectively. Coronary plaques were detected in 80% of patients. Of all plaques, non-calcified plaques, mixed plaques, and calcified plaques were found in 41%, 20%, and 39%, respectively. Importantly, coronary plaques were noted in 56% of patients with no or minimal calcium. Choi et al. performed MDCT and myocardial perfusion imaging (MPI) in 116 asymptomatic diabetic patients [94]. MPI was abnormal in 24% of patients. However 79% had coronary plaques (2 ± 2 segments per subject). They found that the prevalence of coronary plaques, significant stenosis, severe stenosis and plaque type, and high coronary calcium score was not significantly different between patients with normal and abnormal findings on MPI.

Our recent study investigated the prevalence of coronary artery disease in 93 asymptomatic diabetic patients compared with 93 age- and gender- matched asymptomatic nondiabetic patients by 64-MDCT [95]. Clinical characteristics were not significantly different between the two groups. The CACS was significantly higher in diabetic group than that in non-diabetic group (median 117 vs. 53.5, $p<0.0001$). No coronary calcium was detected in 30.0% of non-diabetic group compared with 15.1% of diabetic group ($p=0.0022$). The CACS score >400 was detected in 9.7% of non-diabetic group compared with 36.6% of diabetic group (p<0.0001). Coronary plaques were found in 67.7% of non-diabetic group compared with 91.4% of diabetic group (p<0.0001). Multiple plaques were detected in 57.0% and 77.4% of patients in non-diabetic and diabetic group, respectively (p=0.0030). Significant coronary stenosis was found in 16.1% of non-diabetic group compared with 33.3% of diabetic group (p=0.0065).

Taken together, these studies demonstrate that the prevalence of coronary plaques in asymptomatic diabetic patients is very high and diabetic patients deserve imaging by MDCT to detect subclinical atherosclerosis. Also these results underscore the circumstance that cardiovascular disease is the principal cause of death in patients with type 2 diabetes.

Representative cases are shown in Figure 8 and 9.

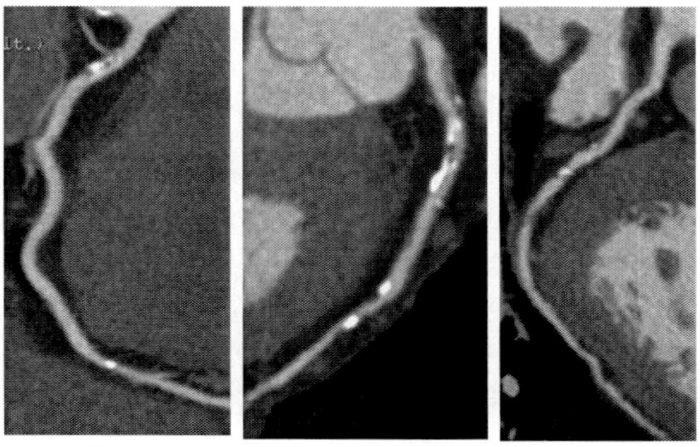

Figure 8. Representative case of asymptomatic diabetic patient. A 65-years-old man receives oral hypoglycemic therapy and statin therapy for more than 20 years. His blood pressure is 136/72mmHg, HDL-cholesterol is 40mg/dl、LDL-cholesterol is 123mg/dl, and triglyceride is 185mg/dl. His diabetes control is good with HbA1c of 6.2%. 64-MDCT demonstrated mixed plaques with moderate stenosis in the proximal portion of the three coronary arteries. Also the plaques in the left main coronary artery and left anterior descending coronary artery showed positive remodeling. Thus his medication is not sufficient to prevent plaque progression and his LDL-cholesterol value should be kept as 70 to 80mg/dl.

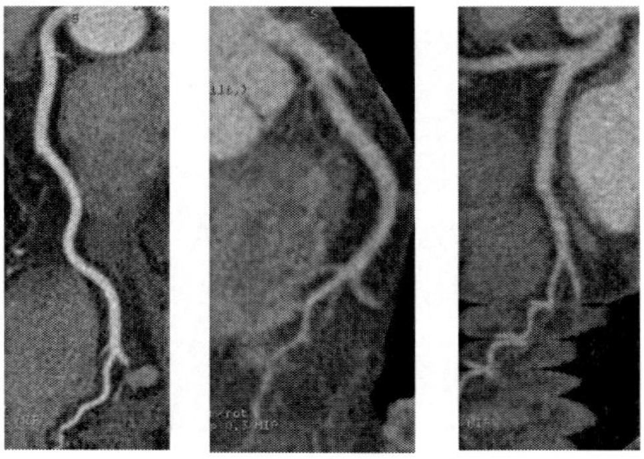

Figure 9. Representative case of asymptomatic diabetic patient. A 73-years-old woman receives insulin therapy for more than 10 years. She also receives statin therapy. Her blood pressure is 140/84mmHg, HDL-cholesterol is 83mg/dl、LDL-cholesterol is 108mg/dl, and triglyceride is 213mg/dl. But her diabetes control is poor, whose blood sugar is 217 to 356mg/dl and HbA1c is 7.9 to 8.9%. She seems to be at high-risk for coronary artery disease. However 64-MDCT showed normal coronary artery. Thus we advised her physician to continue statin therapy and intensify blood sugar control. Abbreviations are the same as Figure 1.

Prevalence of Coronary Artery Disease in Asymptomatic Patients with Abnormal Intima-Media Thickness by MDCT

Intima-media thickness (IMT) meets the criteria for an ideal screening tool in coronary artery disease. It is noninvasive and quantitative and correlates with clinical outcome [96-99]. Also a significant association between an abnormality of the carotid IMT and evidence of established coronary artery disease has been demonstrated [100].

Although atherosclerosis is predominantly a disease of the intima, carotid IMT correlates with the degree of carotid atherosclerosis measured at autopsy [101]. And the latter has been found to correlate with atherosclerotic vascular disease in other arterial beds [102]. Thus, ultrasound-derived carotid IMT is considered a surrogate for systemic atherosclerotic disease burden [103] IMT findings have been demonstrated to correlate with cardiac and cerebrovascular outcomes [81, 96-99]. Recent meta-analysis by Lorenz et al. [104] showed that the age- and sex-adjusted overall estimates of the relative risk of myocardial infarction were 1.26 per 1-standard deviation common carotid artery IMT difference and 1.15 per 0.10-mm common carotid artery IMT difference.

Many studies demonstrate the significant association of a quantitative abnormality of the carotid IMT with angiographic severity and extent of coronary artery disease, although some studies found a weak relationship between the two indices [105-108]. Also recent studies found that coronary calcification had significant correlations with carotid IMT [109-112]. In a substudy of Cardiovascular Health Study, Newman et al. [113] found that internal carotid IMT was most closely related to coronary artery calcium. We studied the prevalence of coronary plaque in 100 asymptomatic patients with IMT >1.0mm [114]. Coronary calcium was detected in 74.0% of patients and coronary plaque was detected in 77.0% of them. Median value of CACS was 21 and 140 in patients with maximum IMT<1.7mm and >1.8mm, respectively, ($p=0.0026$). Median number of coronary plaque was 3 and 6 in patients with maximum IMT<1.7mm and >1.8mm, respectively ($p=0.0482$). Significant coronary stenosis was found in 29% of patients. This study suggests that the prevalence of coronary artery disease in asymptomatic patients with abnormal carotid findings is high and that the severity of IMT and carotid plaques are well correlated with the severity of coronary calcium and coronary plaques.

Prevalence of Subclinical Atherosclerosis in Asymptomatic Patients with Low to Intermediate Risk by MDCT

There are few studies which investigated the prevalence of coronary plaques in patients with low to intermediate risk for coronary artery disease.

Hausleiter et al. performed a 64-MDCT scan in 161 patients with an intermediate risk for having coronary artery disease [115]. They found non-calcified plaques in 10 patients (6.2%) and calcified plaques in 98 patients (60.9%). Thus the prevalence of coronary plaques was 67.1%. Choi et al. studied 1,000 middle-aged asymptomatic subjects with 64-MDCT [116]. They found that atherosclerotic plaques were identified in 215 (22%) individuals and 40 individuals (4%) had only non-calcified plaques.

We studied the prevalence of subclinical atherosclerosis in 415 asymptomatic patients with low to intermediate risk by 64-MDCT [117]. We detected coronary plaques in 295 patients (71.1%). Of 135 patients with negative scan for coronary calcification, non-calcified plaques were detected in 15 patients (11.1%). Two hundred and thirty-five patients (79.7%) had multiple plaques and on average one patient had 4.6 plaques. Sixty-seven patients (18.3%) had high risk CACS (10.8% had CACS 400 to 999 and 7.5% had CACS >1,000). Significant coronary stenosis was detected in 91 patients (21.9%) and 85 patients underwent stress myocardial perfusion imaging. Myocardial ischemia was found in 27 patients (31.8%) and 21 patients underwent percutaneous coronary intervention. For a mean follow-up period of 2.8 years, four patients developed acute coronary syndrome. Thus these studies demonstrate that the prevalence of subclinical atherosclerosis in asymptomatic patients with low to intermediate risk is high. Importantly, these studies also suggest that the finding of no calcium does not guarantee good endothelial/ coronary health and such patients may still be at risk. Individuals with zero coronary calcium scores have not yet developed detectable, calcified coronary plaque, but they may have fatty streaking and early stages of plaque, and may have obstructive disease. Noncalcified plaques are present in many young adults [118].

There are several studies that investigated the prevalence of non-calcified plaque in patients without coronary calcium. Cheng et al. studied 416 low-intermediate risk patients without coronary calcium and found non-calcified plaque in 6.5% of them [119]. Hausleiter et al. found non-calcified plaque in 15.9% of patients with intermediate risk and no coronary calcium [115]. Schroeder et al. found non-calcified plaque in 10% of 29 patients with multiple risk factors [120]. Gottlieb et al. found non-calcified plaque in 19% of 72 patients without coronary calcium in a substudy of CORE64 (Coronary Evaluation Using Multi-Detector Spiral Computed Tomography Angiography Using 64 Detectors) [121]. A recent study by Schenker et al, using hybrid positron emission tomography/computed tomography scanner, showed that in even patients with no coronary calcium the frequency of ischemia was 16.0%, and its absence only afford a negative predictive value of 84.0% [122]. Taken together, these studies demonstrate that the prevalence of subclinical atherosclerosis in asymptomatic patients with low to intermediate risk is high and MDCT has a potential to contribute significantly to detect subclinical atherosclerosis.

Representative cases are shown in Figure 10 and 11.

MDCT and Prognosis

Prognostic value of coronary calcium score is described in the section of "Multidetector computed tomography (MDCT)".

Recent studies investigated the prognostic value of CCTA.

Pundziute et al. studied 100 patients with suspected coronary artery disease [123]. In patients with normal coronary arteries, event rate was 0% vs. 30% in patients with any evidence of coronary artery disease. The event rate was highest in the presence of obstructive lesions (63%) and when obstructive lesions were located in the left main or left anterior descending coronary arteries (77%). Importantly, in patients with non-obstructive coronary artery disease, event rate was 8%. Min et al. studied the prognostic significance of MDCT-defined extent and severity of coronary artery disease in 1,127 patients [124]. They found that

MDCT predictors of death included proximal left anterior descending coronary artery stenosis and number of vessels with >50% and >70% stenosis. Patients with <50% stenosis had the highest survival at 99.7%. Survival ranged from 96% survival for one stenosis >70% or two stenoses >50% to 85% survival for >50% left main coronary artery stenosis. Ostrom et al. studied 2,538 consecutive patients without known coronary artery disease [125]. Risk-adjusted hazard ratio was 1.7, 1.8, 2.3, 2.6 for 3-vessel non-obstructive, 1-vessel obstructive, 2-vessel obstructive, and 3-vessel obstructive, respectively, when compared with patients without coronary artery disease. Van Werkhoven et al. performed both MDCT and myocardial perfusion imaging (MPI) in 517 patients [126]. The annualized hard event rate in patients with none or mild coronary artery disease (<50% stenosis) was 1.8% vs. 4.8% in patients with significant (>50%) coronary artery disease. A normal MPI and abnormal MPI were associated with an annualized hard event rate of 1.1% and 3.8%, respectively.

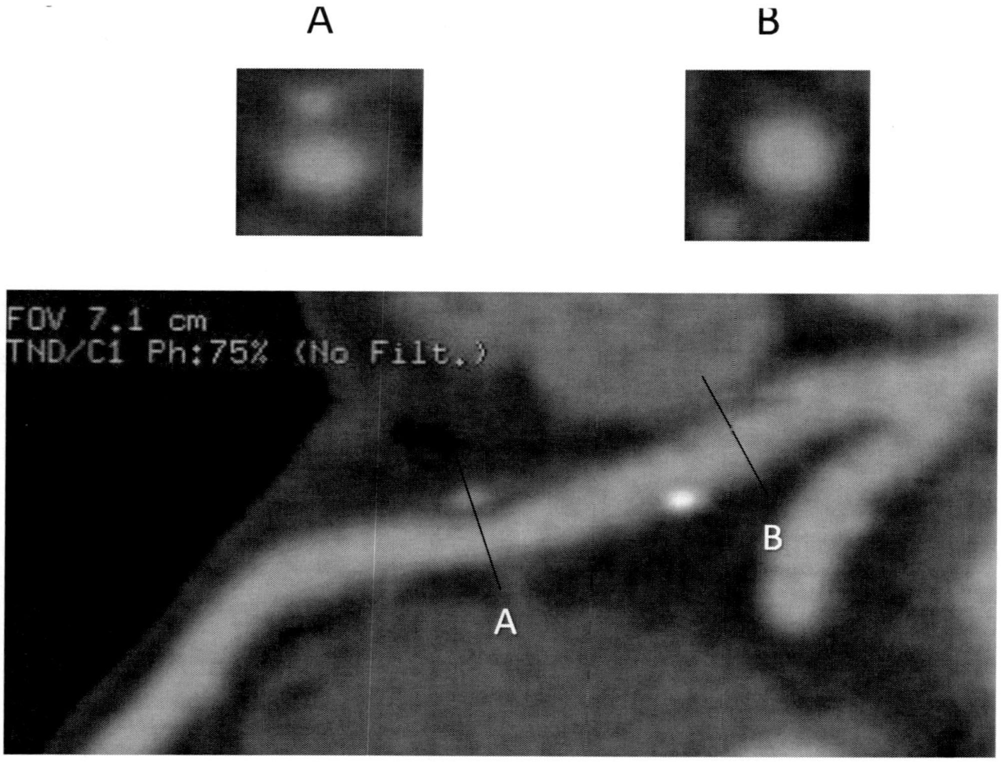

Figure 10. Representative case of asymptomatic patient with intermediate risk. A 61-years-old man underwent 64-MDCT. He has a strong family history of coronary artery disease but does not have hypertension, hyperlipidemia, or diabetes. He takes aspirin and statin and his HDL-cholesterol is 45mg/dl、 and LDL-cholesterol is 82mg/dl, and triglyceride is 90mg/dl. 64-MDCT showed non-calcified plaques with positive remodeling and CT value of 30-40 HU. Thus his medication is not sufficient to prevent plaque formation and his LDL-cholesterol value should be kept as 50 to 60mg/dl.

Taken together, these studies show that the severity of coronary artery disease is a major determinant of prognosis of patients with coronary artery disease.

Chow et al. studied the prognostic value of severity of coronary artery disease, total plaque score, and left ventricular ejection fraction (LVEF) in 2,076 patients [127].

Multivariate analysis showed that coronary artery disease severity was a major predictor of major adverse cardiac events (hazard ratio [HR] 3.02). In addition, LVEF and total plaque score had incremental value over coronary artery disease severity (HR 1.47 and 1.17, respectively).

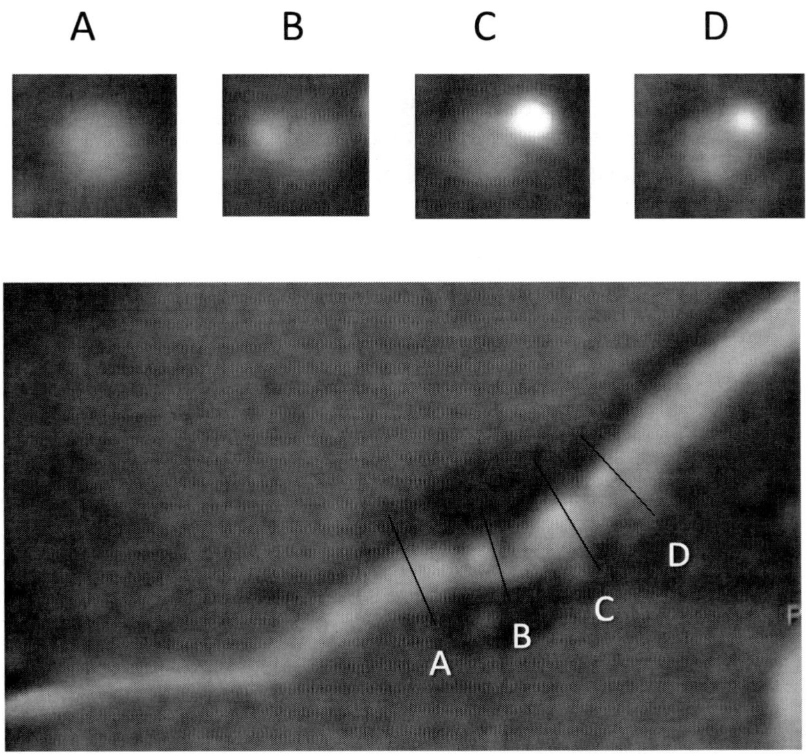

Figure 11. Representative case of asymptomatic patient with intermediate risk. A 75-years-old woman receives medication for hypertension and hyperlipidemia. Her blood pressure is 130/82mmHg, HDL-cholesterol is 66mg/dl、LDL-cholesterol is 108mg/dl, and triglyceride is 74mg/dl. So she seems to be in good control of her risk factors. However 64-MDCT found a mixed plaque with significant stenosis in the middle portion of the left anterior descending coronary artery. Stress myocardial perfusion imaging showed no ischemic findings. Thus she was advised to intensify her medication and her LDL-cholesterol should be kept as 70 to 80 mg/dl.

Russo et al. studied the prognostic value of MDCT as compared to baseline clinical risk factors in 441 patients with suspected coronary artery disease [128]. Coronary calcium score showed a significant incremental prognostic value as compared to a baseline clinical model, whereas CCTA provided an additional incremental prognostic value as compared with a baseline clinical model plus calcium scoring if considering both nonobstructive vs. obstructive coronary artery disease or, better, plaque composition (calcified vs. noncalcified and/or mixed plaques). The presence of noncalcified or mixed plaques, regardless of lesion severity, was found to be the strongest predictor of events. Thus these studies demonstrate that MDCT provides independent and incremental prognostic value independent of conventional risk factors.

MDCT and Acute Coronary Syndrome

Many studies demonstrate that nearly 70% of acute coronary events result from coronary lesions that are not hemodynamically significant or flow-limiting before the event and coronary revascularization therapy of coronary obstruction in patients with stable angina do not reduce the risk of myocardial infarction or cardiac death [4-8].

From these observations, the concept of vulnerable plaque has been developed. Vulnerable plaque is thrombosis-prone plaques and plaques with high probability of undergoing rapid progression, thus becoming culprit plaques [129]. As underlying pathologies of culprit coronary lesions, plaque rupture accounts for 70~80% and plaque erosion accounts for another 20~40%. Calcified nodule is a rare entity [129, 130].

Plaque rupture is a lesion with a luminal thrombus containing a necrotic core encapsulated by a thin fibrous cap infiltrated by macrophages and T cells [129]. Thin-cap fibroatheroma (TCFA) resembles the plaque rupture in morphology and is regarded as a precursor lesion of plaque rupture. Thin-cap fibroatheroma has three characteristics. These are thin fibrous cap (mean thickness <65μm), large lipid-rich necrotic core (occupies >40% of cross sectional area), and cellular infiltration (with macrophage and T-cell). Expansive remodeling and neovascularization are another characteristics of TCFA [131].

Several studies investigated the lesion characteristics associated with acute coronary syndrome (ACS).

Hoffmann et al. analyzed 40 lesions in 14 patients with ACS and 9 patients with stable angina pectoris (SAP) by 16-MDCT [132]. Culprit lesions in patients with ACS had significantly greater plaque area and higher remodeling index than both stable lesions in patients with ACS and in patients with SAP. The prevalence of non-calcified plaque was 100%, 62%, and 77%, respectively, in culprit lesions in patients with ACS and in stable lesions in patients with ACS or SAP. Meijs et al. analyzed culprit plaque characteristics in 50 patients with unstable angina and 64 with stable angina by 64-MDCT [133]. They found that non-calcified plaques and large non-calcified culprit plaques were more frequently found in patients with unstable angina than in those with stable angina. Sato et al. performed 64-MDCT in 60 patients with acute myocardial infarction and 150 patients with SAP [134]. They found that positive remodeling and low-attenuation plaques (<30 Hounsfield units) were more frequently observed in patients with myocardial infarction than in those with SAP.

Motoyama et al. performed 16-slices or 64-slices CT in 38 patients with ACS and 33 patients with SAP before percutaneous coronary intervention [135]. They found that positive remodeling (87% vs. 12%, $p<0.0001$), non-calcified plaque with CT value of less than 30 HU (79% vs. 9%, $p<0.0001$), and spotty calcification (63% vs. 21%, $p=0.0005$) were significantly more frequent in the ACS lesions compared with the SAP lesions. Presence of all three findings showed a high positive predictive value (95%), and absence of all three showed a high negative predictive value (100%) for the culprit plaques associated with ACS.

These studies suggest that there are specific lesion characteristics associated with acute coronary syndrome, such as positive remodeling and low attenuation plaque.

Recently, Motoyama et al. reported a landmark study, in which they prospectively investigated the predictive relation of MDCT-related features to ACS [136]. They recruited 1,059 patients who underwent 64-MDCT and analyzed for the presence of two features of positive remodeling and attenuation plaque (low non-calcified plaque <30 HU). In 1,059 patients, 45 patients (4.3%) had plaques with these two features (two-feature positive plaques), 27 patients (2.5%) had either feature (one-feature positive plaques), 820 patients (77.4%) had neither features but had plaques (two-feature negative plaques), and 167 patients (15.8%) had no plaques. During the follow-up of 27±10 months, 22.2% of patients with two-feature positive plaques, 3.7% of patients with one-feature positive plaques, and 0.5% of patients with two-feature negative plaques developed ACS. None of patients without plaques had ACS.

Taken together, these studies demonstrate that the coronary plaques that are prone to subsequent ACS are often associated with positive remodeling and low attenuation plaque, suggesting that once a patient is identified to be at high risk of having an adverse cardiac event by clinical risk assessment, imaging with 64-MDCT would help better identify those at greater risk of acute coronary events.

Representative cases are shown in Figure 12.

Thus, these studies suggest that 64-MDCT have a potential ability to identify high risk patients who will develop ACS.

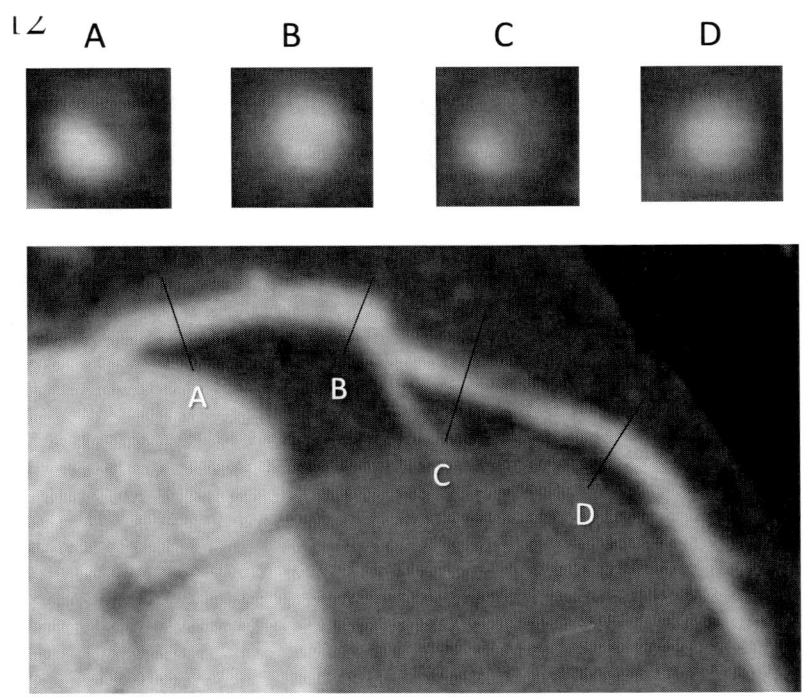

Figure 12. Representative case of asymptomatic patient with vulnerable plaque. A 63-years-old man receives anti-hypertensive therapy with good control. His HDL-cholesterol is 49mg/dl、LDL-cholesterol is 171mg/dl and triglyceride is 88mg/dl. 64-MDCT demonstrated non-calcified plaques in the proximal and middle portion of the left anterior descending coronary artery. These plaques also showed positive remodeling and mean CT value of the plaques was 30 HU. Thus this patient has a typical vulnerable plaque and he should receive aspirin and statin, whose LDL-cholesterol should be kept less than 80mg/dl.

Statin Therapy

The body of clinical trial data testing the effects of statins on coronary artery disease is extensive and convincing. A 1% reduction in low density lipoprotein (LDL)-cholesterol reduces coronary events by approximately 1% [137-142]. With larger doses of potent statins, LDL-cholesterol levels and coronary events can thus be reduced by approximately 50%.

Statins are particularly suited for primary prevention in high risk patients with subclinical atherosclerosis because they not only dramatically decrease LDL-cholesterol but also exert pleiotropic effect on plaque stabilization and atherosclerotic regression [143-145].

Studies using intravascular ultrasound demonstrate that interventions with statins reduce the plaque volume considerably, without significantly influencing the luminal volume [146, 147]. Furthermore, studies using MDCT show that the plaques in fact demonstrate negative remodeling after statin treatment and the reduction in the plaque volume was related to the reduction in low attenuation plaque area [148, 149].

Roberts describes the value of statin therapy as follows [150]; "The statin drugs are the best cardiovascular drugs ever created, in that they have the greatest potential to prevent atherosclerotic plaques and their complications, and they also have the greatest potential to arrest plaque formation, and therefore, to prevent additional atherosclerotic events. The statin drugs are to atherosclerosis what penicillin was to infectious disease."

In the Atherosclerosis Risk in Communities (ARIC) study, approximately 3% had sequence variation in the gene called *PCSK-9* (pro-protein conconvertase subtilisin/kexin type 9 serine protease) [151]. These variants lower LDL-cholesterol by a mean of approximately 19% compared with the general population. Individuals with the *PCSK-9* mutation have had a mean 62% lower rate of cardiac events over the first 15 years of observation. In white subjects, mutations were associated with a 15% reduction in mean LDL- cholesterol and a 47% reduction in the risk of coronary artery disease. In black subjects, mutations were associated with a 28% reduction in mean LDL- cholesterol and an 88% reduction in the risk of coronary artery disease. In contrast a 28% drop in LDL-cholesterol in 5-year statin trial is associated with a 25% to 35% drop in coronary artery disease risk.

These data suggest that an early and long-term reduction in LDL- cholesterol lead to a substantial reduction in coronary events, namely the efficacy of a lifetime lowering of LDL-cholesterol level. If therapeutic lowering of LDL-cholesterol had a similar long-term impact in higher risk asymptomatic individuals, this could result in a major reduction in cardiac events.

Perspective

It is time to change the paradigm of testing for coronary artery disease from detection of a symptomatic luminal obstruction to preclinical arterial wall atherosclerosis [152-154].

The major limitation of MDCT is high radiation dose in initial studies, a concern in the widespread application of the technique. However, a number of measures such as ECG-controlled tube current modulation, prospective gating, and use of lower tube voltage in patients with normal body mass index have reduced the radiation burden of CCTA significantly without compromising image quality [155, 156]. Using prospective gating,

CCTA can be performed with a lower radiation dose than conventional catheter-based coronary angiography [157, 158]. Recently introduced dual source CT scanners with high pitch scanning report effective radiation dose of less than 1mSv in patients with heart rate <60bpm [159].

Contrast-induced nephropathy is another limitation of MDCT. Initially between 50 and 100ml of contrast agent was needed. Recent advances in scanning technology reduced the contrast media dose as low as 40 ml [160].

Whereas radiation exposure sets a limit to increases in spatial resolution, temporal resolution will most likely be increased considerably, which will reduce artifact, especially in the context of coronary artery visualization. Careful clinical studies of appropriate size and design will be needed to clarify the role of CCTA.

References

[1] Third Report of National Cholesterol Educational Program (NCEP) Expert Panel on Detection, Evaluation, and Treatment of High Blood Cholesterol in Adults (Adult Treatment Panel III final report. *Circulation* 2002; 106: 3143-421.

[2] Schatzkin A, Cupples LA, Heeren T, Morelock S, Kannel WB. Sudden death in the Framingham Heart Study, Differences in incidence and risk factors by sex and coronary disease status. *Am J Epidemiol* 1984; 120: 888-99.

[3] Gibbons RJ, Jones DW, Gardner TJ, Goldstein LB, Moller JH, Yancy CW. The American Heart Association's 2008 statement of principles for healthcare reform. *Circulation* 2008; 118: 2209-18.

[4] Falk E, Shah PK, Fuster V. Coronary plaque disruption. *Circulation* 1995; 92: 657-71.

[5] Alderman EL, Corley SD, Fisher LD, Chaitman BR, Faxon DP, Foster ED, Killip T, Sosa JA, Bourassa MG. Five-year angiographic follow-up of factors associated with progression of coronary artery disease in the Coronary Artery Surgery Study (CASS). *J Am Coll Cardiol* 1993; 22: 1141-54.

[6] Miller GL, Herman SD, Heller GV, Kalla S, Levin WA, Stilwell KM, Travin MI. Relation between perfusion defects on stress technetium-99m sestamibi SPECT scintigraphy and the location of a subsequent acute myocardial infarction. *Am J Cardiol* 1996; 78: 26-30.

[7] Kolodgie FD, Burke AP, Skorija KS, Ladich E, Kutys R, Makuria AT, Virmani R. Lipoprotein-associated phospholipase A2 protein expression in the natural progression of human coronary atherosclerosis. *Arterioscler Thromb Vasc Biol* 2006; 26: 2523-9.

[8] Parisi AF, Folland ED, Hartigan P, For the Veterans Affairs ACME Investigators. A comparison of angioplasty with medical therapy in the treatment of single-vessel coronary artery disease. *N Engl J Med* 1992; 326: 10-6.

[9] Shaw LJ, Taylor A, Raggi P, Berman DS. Role of noninvasive imaging in asymptomatic high-risk patients. *J Nucl Cardiol* 2006; 13: 156-62.

[10] Grundy S. Promise of low-density lipoprotein-lowering therapy for primary and secondary prevention. *Circulation* 2008; 117: 569-57.

[11] Abdulla J, Abildstrom SZ, Gotzsche O, Christensen E, Kober L, Torp-Pedersen C. 64-Multisclice detector computed tomography coronary angiography as potential

alternative to conventional coronary angiography: a systematic review and meta-analysis. *Eur Heart J* 2007; 28: 3042-50.
[12] Hamon M, Biondi-Zoccai GG, Malagutti P, Agostoni P, Morello R, ValgimigliM, Hamon M. Diagnostic performance of multislice spiral computed tomography of coronary arteries as compared with conventional invasive coronary angiography: a meta-analysis. *J Am Coll Cardiol* 2006; 48: 1896-910.
[13] Hamon M, Morello R, Riddle JW, Hamon M. Coronary arteries: diagnostic performance of 16- versus 64-section spiral CT compared with invasive coronary angiography- meta-analysis. *Radiology* 2007; 245: 720-31.
[14] Mowatt G, Cook JA, Hillis GS, Walker S, Fraser C, Jia X, Waugh N. 64-slice computed tomography angiography in the diagnosis and assessment of coronary artery disease; systemic review and meta-analysis. *Heart* 2008; 94: 1386-93.
[15] Leber AW, Becker A, Knez A, von Zieger F, Sirol M, Nikolaou K, Ohnesorge B, Fayad ZA, Becker CR, Reiser M, Steinbeck G, Boekstegers P. Accuracy of 64-slice computed tomography to classify and quantify plaque volumes in the proximal coronary system. *J Am Coll Cardiol* 2006; 47: 672-7.
[16] Carrascosa PM, Capuñay CM, Garcia-Merletti P, Carrascosa J, Garcia MJ. Characterization of coronary atherosclerotic plaques by multidetector computed tomography. *Am J Cardiol* 2006; 97: 598-602.
[17] Ferencik M, Nieman K, Achenbach S. Noncalcified and calcified coronary plaque detection by contrast-enhanced multi-detector computed tomography: a study of interobserver agreement. *J Am Coll Cariol* 2006; 47: 207-209.
[18] Achenbach S, Moselewski F, Ropers D, Ferencik M, Hoffmann U, MacNeill B, Pohle K, Baum U, Anders K, Jang IK, Daniel WG, Brady TJ. Detection of calcified and noncalcified coronary atherosclerotic plaque by contrast-enhanced, submillimeter multidetector spiral computed tomography. A segment-based comparison with intravascular ultrasound. *Circulation* 2004; 109: 14-17.
[19] Leber AW, Knez A, Becker A, Becker C, von Zieger F, Nikolaou K, Rist C, Reiser M, White C, Steinbeck G, Boekstegers P. Accuracy of multidetector spiral computed tomography in identifying and differentiating the composition of coronary atherosclerotic plaques: a comparative study with intravascular ultrasound. *J Am Coll Cardiol* 2004; 43: 1241-7.
[20] Leber AW, Knez A, von Zieger F, Becker A, Nikolaou K, Paul S, Wintersperger B, Reiser M, Becker CR, Steinbeck G, Boekstegers P. Quantitation of obstructive and nonobstructive coronary lesions by 64-slice computed tomography. A comparative study withquantitative coronary angiography and intravascular ultrasound. *J Am Coll Cardiol* 2005; 46: 147-54.
[21] Schroeder S, Kopp AF, Baumbach A, Meisner C, Kuettner A, Georg C, Ohnesorge B, Herdeg C, Claussen CD, Karsch KR. Noninvasive detection and evaluation of atherosclerotic coronary plaques with multislice computed tomography. *J Am Coll Cardiol* 2001; 37:1430-5.
[22] de Graaf FR, Scuijf JD, van Celzen JE, Kroft LJ, de Roos A, Reiber JHC, Boersma E, Schalij MJ, Spanó F, Jukema JW, van der Wall EE, Bax JJ. Diagnostic accuracy of 320-row multidetector computed tomography coronary angiography in the non-invasive evaluation of significant coronary artery disease. *Eur Heart J* 2010; 31: 1908-15.

[23] Heuschmid M, Burgstahler C, Reimann A, Brodoefel H, Mysal I, Haeberle E, Tsiflikas I, Calussen CD, Kopp AF, Schroeder S. Usefulness of noninvasive cardiac imaging using dual-source computed tomography in an unselected population with high prevalence of coronary artery disease. *Am J Cardiol* 2007; 100: 587-92.

[24] Agatston AS, Janowitz WR, Hildner FJ, Zusmer NR, Viamonte M Jr., Detrano R. Quantification of coronary artery calcium using ultrafast computed tomography. *J Am Coll Cardiol* 1990; 15: 827-32.

[25] Rumberger JA, Simons DB, Fitzpatrick LA, Sheedy PF, Schwartz RS. Coronary artery calcium area by electron-beam computed tomography and coronary atherosclerotic plaque area. A histopathologic correlative study. Circulation 1995; 92: 2157-62.

[26] Sangiorgi G, Rumberger JA, Severson A, Edwards WD, Gregorie J, Fitzpatrick LA, Schwartz RS. Arterial calcification and not lumen stenosis is highly correlated with atherosclerotic plaque burden in humans: a histologic study of 723 coronary artery segments using nondecdalcifying methodology. *J Am Coll Cardiol* 1998; 31: 126-33.

[27] Rumberger JA, Simons DB, Fitzpatrick LA, Sheedy PF, Schwartz RS. Coronary artery calcium area by electron-beam computed tomography and coronary atherosclerotic plaque area. A histopathologic correlative study. *Circulation* 1995; 92: 2157-62.

[28] Baumgart D, Schmermund A, Görge G, Haude M, Ge J, Adamzik M, Sehnert C, Altmaier K, Grönemeyer D, Seibel R, Erbel R. Comparison of electron-beam computed tomography with intracoronary ultrasound and coronary angiography for detection of coronary atherosclerosis. *J Am Coll Cardiol* 1997; 30: 57-64.

[29] Schmermund A, Baumgart D, Görge G, Seibel R, Grönemeyer D, Ge J, Haude M, Rumberger J, Erbel R. Coronary artery calcium in acute coronary syndrome: a comparative study of electron-beam computed tomography, coronary angiography, and intracoronary ultrasound in survivors of acute myocardial infarction and unstable angina. *Circulation* 1997; 96: 1461-9.

[30] Arad Y, Spadaro LA, Goodman K, Newstein D, Guerci AD. Prediction of coronary events with electron beam computed tomography. *J Am Coll Cardiol* 2000; 36: 1253-60.

[31] Kondos GT, Hoff JA, Sevrukov A, Daviglus ML, Garside DS, Devries SS, Chomka EV, Liu K. Electron-beam tomography coronary artery calcium and cardiac events: a 37-months follow-up of 5635 initially asymptom atic low- to intermediate-risk adults. *Circulation* 2003; 107: 2571-6.

[32] Raggi P, Callister TQ, Cooil B, He ZX, Lippolis NJ, Russo DJ, Zelinger A, Mahmarian JJ. Identification of patients at increased risk of first unheralded acute myocardial infarction by electron-beam computed tomography. *Circulation* 2000; 101: 850-5.

[33] Arad Y, Spadaro LA, Goodman K, Newstein D, Guerci AD. Prediction of coronary events with electron beam computed tomography. *J Am Coll Cardiol* 2000; 36: 1253-60.

[34] Kondos GT, Hoff JA, Sevrukov A, Daviglus ML, Garside DB, Devries SS, Chomka EV, Liu K. Electron-beam tomography coronary artery calcium and cardiac events: a 37-months follow-up of 5635 initially asymptomatic low- to intermediate-risk adults. *Circulation* 2003; 107: 2571-6.

[35] Greenland P, LaBree L, Azen SP, Doherty TM, Detrano RC. Coronary artery calcium score combined with Framingham score for risk prediction in asymptomatic individuals. *JAMA* 2004; 291: 210-5.

[36] Arad Y, Goodman KJ, Roth M, Newstein D, Guerci AD. Coronary calcification, coronary disease risk factors, C-reactive protein, and atherosclerotic cardiovascular disease events: the St. Francis Heart Study. *J Am Coll Cardiol* 2005; 46: 158-65.

[37] Greenland P, Bonow RO, Brundage BH, Budoff MJ, Eisenberg MJ, Grundy SM, Lauer MS, Post WS, Raggi P, Redberg RF, Rodgers GP, Shaw LJ, Taylor AJ, Weintraub WS. ACCF/AHA 2007 Clinical Expert Consensus Document on Coronary Artery Calcium Scoring by Computed Tomography in Global Cardiovascular Risk Assessment and in Evaluation of Patients With Chest Pain. *J Am Coll Cardiol* 2007; 49: 378-402.

[38] Pham PH, Rao DS, Vasunilashorm F, Fishbein MC, Goldin JG. Computed tomography calcium quantitation as a measure of atherosclerotic plaque morphology and stability. *Invest Radiol* 2006; 41:674-80.

[39] Marwan M, Ropers D, Pflederer T, Daniel WG, Achenbach S. Clinical characteristics of patients with obstructive coronary lesions in the absence of coronary calcification: an evaluation by coronary CT angiography. *Heart* 2009; 95: 1056-60.

[40] Gottlieb I, Miller JM, Arbab-Zadeh A, Dewey M, Clouse ME, Sara L, Niinuma H, Bush DE, Paul N, Varere AL, Texter J, Brinker J, Lima JA, Rochitte CE. The absence of coronary calcification does not exclude obstructive coronary artery disease or the need for revascularization in patients referred for conventional coronary angiography. *J Am Col Cardiol* 2010; 55: 627-34.

[41] Lima RS, Watson DD, Goode AR, Siadaty MS, Ragosta M, Beller GA, Samady H. Incremental value of combined perfusion and function over perfusion alone by gated SPECT myocardial perfusion imaging for detection of severe three-vessel coronary artery disease. *J Am Coll Cardiol* 2003; 42: 64-70.

[42] Berman DS, Kang X, Siomka PJ, Gerlach J, de Yang L, Hayes SW, Friedman JD, Thompson LE, Germano G. Underestimation of extent of ischemia by gated SPECT myocardial perfusion imaging in patients with left main coronary artery disease. *J Nucl Cardiol* 2007; 14: 521-8.

[43] Pohle K, Achenbach S, MacNeill B, Ropers D, Ferencik M, Moselewski F, Hoffmann U, Brady TJ, Jang IK, Daniel WG. Characterization of non-calcified coronary atherosclerotic plaque by multi-detector row CT: Comparison to IVUS. *Atherosclerosis* 2007; 190: 174-80.

[44] Petranovic M, Soni A, Bezzera H, Loureiro R, Sarwar A, Raffel C, Pomerantsev E, Jang IK, Brady TJ, Achenbach S, Cury RC. Assessment of nonstenotic coronary lesions by 64-slice multidetector computed tomography in comparison to intravascular ultrasound: evaluation of nonculprit coronary lesions. *J Cardiovasc Comput Tomogr* 2009; 3: 24-31.

[45] Cademartiri F, Mollet NR, Runza G, Bruining N, Hamers R, Somers P, Knaapan M, Verheye S, Midiri M, Krestin GP, de Feyter PJ. Influence of intracoronary attenuation on coronary plaque measurements using multislice computed tomography: observation in an ex vivo model of coronary computed tomography angiography. *Eur Radiol* 2005; 15: 1426-31.

[46] Achenbach S, Boehmer K, Pflederer T, Ropers D, Seltmann M, Lell M, Anders K, Luettner A, Uder M, Daniel WG, Marwan M. Influence of slice thickness and

reconstruction kernel on the computed tomographic attenuation of coronary atherosclerotic plaque. *J Cardiovasc Comput Tomogr* 2010; 4: 110-5.

[47] Gaeber TC, Jeffrey CJ, Arai AE, Dixon RL, Ferrari VA, Gomes AS, Heller GV, McCollough CH, McNitt-Gray MF, Mettler FA, Mieres JH, Morin RL, Yester MV. Ionizing Radiation in Cardiac Imaging. A Society Advisory from the American Heart Association Committee on Cardiac Imaging of the Council on Clinical Cardiology and Committee on Cardiovascular Imaging and Intervention of the Council on Cardiovascular Radiology and Intervention. *Circulation* 2009; 119: 1056-65.

[48] Ge J, Erbel R, Gerber T, Görge G, Koch L, Haude M, Meyer J. Intravascular ultrasound imaging of angiographically normal coronary arteries: a prospective study in vivo. *Br Heart J* 1994; 71: 572-8.

[49] Glagov S, Weisenberg E, Zarins CK, Stankunavicius R, Kolettis GJ. Compensatory enlargement of human coronary arteries. *N Engl J Med* 1987; 316: 1371-5.

[50] Grodin CM, Dyrda I, Pasternac A, Campeu L, Bourassa MG. Discrepancies between cineangiographic and post-mortem findings in patients with coronary artery disease and recent myhocardial revascularization. *Circulation* 1974; 49: 703-9.

[51] Roberts WC, Jones AA. Quantitation of coronary arterial narrowing at necropsy in sudden coronary death. *Am J Cardiol* 1979; 44: 39-44.

[52] Hausmann D, Johnson JA, Sudhir K, Mullen WL, Friedrich G, Fitzgerald PJ, Chou TM, Ports TA, Kane JP, Malloy MJ, Yock PG. Angiographically silent atherosclerosis detected by intravascular ultrasound in patients with familial hypercholesterolemia and familial combined hyperlipidemia: correlation with high density lipoprotein. *J Am Coll Cardiol* 1996; 27: 1562-70.

[53] Alfonso F, Macaya C, Goicolea J, Iñiguez A, Hernandez R, Zamorano J, Perez-Vizcayne MJ, Zarco P. Intravascular ultrasound imaging of angiographically normal coronary segments in patients with coronary artery disease. *Am Heart J* 1994; 127: 536-44.

[54] Porter TR, Sears T, Xie F, Michels A, Mata J, Welsh D, Shurmur S. Intravascular ultrasound study of angiographically mildly diseased coronary arteries. *J Am Coll Cardiol* 1993; 22: 1858-65.

[55] Manning WJ, Li W, Edelman RR. A preliminary report comparing magnetic resonance coronary angiography with conventional angiography. *N Engl J Med* 1993; 328: 828-32.

[56] Pennel DJ, Bogren HG, Keegan J, Firmin DN, Underwood SR. Assessment of coronary artery stenosis by magnetic resonance imaging. *Heart* 1996; 75: 127-33.

[57] Post JC, van Rossum AC, Hofman MBM, de Cock CC, Valk J, Visser CA. Clinical utility of two-dimensional magnetic resonance angiography in detecting coronary artery disease. *Eur Heart J* 1997; 18: 426-33.

[58] Mohiaddin RH, Bogren HG, Lazim F, Keegan J, Gatehouse PD, Barbir M, Firmin DN, Yacoub MH. Magnetic resonance coronary angiography in heart transplant recipients. *Coron Artery Dis* 1996; 7: 591-7.

[59] Kim WY, Spuentrup E, Buecker A, Manning WJ, Botnar RM. Cardiovascular magnetic resonance imaging of coronary atherothrombosis. *J Nucl Cardiol* 2005; 12: 337-44.

[60] Yock PG, Johnson EL, Linker DT. Intravascular ultrasound: development and clinical potential. *Am J Cardiol Imaging* 1988; 2: 185-93.

[61] Nissen SE, Yock P. Intravascular ultrasound: Novel pathophysiological insights and current clinical application. *Circulation* 2001; 103: 604-16.

[62] DeMaria AN, Narula J, Mahmud E, Tsimikas S. Imaging vulnerable plaque by ultrasound. *J Am Coll Cardiol* 2006; 47: C32-9.

[63] Kotani J, Mintz GS, Castagna MT, Pinnow E, Berzingi CO, Bui AB, Pichard AD, Satler LF, Suddath WO, Waksman R, Laird JR Jr, Kent KM, Weissman NJ. Intravascular ultrasound analysis of infarct-related and non-infarct-related arteries in patients who presented with an acute myocardial infarction. *Circulation* 2003; 107: 2889-93.

[64] Maehara A, Mintz GS, Bui AB, Walter OR, Castagna MT, Canos D, Pichard AD, Satler LF, Waksman R, Suddath WO, Laird JR Jr, Kent KM, Weissman NJ. Morphologic and angiographic features of coronary plaque rupture detected by intravascular ultrasound. *J Am Coll Cardiol* 2002; 40: 904-10.

[65] Nair A, Kuban BD, Tuzcu EM, Schoenhagen P, Nissen SE, Vince DG. Coronary plaque classification with intravascular ultrasound radiofrequency data analysis. *Circulation* 2002; 106: 2200-6.

[66] Stone GW, Maehara A, Lansky AJ, de Bruyne B, Cristea E, Maintz GS, Mehran R, McPherson J, Farhat N, Marso SP, Parise H, Templin B, White R, Zhang Z, Serruys PW, For the PROSPECT investigators. A prospective natural-history study of coronary atherosclerosis. *N Engl J Med* 2011; 364: 226-35.

[67] Yabushita H, Bouma BE, Houser SL, Aretz HT, Jang IK, Schlendorf KH, Kauffman CR, Shishkov M, Kang DH, Halpern EF, Tearney GJ. Characterization of human atherosclerosis by optical coherence tomography. *Circulation* 2002; 106: 1640-5.

[68] Prati F, Regar E, Mintz GS, Arbustini E, Di Maria C, Jang IK, Akasaka T, Costa M, Guagliumi G, Grube E, Ozaki Y, Pinto F, Serruys PWJ, For the Expert's OCT Review Document. Expert review document on methodology, terminology, and clinical applications of optical coherence tomography: physical principles, methodology of image acquisition, and clinical application for assessment of coronary arteries and atherosclerosis. *Eur Heart J* 2010; 31: 401-15.

[69] Takano M, Jang IK, Inami S, Yamamoto M, Murakami D, Okamatsu K, Seimiya K, Ohba T, Mizuno K. In vivo comparison of optical coherence tomography and angioscopy for the evaluation of coronary plaque characteristics. *Am J Cardiol* 2008; 101: 471-6.

[70] Wilson PW, D'Agostino RB, Levy D, Balanger AM, Silbershatz H, Kannel WB. Prediction of coronary artery disease using risk factor categories. *Circulation* 1998; 97: 1837-47.

[71] D'Agostino RB, Vasan RS, Pencina MJ, Wolf PA, Cobain M, Massaro JM, Kannel WB. General cardiovascular risk profile for use in primary care: the Framingham Heart Study. *Circulation* 2008; 117: 743-53.

[72] D'Agostino RB, Grundy SM, Sullivan LM, Wilson P, for the CHD Risk Prediction Group. Validation of the Framingham coronary heart disease prediction scores: results of a multiple ethnic groups investigation. *JAMA* 2001; 286: 180-7.

[73] Karim R, Hodis HN, Detrano R, Liu CR, Liu CH, Mack WJ. Relation of Framingham risk score to subclinical atherosclerosis evaluated across three arterial sites. *Am J Cardiol* 2008; 102: 825-30.

[74] Nasir K, Michos ED, Blumenthal RS, Raggi P. Detection of high-risk young adults and women by coronary calcium and National Cholesterol Educational Program Panel III guidelines. *J Am Coll Cardiol* 2005; 46: 1931-6.
[75] Armadi N, Hajsadeghi F, Blumenthal RS, Budoff MJ, Stone GW, Ebrahimi R. Mortality in individuals without known coronary artery disease but with discordance between the Framingham risk score and coronary artery calcium. *Am J Cardiol* 2011; 107: 799-804.
[76] Hadamizky M, Freissmuth B, Meyer T, Hein F, Kastrati A, Martinoff S. Prognostic value of coronary computed tomographic angiography for prediction of cardiac events in patients with suspected coronary artery disease. *J Am Coll Cardiol Imaging* 2009; 2; 404-11.
[77] Schlendorf KH, Nasir K, Blumenthal RS. Limitations of Framingham risk score are now much clearer. *Prev Med* 2009; 110: 227-239.
[78] Shaw LJ, Blumenthal RS, Raggi P. Screening asymptomatic low-risk individuals for coronary artery disease: issues and controversies. *J Nucl Cardiol* 2004; 11: 382-7.
[79] Kullo IJ, Ballantyne CM. Conditional risk factors for atherosclerosis. *Mayo Clin Proc* 2005; 80: 219-30.
[80] Lauer MS. Primary prevention of atherosclerotic cardiovascular disease: the high public burden of low individual risk. *JAMA* 2007; 297: 1376-8.
[81] Greenland P, Abrama J, Aurigemma GP, Bond MG, Clark LT, Criqui MH, Crouse JR 3rd, Friedman L, Fuster V, Herrington DM, Kuller LH, Ridker PM, Roberts WC, Stanford W, Stone N, Swan HJ, Taubert KA, Wexler L. Prevention Conference V:Beyond secondary prevention: identifying the high-risk patient for primary prevention: noninvasive tests of atherosclerotic burden: Writing Group III. *Circulation* 2000; 101: E16-22.
[82] Berger JS, Jordan CO, Lloyd-Jones D, Blumenthal RS. Screening for cardiovascular risk in asymptomatic patients. *J Am Coll Cardiol* 2010; 55: 1169-77.
[83] Jaffer FA, O'Donnell CJ, Larson MG, Chan SK, Kissinger KV, Kupta MJ, Salton C, Botnar RM, Levy D, Manning WJ. Age and sex distribution of subclinical aortic atherosclerosis: a magnetic resonance imaging examination of the Framingham Heart Study. *Atheroscler Thromb Vasc Biol* 2002; 22: 849-54.
[84] Grundy SM. Age as a risk factor: you are as old as your arteries. *Am J Cardiol* 1999; 83: 1455-7.
[85] Grobbee DE, Bots ML. Statin treatment and progression of atherosclerotic plaque burden. *Drugs* 2003; 63: 893-911.
[86] Redberg RF, Greenland P, Fuster V, Pyorala K, Blair SN, Foisom AR, Newman AB, O'Leary DH, Orchard TJ, Psaty B, Schwartz JS, Starke R, Wilson PW. Prevention Conference VI: Diabetes and Cardiovascular Disease; Writing Group III: risk assessment in persons with diabetes. *Circulation* 2002; 105: e144-52.
[87] Haffner SM, Lehto S, Ronnemaa T, Pyorala K, Laakso M. Mortality from coronary heart disease in subjects with type diabetes and in nondiabetic subjects with and without prior myocardial infarction. *N Engl J Med* 1998; 339: 229-34.
[88] Expert Panel on Detection, Evaluation, and Treatment of High Blood Cholesterol in Adults. Executive Summary of The Third Report of The National Cholesterol Education Program (NCEP) Expert Panel on Detection, Evaluation, and Treatment of

High Blood Cholesterol in Adults (Adult Treatment Panel III). *JAMA* 2001; 285: 2486-97.

[89] The BARI investigators. Influence of diabetes on 5-year mortality and morbidity in a randomized trial comparing CABG and PTCA in patients with multivessel disease: the Bypass Angioplasty Revascularization Investigation (BARI). *Circulation* 1997; 96: 1761-9.

[90] Carli Di, Hachamovitch R. Should we screen for occult coronary artery disease among asymptomatic patients with diabetes? *J Am Coll Cardiol* 2005; 45: 50-3.

[91] Wackers FJT, Young LH, Inzucchi SE, Chyun DA, Davey JA, Barrett E, Taillefer R, Wittlin SD, Heller GV, Filipchuk N, Engel S, Ratner RE, Iskandrian AE, For the Detection of Ischemia in Asymptomatic Diabetic Investigators. Detection of silent myocardial ischemia in asymptomatic diabetic subjects: the DIAD study. *Diabetes Care* 2004; 27: 1954-61.

[92] Khaleeli E, Peters SR, Bobrowsky K, Oudiz RJ, Ko JY, Budoff MJ. Diabetes and the associated incidence of subclinical atherosclerosis and coronary artery disease: Implication for management. *Am Heart J* 2001; 141: 637-44.

[93] Scholte AJH, Scuijf JD, Kharagjitsingh AV, Jukema JW, Pundziute G, van der Wall EE, Bax JJ. Prevelence of coronary artery disease and plaque morphology assessed by multi-slice computed tomography angiography and calcium scoring in asymptomatic patients with type 2 diabetes. *Heart* 2008; 94: 29-5.

[94] Choi EK, Chun EJ, Choi SI, Chang SA, Choi SH, Lim S, Rivera JJ, Nasir K, Blumenthal RS, Jang HC, Chang HJ. Assessment of subclinical atherosclerosis in asymptomatic patients with type 2 diabetes mellitus with single photon emission computed tomography and coronary computed tomography angiography. *Am J Cardiol* 2009; 104: 890-6.

[95] Iwasaki K, Matsumoto T, Aono H, Furukawa H, Samukawa M. Prevalence of subclinical atherosclerosis in asymptomatic diabetic patients by 64-slice computed tomography. *Coron Artery Dis* 2008; 19: 195-202.

[96] Bots ML, Hoes AW, Koudstaal PJ, Hofman A, Grobbee DE. Common carotid intima-media thickness and risk of stroke and myocardial infarction: the Rotterdam Study. *Circulation* 1997; 96: 1432-7.

[97] Blankenborn DH, Seizer RH, Crawford DW, Barth JD, Liu CR, Liu CH, Mack WJ, Alaupovic P. Beneficial effects of colstestipol-niacin therapy on the common carotid artery. Two- and four-year reduction of intima-media thickness measured by ultrasound. *Circulation* 1993; 88: 20-8.

[98] Hodis HN, Mack WJ, LaBree L, Seizer RH, Liu CR, Liu CH, Azen SP. The role of carotid arterial intima-media thickness in predicting clinical coronary events. *Ann Intern Med* 1998; 128: 262-9.

[99] Hoeg JM. Evaluating coronary heart disease risk. Tiles in the mosaic. *JAMA* 1997; 277: 1387-90.

[100] Devine PJ, Carlson DW, Taylor AJ. Clinical vale of carotid intima-media thickness testing. *J Nucl Cardiol* 2006; 13: 710-8.

[101] Pignoli P, Tremoli E, Poli A, Oreste P, Paoletti R. Intimal plus medial thickness of the arterial wall: a direct measurement with ultrasound imaging. *Circulation* 1986; 74: 1399-406.

[102] Michell JR, Schwartz CJ. Relationship between arterial disease in different sites. A study of the aorta and coronary, carotid, and iliac arteries. *Br Med J* 1962; 1: 1293-301.

[103] Kullo IJ, Malik AR. Arterial ultrasonography and tonometry as an adjuncts to cardiovascular risk stratification. *J Am Coll Cardiol* 2007; 49: 1413-26.

[104] Lorenz MW, Markus HS, Bots ML, Rosvall M, Sitzer M. Prediction of clinical cardiovascular events with carotid intima-media thickness. A systematic review and meta-analysis. *Circulation* 2007; 115: 459-67.

[105] Crouse JRⅢ, Craven TE, Hagaman AP, Bond MG. Association of coronary disease with segment-specific iintimal-medial thickening of the extracranial carotid artery. *Circulation* 1995; 92: 1141-7.

[106] Kabiak-Ziembicka A, Tracz W, Przewiocki T, Pieniazek P, Sokolowski A, Konieczynska M. Association of increased carotid intima-media thickness with the extent o coronary artery disease. *Heart* 2004; 90: 1286-90.

[107] Granér M, Varjut M, Kahri J, Salonen RM, Nyyssönen K, Nieminen MS, Taskinen MR, Syvänne M. Association of carotid intima-media thickness with angiographic severity and extent of coronary artery disease. *Am J Cardiol* 2006; 97: 624-9

[108] Adams MR, Nakagomi A, Keech A, Robinson J, McCredie R, Bailey BP, Freedman SB, Celermajer DS. Carotid intima-media thickness is only weakly correlated with the extent and severity of coronary artery disease. *Circulation* 1995; 92: 2127-34.

[109] Davis PH, Dawson JD, Mahoney LT, Lauer RM. Increased carotid intimal-media thickness and coronary calcification are related in young and middle-aged adults. The Muscatine Study. *Circulation* 1999; 100: 838-42.

[110] Newman AB, Naydeck BL, Sutton-Tyrrell K, Edmundowicz D, O'Leary D, Kronmal R, Burke GL, Kuller LH. Relationship between coronary artery calcification and other measures of subclinical cardiovascular disease in older adults. *Arterioscler Thromb Vasc Biol* 2002; 22: 1674-9.

[111] Terry JG, Carr JJ, Tang R, Evans GW, Kouba EO, Shi R, Cook DR, Vieira JL, Espeland MA, Mercuri MF, Crouse JR 3rd. Coronary artery calcium outperforms carotid artery intima-media thickness as a noninvasive index of prevalent coronary artery stenosis. *Arterioscler Thromb Vasc Biol* 2005; 25: 1723-8

[112] Barrett-Conner E, Laughlin GA, Conner C. Coronary artery calcium versus intima-media thickness as a measure of cardiovascular disease among asymptomatic adults (from The Rancho Bernardo Study). *Am J Cardiol* 2007; 99: 227-31.

[113] Newman AB, Naydeck BL, Sutton-Tyrrell K, Edmundowicz D, O'Leary D, Kronmal R, Burke GL, Kuller LH. Relationship between coronary artery calcification and other measures of subclinical cardiovascular disease in older adults. *Arterioscler Thromb Vasc Biol* 2002; 22: 1674-9.

[114] Iwasaki K, Matsumoto T, Furukawa H, Samukawa M. Prevalence of coronary artery disease in asymptomatic patients with abnormal intima-media thickness by 64-slice computed tomography. *Int J Cardiol* online 24 April 2009.

[115] Hausleiter J, Meyer T, Hadamitzky M, Kastrati A, Martinoff S, Schömig A. Prevalence of noncalcified coronary plaques by 64-slice computed tomography in patients with an intermediate risk for significant coronary artery disease. *J Am Coll Cardiol* 2006; 48: 312-8.

[116] Choi EK, Choi SI, Rivera JJ, Nasir K, Chang SA, Chun EJ, Kim HK, Choi DJ, Blumenthal RS, Cahng HJ. Coronary computed tomography angiography as a screening tool for the detection of occult coronary artery disease in asymptomatic individuals. J Am Coll Cardiol 2008; 52: 357-65.

[117] Iwasaki K, Matsumoto T, Aono H, Furukawa H, Samukawa M. Prevalence of subclinical atherosclerosis in asymptomatic patients with low to intermediate risk by 64-slice computed tomography. *Coron Artery Dis* 2011; 22:18-25.

[118] Tuzcu EM, Kapadia SR, Tutar E, Ziada KM, Hobbs RE, McCarthy PM, Young JB, Nissen SE. High prevalence of coronary atherosclerosis in asymptomatic teenagers and young adults: evidence from intravascular ultrasound. *Circulation* 2001; 103: 2705-10.

[119] Cheng VY, Lepor NE, Madyoon H, Fshaghian S, Naraghi AL, Shah PK. Presence and severity of noncalcified coronary plaque on 64-slice computed tomographic coronary angiography in patients with zero and low coronary artery calcium. *Am J Cardiol* 2007; 99: 1183-6.

[120] SchroederS, Kuettner A, Kopp AF, Heuschmidt M, Burgstahler C, Herdeg C, Claussen CD. Noninvasive evaluation of the prevalence of noncalcified atherosclerotic plaques by multi-slice detector computed tomography: results of a pilot study. *Int J Cardiol* 2003; 92: 151-5.

[121] Gottlieb I, Miller JM, Arbab-Zadeh A, Dewey M, Clouse ME, Sara L, Niinuma H, Bush DE, Paul N, Vavere AL, Texter J, Brinker PA-CJ, Lima JAC, Rochitte CE. The absence of coronary calcification does not exclude obstructive coronary artery disease or the need for revascularization in patients referred for conventional coronary angiography. *J Am Coll Cardiol* 2010; 55: 627-34.

[122] Schenker MP, Dorbala S, Hong ECT, Rybicki F, Hachamovitch, Kwong RY, Di Carli MF. Interrelation of coronary calcification, myocardial ischemia, and outcomes in patients with intermediate likelihood of coronary artery disease. A combined positron emission tomography/ computed tomography study. *Circulation* 2008; 117: 1693-700.

[123] Pundziute G, Schuijf JD, Jukema JW, Boersma E, de Roos A, van der Wall EE, Bax JJ. Prognostic value of multislice computed tomography coronary angiography in patients with known or suspected coronary artery disease. *J Am Coll Cardiol* 2007; 49: 62-70.

[124] Min JK, Shaw LJ, Devereux RB, Okin PM, Weinsaft JW, Russo DJ, Lippolis NJ, Berman DS, Callister TG. Prognostic value of multidetector coronary computed tomographic angiography for prediction of all-cause mortality. *J Am Coll Cardiol* 2007; 50: 1161-70.

[125] Ostrom MP, Gopal A, Ahmadi N, Nasir K, Yang E, Karadiaris I, Flores F, Mao SS, Budoff MJ. Mortality incidence and the severity of coronary atherosclerosis assessed by computed tomography angiography. *J Am Coll Cardiol* 2008; 52: 1335-43.

[126] Van Werkhoven JM, Schuijf JD, Gaemperli O, Jukema JW, Boersma P, Alkadhi H, Valenta I, Stokkel MP, Kroft LJ, de Roos A, Pundziute G, Scholte A, van der Wall EE, Kaufmann PA, Bax JJ. Prognostic value of multislice computed tomography and gated single-photon emission computed tomography in patients with suspected coronary artery disease. *J Am Coll Cardiol* 2009; 53: 623-32.

[127] Chow BJW, Wells GA, Chen L, Yam Y, Galiwango P, Abraham A, Sheth T, Dennie C, Beablabds RS, Ruddy TD. Prognostic value of 64-slice cardiac computed tomography. Severity of coronary artery disease, coronary atherosclerosis, and left ventricular ejection fraction. *J Am Coll Cardiol* 2010; 55: 1017-28.

[128] Russo V, Zavalloni A, Reggiani MLB, Buttazi K, Gostoli V, Bartolini S, Fattori R. Incremental prognostic value of coronary CT angiography in patients with suspected coronary artery disease. *Cir Cardiovasc Imaging* 2010; 3: 351-9.

[129] Naghavi M, Libby P, Falk E, Casscells SW, Litovsky S, Rumberger J, Badimon J,Stefanadis C, Moreno P, Pasterkamp G, Fayad Z, Stone PH, Waxman S, Raggi P, Madjid M, Zarrabi A, Burke A, Yuan C, Fitzgerald PJ, Siscovick DS, de Korte CL, Aikawa M, Airaksinen KEJ, Assmann G, Becker CR, Chesebro JH, Farb A, Galis ZS, Jackson C, Jang IK, Koenig W, Lodder RA, March K, Demirovic J, Navab M, Priori SG, Rekhter MD, Bahr R, Grundy SM, Mehran R, Colombo A, Boerwinkle E, Ballantyne C, Insull W, Schwartz RS, Vogel R, Serruts PW, Hansson GK, Faxon DP, Kaul S, Drexler H, Greenland P, Muller JE, Virmani R, Ridker PM, Zipes DP, Shah PK, Willerson JT. From vulnerable plaque to vulnerable patient. A Call for new definitions and risk assessment strategies: Part I . *Circulation* 2003;108:1664-72

[130] Falk E. Pathogenesis of atherosclerosis. *J Am Coll Cardiol* 2006; 47: C7-12.

[131] Virmani R, Burke AP, Farb A, Kolodgie FD. Pathology of the vulnerable plaque. *J Am Coll Cardiol* 2006; 47: C13-8.

[132] Hoffmann U, Moselewski F, Nieman K, Jang IK, Ferencik M, Rahman AM, Cury RC, Abbara S, Joneidi-Jafari H, Achenbach S, Brady TJ. Noninvasive assessment of plaque morphology and composition in culprit and stable lesions in acte coronary syndrome and stable lesions in stable angina by multidetector computed tomography. J Am Coll Cardiol 2006; 47: 1655-62.

[133] Meijs MFL, Meijboom WB, Bots ML, Kyrzopoulus S, Eu RN, Prokop M, Doevendans PA, de Feyter PJ, Cramer MJ. Comparison of frequency of calcified versus non-calcified coronary lesions by computed tomographic angiography in patients with stable versus unstable angina pectoris. *Am J Cardiol* 2009; 104: 305-11.

[134] Sato A, Ohigashi H, Nozato T, Hikita H, Tamura M, Miyazaki S, Takahashi Y, Kuwahara T, Takahashi A, Hiroe M, Aonuma K. Coronary artery spatial distribution, morphology, and composition on nonculprit coronary plaques by 64-slice computed tomographic angiography in patients with acute myocardial infarction. *Am J Cardiol* 2010; 105: 930-5.

[135] Motoyama A, Kondo T, Sarai M, Sugiura A, Harigaya H, Sato T, Inoue K, Okumura M, Ishii J, Anno H, Virmani R, Ozaki Y, Hishida H, Narula J. Multislice computed tomographic characteristics of coronary lesions in acute coronary syndromes. *J Am Coll Cardiol* 2007; 50: 319-26.

[136] Motoyama A, Sarai M, Harigaya H, Anno H, Inoue K, Hara T, Naruse H, Ishii J, Hishida H, Wong ND, Virmani R, Kondo T, Ozaki Y, Narula J. Computed tomographic angiography characteristics of atherosclerotic plaques subsequently resulting in acute coronary syndromes. *J Am Coll Cardiol* 2009; 54: 49-57.

[137] Scandinavian Simvastatin Survival Study (4S) Group. Randomized trial of cholesterol lowering in 4444 patients with coronary heart disease: Scandinavian Simvastatin Survival Study (4S). *Lancet* 1994; 344: 1383-9.

[138] Shepherd J, Cobbe SM, Ford I, Isles CG, Lorimer AR, Macfarlane PW, McKillop JH, Packard CJ, For the West of Scotland Coronary Prevention Study Group. Prevention of coronary heart disease with pravastatin in men with hypercholesterolemia. *N Engl J Med* 1995; 333: 1301-7.

[139] Sacks FM, Pfeffer MA, Moye LA, Rouleau JL, Rutherford JD, Cole TG, Brown LMPH, Warnica JW, Arnold JMO, Wun CC, Davis BR, Braunwald E, For the Cholesterol AND Recurrent Events Trial Investigators. The effect of pravastatin on coronary events after myocardial infarction in patients with average cholesterol levels. *N Engl J Med* 1996; 335: 1001-9.

[140] Downs JR, Clearfield M, Weis S, Whitney E, Shapiro DR, Beere PA, Langendorfer A, Stein EA, Kruyer W, Gotto AM, For the AFCAPS/TexCAPS Research Group. Primary prevention of acute coronary events with lovastatin in men and women with average cholesterol levels. *JAMA* 1998; 279: 1615-22.

[141] Waters DD. What the statin trials taught us. *Am J Cardiol* 2006; 98: 129-34.

[142] Cholesterol Treatment Trialists' (CTT) Collaboration Efficacy and safety of more intensive lowering of LDL cholesterol: a meta-analysis of data from 170,000 participants in 26 randomized trials. *Lancet* 2010; 376: 1670-81.

[143] Halcox JPJ, ion. Deanfield JE. Beyond the laboratory. Clinical implications for stain pleiotropy. *Circulation* 2004; 109[suppl Ⅱ]; Ⅱ-42-8.

[144] Davignon J. Beneficial cardiovascular pleiotropic effects of statins. *Circulation* 2004; 109[supplⅢ]; Ⅲ-39-43.

[145] Libby P, Sasiela W. Plaque stabilization: Can we turn theory into evidence? Am J Cardiol 2006; 98[suppl]: 26-33P.

[146] Jensen LO, Thayssen P, Pedersen KE, Stender S, Haghfelt T. Regression of coronary atherosclerosis by simvastatin. A serial intravascular ultrasound study. *Circulation* 2004; 110: 265-70.

[147] Schoenhagen P, Tuzcu M, Apperson-Hansen C, Wang C, Wolski K, Lin S, Sipahi I, Nicholls SJ, Magyar WA, Loyd A, Churchill T, Crowe T, Nisse SE. Determinants of arterial wall remodeling during lipid-lowering therapy. Serial intravascular ultrasound observation from the Reversal of Atherosclerosis with Aggressive Lipid Lowering Therapy (REVERSAL) Trail. *Circulation* 2006; 113: 2826-34.

[148] Inoue K, Motoyama S, Sarai M, Sato T, Harigaya H, Hara T, Sanda Y, Anno H, Kondo T, Wong ND, Narula J, Ozaki Y. Serial coronary CT angiography- verified changes in plaque characteristics as an end point. *J Am Coll Cardiol Img* 2010; 3: 691-8.

[149] Kunita E, Fujii T, Urabe Y, Tsujiyama S, Maeda K, Tasaki N, Sekiguchi Y. Coronary plaque stabilization followed by color code plaque analysis with 64-slice multidetector row computed tomography. *Circ J* 2009; 73: 772-5.

[150] Roberts WC. Atherosclerosis: its cause and its prevention. *Am J Cardiol* 2006: 98; 1550-5.

[151] Cohen JC, Boerwinkle E, Mosley TH Jr., Hobbs HH. Sequence variations in PCSK9, low LDL-C, and protection against coronary heart disease. *N Engl J Med* 2006; 354: 1264-72.

[152] Shaw LJ, Taylor A, Raggi P, Berman DS. Role of noninvasive imaging in asymptomatic high-risk patients. *J Nucl Cardiol* 2006;13:156-62.

[153] Berman DS. Fourth Annual Mario S. Verani, MD Memorial Lecture: Noninvasive imaging in coronary artery disease: Changes roles, changing players. *J Nucl Cardiol* 2006;13:457-473

[154] Jay N. Cohn. Time to foster a rational approach to preventing cardiovascular morbid events. *J Am Coll Cardiol* 2008; 52: 327-9.

[155] Hausleiter J, Meyer T, Hermann F, Hadamitzky M, Krebs M, Gerber TC, McCollough C, Martinoff S, Kastrati A, Schömig A, Achenbach S. Estimated radiation dose associated with cardiac CT angiography. *JAMA* 2009; 301: 500-7.
[156] Raff GL, Chinnaiyan KM, Share DA, Goraya TY, Kazerooni EA, Moscucci M, Gentry RE, Abidov A, Advanced cardiovascular imaging consortium co-investigators. Radiation dose from cardiac computed tomography before and after implementation of radiation dose-reduction techniques. *JAMA* 2009; 301: 2340-8.
[157] Herzog BA, Wyss CA, Husmann L, Gaemperli O, Valenta I, Treyer V, Land messer U, Kaufmann PA. First head-to-head comparison of effective radiation dose from low-dose 64-slice CT with prospective ECG-triggering versus invasive coronary angiography. *Heart* 2009; 95: 1656-61.
[158] Buechel RR, Husmann L, Herzog BA, Pazhenkottil AP, Nkoulou R, Ghadri JR, Treyer V, von Schulthess P, Kaufmann PA. Low-dose computed tomography coronary angiography with prospective electrocardiogram triggering. Feasibility in a large population. *J Am Coll Cardiol* 2011; 57: 332-6.
[159] Achenbach S, Marwan M, Ropers D, Schepis T, Pflederer T, Anders K, Keuttner A, Daniel WG, Uder M, Lell MM. Coronary computed tomography angiography with a consistent dose below 1 mSv using prospectively electrocardiogram-triggered high-pitch spiral acquisition. *Eur Heart J* 2010; 31: 340-6.
[160] Achenbach S. Current and future status on cardiac computed tomography imaging for diagnosis and risk stratification. *J Nucl Cardiol* 2005; 12: 703-13.

Index

A

B

C

D

E

F

G

H

I

N

O

P

Q

R

S

T

U

V

W

Y

Z